Shock

Monographs in Anaesthesiology

VOLUME 4

Editor-in-Chief

A. R. HUNTER

Shock

Clinical and experimental aspects

Edited by

IAIN McA. LEDINGHAM

Senior Lecturer in Surgery, University of Glasgow;
Consultant Clinical Physiologist, Intensive Thérapy Unit, Western Infirmary, Glasgow, Scotland.

Excerpta Medica – Amsterdam – Oxford – New York
American Elsevier Publishing Co. – New York

ISBN Excerpta Medica 90 219 2076 X
ISBN American Elsevier 0 444 16713 7

Sole distributors for the U.S.A. and Canada

American Elsevier Publishing Company, Inc.
52 Vanderbilt Avenue
New York, N.Y. 10017

Library of Congress Cataloging in Publication Data

Main entry under title:

Shock.

(Monographs in anaesthesiology; v. 4)
Includes index.
1. Shock. I. Ledingham, Iain McAllan.
II. Series. [DNLM: 1. Shock, Surgical. W1 M0567G
v. 4/W0149 S5584]
RD59.S55 617'.21 75-33985
ISBN 0-444-16713-7

Printed in The Netherlands.

Foreword

Progress in the understanding and management of the shocked patient has been hindered by the widespread and indiscriminate use of the word 'shock'; by our failure to appreciate that this is not a single clinical entity amenable to specific therapy but a variety of syndromes in which precision in the delineation of the clinical picture presented by the individual patient is of the utmost importance; by a tendency to concentrate on a study of terminal events; and by a failure to grasp the many clinical opportunities which present to make the various measurements which are required to aid in the definition of the various shock syndromes and thereby to clarify the underlying physiological mechanisms.

In recent years, the international team of contributors to this book have been among the foremost in correcting this situation. They have stimulated the pace and quality of research and have shown that the obstinately high mortality in the shocked patient is amenable to reduction. The regular use of reliable techniques for physiological measurements by experienced clinical investigators, not only in established shock but at the stage when clinical changes are scarcely perceptible, is helping to elucidate the natural history of the various types of shock; distinctive patterns are beginning to emerge according to causation and time, therapeutic action is being initiated before it is too late, and clinicians are gradually being educated to recognise the dangers of a situation before they are made manifest.

This is a subject of the greatest importance to all doctors, but to most it is still a complex field in which difficulty is encountered in integrating new knowledge into clinical management. This volume provides a wider view of the subject than has hitherto been available and has thus made it possible for the relatively inexpert such as myself to perceive the complexity of the disturbances which occur in the shocked patient and, at the same time, indicate where we can hope for advances in understanding and therapy in the future. A text of this kind does not require a foreword – its value is self-evident, but I suspect that the pace now set by the contributors and others in the field will, with the additional stimulus provided by this synthesis of ideas, soon call for another volume.

Andrew Watt Kay
Professor of Surgery
Western Infirmary, Glasgow, Scotland

Preface

The publication of another monograph on shock needs little justification. The acute disruption of coordinated organ function associated with severe hypoperfusion and hypoxia remains one of the most challenging conditions to which the clinician may be exposed. The anaesthetist in particular, may be confronted with this problem in the emergency room after trauma, haemorrhage or burns; in the operating theatre when unexpected blood loss or hypoxaemia occurs; and in the intensive therapy unit when protracted resuscitation of a patient with septicaemia or after a major surgical procedure or drug overdose may be required. It is becoming increasingly appreciated that prompt and efficient management during the phase of acute collapse significantly influences the subsequent clinical course of the shocked patient. In metabolic terms, diminution in the severity of the initial injury by avoiding the complication of shock makes good sense.

During recent years new physiological tools and improved monitoring techniques, including sophisticated computer systems, have led to a clearer understanding of the shock process and thus a more logical approach to therapy. The advent of well-equipped emergency rooms and intensive therapy units has increased the opportunity for resuscitation of shocked patients but the ready availability of skilled, experienced personnel remains the factor most compatible with consistent success.

This monograph has been compiled with an anaesthetic readership in mind, although, as many of the authors have indicated, shock is a condition which demands the knowledge and expertise of several disciplines. No attempt has been made to provide a comprehensive review and account has been taken of topics adequately covered in previous volumes on the subject of shock. Most of the contributions are clinical in orientation and cover a wide range of medical, surgical, obstetric and paediatric emergencies. A few of the experimental growth areas have been included e.g. the biochemical and metabolic disturbances of shock, humoral effects, and disseminated intravascular coagulation.

Each of the authors is a recognised authority in his own field. It is hoped that the results of their combined endeavour will be of value to clinicians and scientists involved in the care of shocked patients.

Iain McA. Ledingham

Contributors

John Bonnar
Professor and Head, Department of Obstetrics and Gynaecology, University of Dublin, Trinity College Medical School, Rotunda Hospital, Dublin 1, Eire

Adam Fleck
Senior Lecturer in Pathological Biochemistry. Consultant Biochemist and Head of Biochemistry Department, Western Infirmary, Glasgow, Scotland

Ulrich F. Gruber
Leitender Arzt Allgemeinchir., Department of Surgery, University of Basle, Division for General Surgery, Kantonsspital, Basle, Switzerland

Rolf M. Gunnar
Professor of Medicine and Chief, Section of Cardiology, Loyola University Stritch School of Medicine, Maywood, Ill., U.S.A.

Denis F.J. Halmagyi
114 Lexow Avenue, Upper Nyack, New York, U.S.A.

David M. Heimbach
Assistant Professor of Surgery, Department of Surgery, University of Washington, Seattle, Wash., U.S.A.

Mark Hilberman
Resident in Anesthesia, Department of Anesthesia, Stanford University Medical Center, Stanford, Calif., U.S.A.

Dennis W. Hill
Reader in Medical Physics, The Royal College of Surgeons of England, Lincoln's Inn Fields, London, England

Iain McA. Ledingham
Senior Lecturer, Department of Surgery, University of Glasgow. Consultant Clinical Physiologist, Intensive Therapy Unit, Western Infirmary, Glasgow, Scotland

Henry S. Loeb
Program Director in Cardiology, Veterans Administration Hospital, Hines, Ill., and Associate Professor of Medicine, Loyola University Stritch School of Medicine, Maywood, Ill., U.S.A.

Rita McConn
Associate Professor of Surgery, Albert Einstein College of Medicine, Yeshiva University, Bronx, N.Y., U.S.A.

Konrad Messmer
Professor, Department of Surgery, Institute of Surgical Research, University of Munich, Nussbaumstrasse 20, 8000 Munich 2, West Germany

J.G. Mone
Consultant Anaesthesist, Division of Anaesthesia and Intensive Therapy Unit, Western Infirmary, Glasgow, Scotland

Arnold L. Nagler
Associate Professor of Surgery and Pathology, Albert Einstein College of Medicine, Yeshiva University, 1300 Morris Park Avenue, Bronx, N.Y., U.S.A.

Per Olsson
Associate Professor of Experimental Surgery, Surgical Research Laboratory, Thoracic Clinics, Karolinska Sjukhuset, Stockholm, Sweden

John J. Osborn
Director, Intensive Care Services, Pacific Medical Center, Senior Research Scientist, Institutes of Medical Sciences, San Francisco, Calif., U.S.A.

James R. Parratt
Professor, Department of Physiology and Pharmacology, Royal College, Strathclyde University, Glasgow, Scotland

J. Douglas Sleigh
Senior Lecturer in Bacteriology and Immunology, University of Glasgow, and Honorary Consultant Bacteriologist, Western Infirmary, Glasgow, Scotland

Verena Sturm
Kastelstrasse 38, CH 4000, Basle, Switzerland

M.K. Sykes
Professor of Clinical Anaesthesia, Royal Postgraduate Medical School, and Consultant Anaesthetist, Hammersmith Hospital, London, England

Michael Thomas
Consultant Cardiologist, Midhurst Medical Research Institute, King Edward VII Hospital, Midhurst, Sussex, England

Andrew W. Wilkinson
Nuffield Professor of Paediatric Surgery, Institute of Child Health, University of London, and Surgeon, The Hospital for Sick Children, Great Ormond Street, London, England

Contents

Ledingham (ed.). Shock

Pathophysiology of shock

I.McA. LEDINGHAM and J.R. PARRATT

Shock is more easily recognised as a clinical entity than defined as a pathological process. The syndrome of hypotension, tachycardia, pallor, sweating, peripheral cyanosis, hyperventilation, clouding of consciousness and oliguria is universally accepted as the clinical expression of the shock state but post-mortem examination of patients dying in shock reveals only non-specific changes. Almost any insult to the body can lead to shock and when the syndrome is fully developed, few physiological processes remain unaffected although the most striking abnormalities are haemodynamic and respiratory in character. Inadequate perfusion of the tissues with oxygenated blood is believed to be common to most forms of shock, and the resultant disturbance in cell function ultimately causes death of the patient in the absence of adequate treatment.

This chapter summarises current views on some of the physiological and biochemical disturbances of shock and serves as an introduction to subsequent chapters which deal with specific topics in greater detail.

General Haemodynamic Disturbances in Shock

The basic feature of shock is that flow through the vessels of the microcirculation is so impaired as to result in cellular damage. The most obvious cause of inadequate tissue perfusion is a reduced cardiac output due to failure of the heart to function as a pump (resulting for example, from the loss of myocardial contractility due to cardiac damage by drugs or ischaemia) or to loss of blood or plasma from the intravascular compartment (hypovolaemia). Some of the mechanisms responsible for reduced cardiac output are summarised in Figure 1.

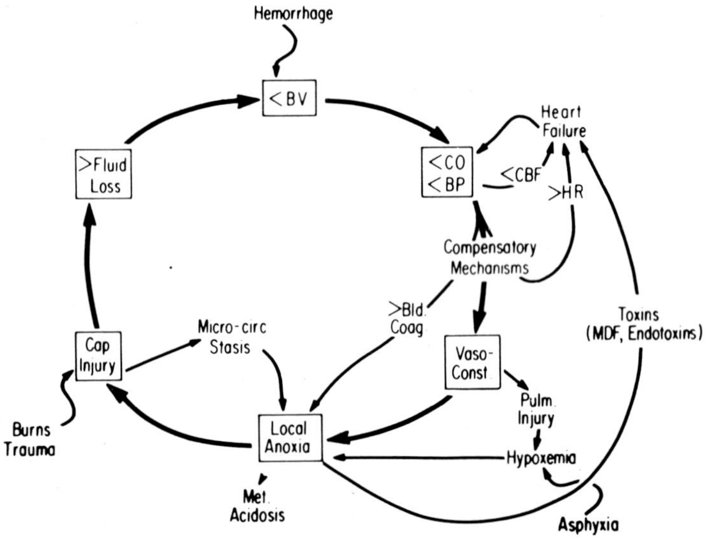

Fig. 1. Mechanisms leading to reduced cardiac output and inadequate tissue perfusion. Some of the vicious cycles of shock. *Abbreviations:* Bld. Coag. = blood coagulability; BP = systemic blood pressure; BV = effective blood volume; Cap. = capillary; CBF = coronary blood flow; CO = cardiac output; HR = heart rate; MDF = myocardial depressant factor; Met. = metabolic; Const. = constriction; Pulm. = pulmonary. (From Hackel et al., 1974.)

Under normal physiological conditions the proportion of the cardiac output available to individual organs is dependent upon the perfusion pressure and the degree of smooth muscle tone in the supplying vessels. This is usually considerable and is due to the activity of sympathetic vasoconstrictor fibres to the arterioles (precapillary resistance vessels) and to the venules (postcapillary resistance vessels) and veins (capacitance vessels). The relationship between perfusion pressure and tissue blood flow varies greatly in individual organs and is illustrated in Figure 2. Some tissues (e.g. skin and, to a certain extent, skeletal muscle) have a passive pressure–flow relationship (convexity towards the pressure axis). Quite a different relationship is seen in the renal, cerebral and coronary vascular beds: steady-state pressure–flow curves are almost

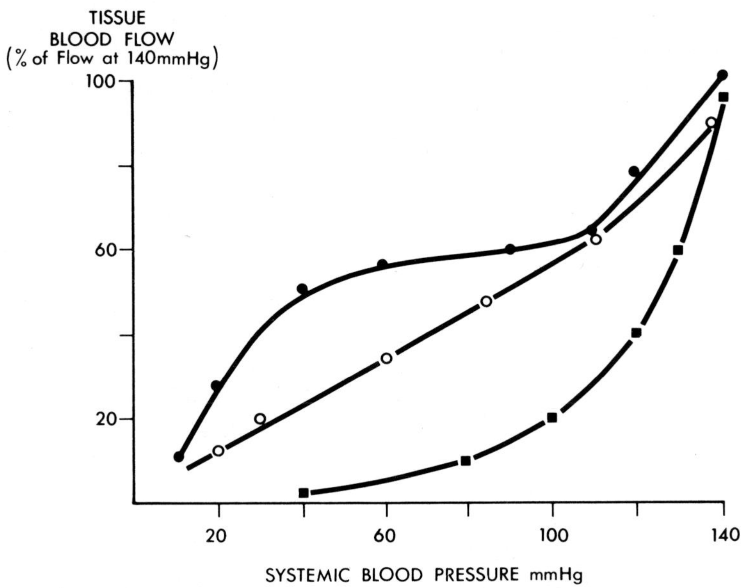

Fig. 2. The relationship between systemic arterial (perfusion) pressure and tissue blood flow in organs demonstrating either a passive pressure–flow pattern (■——■; e.g. skin) or a vascular autoregulation (●——●; e.g. heart and brain). Autoregulation is probably absent in the heart and brain when the major arteries are atheromatous; under these conditions the pressure–flow relationship is probably linear (○——○).

horizontal until a pressure of about 50 mmHg is reached when flow decreases precipitously (and the convexity is then towards the flow axis). This ability of an organ to maintain flow despite changes in perfusion pressure is termed autoregulation. It occurs in the absence of vasomotor nerves and is an intrinsic property of the vascular smooth muscle of the organ concerned. Basically autoregulation is a protective mechanism by which the body attempts to compensate for a reduced perfusion pressure to 'vital' organs. Reduction in tissue blood flow in response to a reduced systemic arterial blood pressure (to levels commonly observed in shocked patients) will clearly be much more marked in tissues and organs that do not exhibit vascular autoregulation. In addition, autoregulation will almost certainly be reduced when the major supplying arteries have a lumen decreased by atheroma; this is probably the reason why the manifestations of reduced coronary blood flow in circulatory shock (myocardial ischaemia) are more common in older patients.

A second compensatory mechanism available to the body during acute pump failure or hypovolaemia is increased sympathoadrenal discharge. This not only increases myocardial contractility but also leads to constriction of the

Table I
Effects of stimulating peripheral vasoconstrictor fibres to skeletal muscle.

	Pre-capillary resistance vessels (arterioles)	Sphincter activity	Post-capillary vessels (venules, capacitance)	Mean capillary pressure	Fluid movement
Normal response and response early in shock	Marked constriction (+ + + +)	Increased (+ + +)	Marked constriction (+ + +)	Decreased	Inward
	There is a decrease in blood flow and transcapillary fluid movement is into the circulation; survival is favoured.				
Response late in shock	(+ or −)	(−)	(+ +)	Increased	Outward
	This change is due to declining vascular reactivity, especially of pre-capillary segment, and to accumulation of metabolites. Fluid leaves circulation and this, with pooling in capacitance vessels, decreases venous return.				

arterioles (thereby tending to restore blood pressure towards normal) and of the capacitance vessels (hence maintaining venous return to the heart). The responses of the vessels of the microcirculation in skeletal muscle to increased sympathetic discharge are summarised in Table 1. Under normal conditions, and early in shock, the effect of sympathetic stimulation results in constriction of the resistance vessels on both sides of the capillary bed. However since precapillary resistance (arteriolar constriction) is increased to a greater extent than postcapillary (venular) resistance mean capillary pressure is decreased and there is a tendency for fluid to move into the circulation from the tissue spaces by osmosis. Late in shock there is a marked change in vascular reactivity; despite the continued release of noradrenaline the response of arteriolar smooth muscle declines much more rapidly than does that of venular smooth muscle. This 'fade' is accentuated by the accumulation of metabolites such as lactic acid which have more profound vasodilator effects on arterioles than on venules. The result of this change in vascular reactivity is that mean capillary pressure is increased which favours transudation of fluid from the plasma into the tissue spaces. Fluid loss is also accentuated by circulating vasoactive substances (such as histamine and the plasma kinins) which increase capillary permeability. From their animal experiments Mellander and Lewis (1963) estimated that in a 70 kg man in shock (with 30 kg skeletal muscle mass) this change in vascular reactivity could result in a decrease of circulating blood volume of more than 600 ml/hour. This would be achieved by filtering only 2 ml of fluid into the interstitial spaces of every 100 g of muscle – a volume hardly detectable as oedema.

One of the consequences of continuing postcapillary vasoconstriction and loss of intravascular fluid is haemoconcentration; this leads to an increase in blood viscosity and therefore a higher resistance to blood flow, since, from the Poiseuille relationship

$$\text{flow} = \frac{\pi(P_1 - P_2)r^4}{8\,l\,\eta}$$

where $P_1 - P_2$ is the pressure drop across vessels of length l and radius r; η is the viscosity of the perfusing fluid.

Additional factors which influence blood viscosity are the fibrinogen level and the haematocrit, both of which are raised in the early stages of shock. These changes in the characteristics of the blood lead to widespread aggregation ('sludging') of red cells and of platelets. Platelet aggregation can be induced by the presence of thrombin, noradrenaline, endotoxin and particulate matter (for example, fibres of collagen released from injured vessels). These appear to release adenosine diphosphate (ADP) from the platelets themselves and this substance is known as the most active platelet aggregating agent. Although platelet aggregation may be beneficial to the organism (haemostasis, phagocytosis of foreign material and interaction with bacteria and viruses) under conditions of decreased tissue perfusion platelet aggregation may obstruct flow (by mechanical plugging of key vessels) and this may lead to infarction of the tissue supplied by the obstructed vessel. Platelet agglutination is accelerated by bacterial endotoxins and hence the deposition of intravascular fibrin is particularly marked in septic shock. The presence of intravascular fibrin stimulates the process of fibrinolysis whereby fibrin is broken down by plasmin, a protease of broad specificity, to produce several degradation products. If the process of intravascular coagulation is protracted, the blood clotting factors may become depleted producing thrombocytopoenia and occasionally afribrinogenaemia. A bleeding diathesis may emerge which can be fatal. Intravascular coagulation may be present throughout the tissues but in man, the lung, liver and kidney are particularly vulnerable.

A further consequence of increased blood viscosity and resistance to blood flow in the vessels of the microcirculation is a reduction in flow velocity. When velocity in the smaller vessels is reduced to 0.1–0.2 mm/second (about 20% of normal) erythrocytes tend to form long continuous chains of 20–30 cells (rouleaux formation). If the endothelium is damaged wall-adhering thrombi (consisting of fibrin, platelets, erythrocytes and granulocytes) may also form which may obstruct the vessel or be released into the circulation to form emboli. A characteristic feature following injury to the blood vessel wall is the occurrence of wall-adhering granulocytes; the presence of such a wall-adhering granulocyte blocking the capillary system of the human skin is shown in Figure 3.

The Release of Vasoactive Agents in Shock

A pronounced feature of shock is the release into the circulation of a variety of vasoactive agents. These include:

i) *Noradrenaline and adrenaline.* There is a massive outpouring of these catecholamines in shock following myocardial infarction, haemorrhage and sepsis. The initial release of noradrenaline is thought to be from the varicosities of the postganglionic sympathetic fibres; this is followed, at a rather later stage, by the release of both adrenaline and noradrenaline from the adrenal

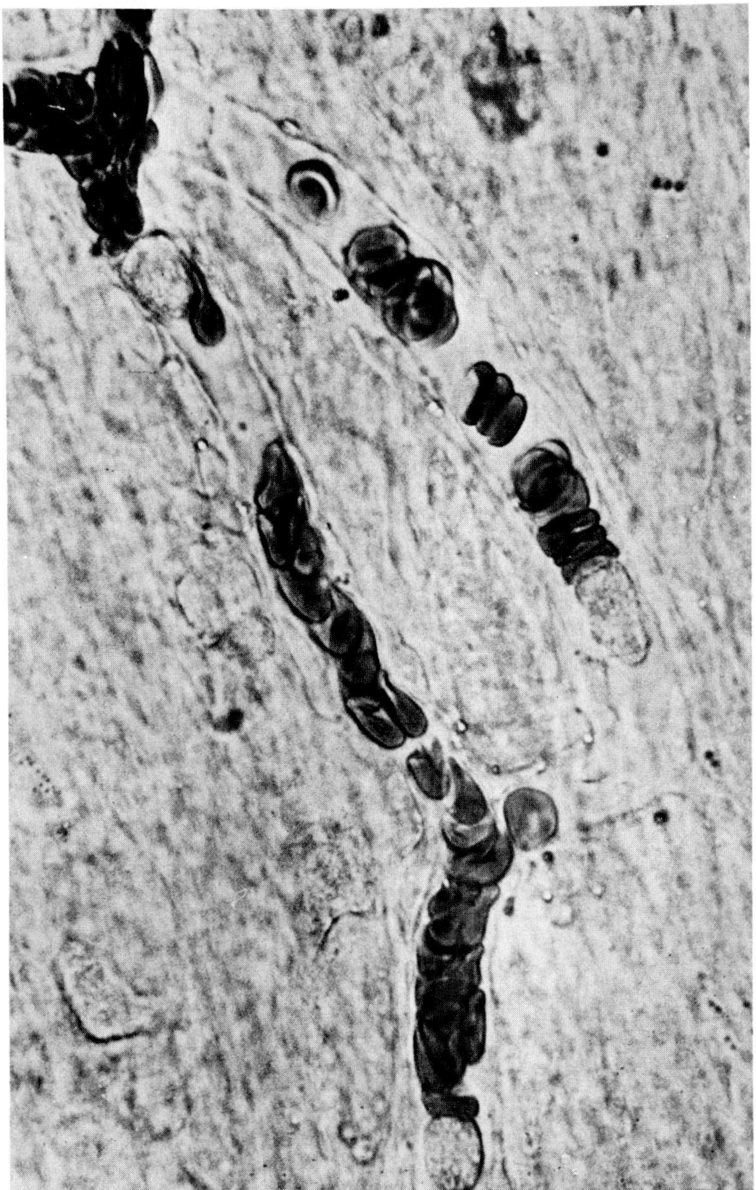

Fig. 3. The capillary system in a human 'skin tube' under conditions of low perfusion. The granulocyte at the bottom of the photograph is circulating and deformable; that at the top left is deformable, wall-adhering and partially blocking and that on the right wall-adhering, rigid and completely blocks the small capillary vessel. Photograph kindly made available by Professor P.-I. Brånemark.

medulla. The levels of plasma catecholamines reached in experimental haemorrhagic and endotoxin shock are sometimes 200 to 500 times normal.

ii) *Histamine.* The release of this vasodilator amine has been demonstrated in experimental endotoxin shock and in septic shock in man, where levels 20 times normal have been reported. The released histamine is derived partly from the mast cell granule (preformed histamine) but there is also evidence that endotoxin stimulates the rate of production of histamine by activating histidine decarboxylase.

iii) *Plasma kinins.* These are vasoactive polypeptides that dilate blood vessels and increase capillary permeability. They are formed from inactive precursors (kininogens) present in the α_2-globulin fraction of the plasma proteins by proteolytic enzymes (kallikreins) released from leucocytes and injured tissues. In some species kallikrein can be released by incubation of blood with endotoxin. Other kinin-releasing proteolytic enzymes (e.g., trypsin) may be released into the circulation from the ischaemic pancreas as a result of lysosomal breakdown.

iv) *Prostaglandins.* These are 20-carbon carboxylic fatty acids, synthesized in the body by cellular microsomes from essential fatty acids. They have a wide range of pharmacological effects on smooth muscle, gastric acid secretion and the cardiovascular system. Prostaglandins of the E series usually dilate blood vessels and increase capillary permeability; those of the F series usually constrict blood vessels, particularly in the pulmonary circulation. The release of prostaglandins of the E series has been demonstrated following haemorrhage and endotoxin administration and substances that inhibit the enzyme responsible for the synthesis of prostaglandins (prostaglandin synthetase) increase peripheral vascular resistance when injected into animals in haemorrhagic or endotoxin shock. These drugs include aspirin, indomethacin and sodium meclofenamate. In some species the release of the prostaglandin F_2 has also been implicated in the pulmonary vasoconstriction, decrease in lung compliance and increase in airways resistance that occur following the administration of endotoxin; these effects are again prevented by antipyretic–analgesic drugs.

v) *Angiotensin I* is a decapeptide formed by the action of renin (a proteolytic enzyme secreted by the kidney) on a protein (angiotensinogen or renin-substrate) found in the α_2-globulin fraction of the plasma proteins. A converting enzyme splits off histidyl-leucine to form the octapeptide angiotensin II (hypertensin or angiotonin) which is the most potent vasoconstrictor agent known. Angiotensin II has been demonstrated in considerable amounts in the blood following haemorrhage and the administration of endotoxin.

It is impossible to predict the effects, at the microcirculatory level, of the combined release of the above humoral agents; it is clear however that a massive release of such potent vasoactive agents must have important consequences in shock states. The initial hypotension which gives rise to the high (or normal) output/low resistance shock often seen in patients with sepsis may well be due to the release by endotoxin of plasma kinins, histamine and vasodilator prostaglandins of the E series. These agents may later contribute (by direct effects on capillary permeability) to the transudation of fluid from capillaries. The increased peripheral resistance which is a characteristic feature of haemorrhagic shock, of cardiogenic shock and of the later stages of sepsis is almost certainly due to the release of catecholamines and of angiotensin.

Management of the Microcirculatory Abnormalities

Whether microvascular constriction occurs alone or in conjunction with intravascular disturbances, the clear priority in treatment is restoration of adequate perfusion of the tissues. The simplest method of achieving this aim is by prompt institution of fluid replacement, the type of fluid being of less importance than the speed with which it is administered. In general, up to 20% deficit of whole blood may be replaced by buffered electrolyte solutions. Losses in excess of 20% may also be corrected using electrolyte solutions but plasma or some form of plasma substitute is usually added to restore normal colloid osmotic pressure. Blood is administered as soon as indicated and available. There is good evidence that optimal oxygen transport to the tissues is achieved when the haematocrit is maintained around 30% (see Chapter 12).

Pharmacological agents with an effect on peripheral blood vessels are used as an adjunct to fluid replacement in the treatment of shock. Provided perfusion pressure remains within the autoregulatory range, vasoconstrictor agents such as noradrenaline and methoxamine are probably of little benefit since the main therapeutic aim should be to improve tissue perfusion by vasodilatation. Thymoxamine, phenoxybenzamine and phentolamine produce this effect by blocking α-adrenoceptors in the small blood vessels; others such as isoprenaline and salbutamol stimulate vascular β-adrenoceptors. It is likely that, at least in shock, these drugs dilate both resistance and capacitance vessels.

This makes repletion of fluid volume with blood or plasma expanders a prerequisite of therapy with these agents. Some of these drugs also stimulate the heart and increase myocardial contractility, either by β-adrenoceptor stimulation (isoprenaline) or by inhibiting the uptake of noradrenaline (phentolamine and phenoxybenzamine).

It is doubtful whether blockade of α-adrenoceptors alone is able to completely overcome the profound vasoconstriction which occurs in shock. One reason for this is the presence in shocked blood of angiotensin II, the vasoconstrictor effects of which are not prevented by α-adrenoceptor blocking agents. It has been suggested that angiotensin antagonists or inhibitors of the angiotensin I converting enzyme, alone or in combination with α-adrenoceptor blockade, may have some potential value in the treatment of shock by restoring adequate tissue perfusion. There is some experimental support for this hypothesis (Jakschik et al., 1974). Dopamine, the precursor of noradrenaline, also has pharmacological properties which has led to its fairly extensive use in shock states. It increases cardiac output (and is rather less likely to induce cardiac dysrhythmias than is isoprenaline), constricts arterioles in certain vascular beds (skin and muscle) by an effect on α-adrenoceptors and dilates the renal and mesenteric vessels by an action on specific dopamine receptors. The increase in renal blood flow leads to increases in glomerular filtration and sodium excretion.

Organ Function in Shock

When different species of animals are subjected to experimental shock the physiological disturbances and thus the mode of death vary considerably. The dog, for instance, is particularly liable to respond to endotoxin with a raised portal venous pressure and a low central venous pressure and may die from effects principally due to splanchnic ischaemia while the cat typically demonstrates pulmonary vasoconstriction and a raised central venous pressure with early cardiac failure. In baboons and probably man the lung, the liver and the kidney appear particularly susceptible to shock. These observations have led over the years to the belief that the failure of a specific organ may account for the eventual refractory nature of shock. There is little evidence to substantiate this belief since it is clear that almost every cell in the body is adversely affected during the shock process. There is merit, however, in appreciating that the shocked patient is susceptible to respiratory failure or renal failure for instance, and that precautions should be taken to reduce the risks of further damage to these organs.

The Heart

It is well recognised that myocardial infarction may be followed by shock in a small proportion of cases (see Chapter 16) but the shock state itself may induce acute cardiac failure thus creating a vicious cycle (Fig. 1). The heart was first implicated in the shock syndrome when Wiggers (1950) demonstrated that dogs subjected to sustained haemorrhagic hypotension eventually required increasing retransfusion of the shed blood to maintain blood pressure. Initially left atrial pressure rose followed by elevation of right atrial pressure and death finally supervened with a progressive fall in cardiac output in spite of replacement of all the shed blood. Since then opinion has varied as to the importance of cardiac failure as a cause of death in clinical shock. There is little doubt that rapid transfusion of blood or other fluids following haemorrhage may be associated with the onset of cardiac failure and the more prolonged the period of shock the more pronounced is this effect. Incipient cardiac failure may not be immediately obvious from measurements of cardiac output in the resting state; special techniques may be required such as those demonstrating the range of left ventricular function (Fig. 4). In the management of

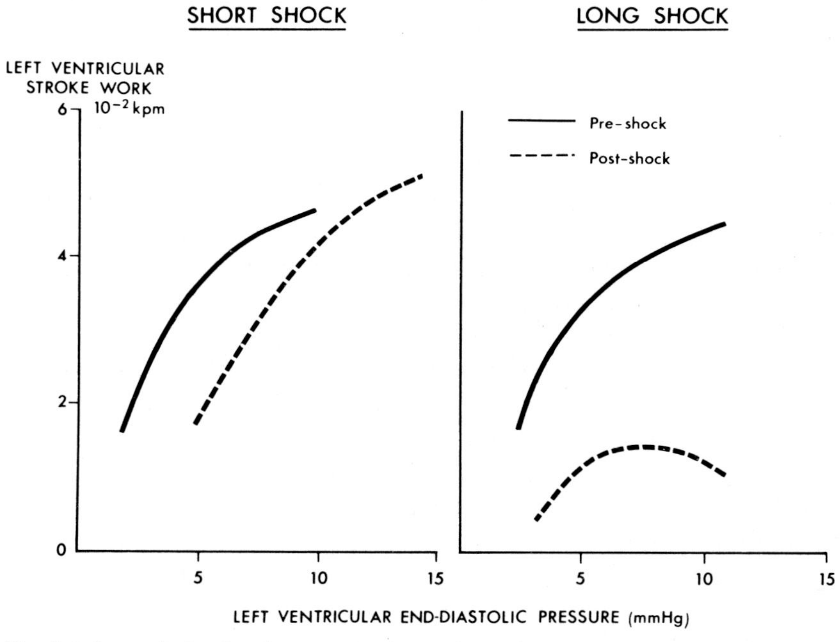

Fig. 4. Left ventricular function curves before and after haemorrhagic shock of short and long duration.

shocked patients a rough assessment of cardiac function may be obtained by noting the relationship between changes in central venous pressure and arterial blood pressure produced by rapid transfusion of small amounts of fluid; the presence of cardiac failure as distinct from hypovolaemia may thus be determined. In a large group of shock patients suffering from trauma, sepsis and haemorrhage, but without evidence of a primary cardiac defect, 20% responded to a test fluid load of 500 ml of dextran in such a way as to indicate cardiac insufficiency, and another 20% had a combination of cardiac insufficiency and peripheral circulatory failure (Shoemaker et al., 1971).

The cause of cardiac failure in shock has evaded precise definition. Since the myocardium has a high oxygen consumption, a discrepancy might be expected to occur between myocardial oxygen availability and consumption during severe hypotension. However, the work of the heart, and therefore myocardial oxygen consumption, falls in most forms of shock. Moreover, the normal heart is able to protect itself to a remarkable degree by autoregulatory vasodilatation during hypotension. These factors account for the difficulty in producing biochemical evidence of myocardial ischaemia. On the other hand, the electrocardiogram during severe hypotension frequently shows changes consistent with ischaemia and, in long term recovery experiments, patchy necrosis of myocardial cells has been demonstrated (Hackel et al., 1974). Another possible explanation of the heart failure present in many patients with shock has recently come to light, in the form of a circulating myocardial depressant factor (MDF) (Lefer, 1973). This substance is thought to originate in the ischaemic pancreas and may reach the systemic circulation via the lymphatic system. In a group of shocked patients who later died of cardiac failure, increased levels of this substance were found in plasma ultrafiltrates (Fisher et al., 1973).

It is also possible that endotoxin may directly damage myocardial cells but clearcut evidence of this effect is lacking and, in any case, is likely to occur only after prolonged endotoxaemia (Hinshaw et al., 1972). In patients with long-standing atheromatous coronary artery disease, cardiac failure may be more readily explained after a period of shock. The patient with diseased coronary arteries may be unable to dilate his vessels in response to hypotension (see Fig. 2) and myocardial ischaemia of greater severity may occur in these patients than in patients with normal coronary arteries for an equivalent degree of hypotension.

The possibility of unsuspected myocardial infarction contributing to the clinical presentation should always be borne in mind in shocked patients, particularly if arrhythmias occur during or after hypotension. The acute onset of myocardial infarction may explain an unexpected failure to respond to resuscitation. Other causes of primary cadiogenic shock include the drugs and agents used by the anaesthetist, e.g., barbiturate and halothane, and, in the late postoperative period, the risk of pulmonary embolism arises.

Drugs which stimulate cardiac action are often advocated in shock and there is little doubt that cardiac output can be increased in this way. Indeed digitalisation is not infrequently specifically indicated to correct uncontrolled atrial fibrillation. Ouabain may be preferred to digoxin if a rapid action is imperative; in either case the intravenous route should be used because of uncertain absorption by other routes. Isoprenaline has the advantage that, in addition to its inotropic action, it dilates the peripheral blood vessels, but its tendency to produce tachycardia and even tachyarrhythmias is a disadvantage. A number of new inotropic drugs are being evaluated e.g., dobutamine, glucagon and dopamine; some of these may prove useful (see Chapter 13).

The Lung

The shocked patient normally has an increased respiratory rate with a variable change in tidal volume. In the early stages a fall in arterial carbon dioxide tension usually occurs with minimal changes in arterial oxygen tension. The increased respiratory rate results from an increase in peripheral chemoreceptor activity and from the stimulant effect of systemic metabolic acidosis.

Investigation of the hyperventilatory response in shock has revealed a discrepancy between the increase in minute ventilation and the decrease in arterial carbon dioxide tension. The arterial carbon dioxide tension which frequently falls to 20–30 mmHg should fall considerably further if there was a corresponding increase in alveolar ventilation. The discrepancy is due to an increase in dead space ventilation, i.e., ventilation of alveoli with diminished or absent blood supply. The diminution in blood flow leads to widespread inequalities in the ventilation/perfusion ratios. In those alveoli where the ventilation greatly exceeds perfusion, alveolar carbon dioxide tension falls to low levels and dilutes the carbon dioxide concentration of more normally perfused alveoli. Thus it is characteristic in shock for the difference between the arterial carbon dioxide tension and the mixed expiratory or end-tidal carbon dioxide tension to increase and this measurement is a useful reflection of changes in pulmonary blood flow. In the early stage of haemorrhagic shock there is remarkably little change in lung mechanics.

In the normal lung up to 3% of the blood reaches the left side of the heart effectively without coming in contact with alveolar gas – so-called pulmonary venous admixture. This includes blood passing through poorly ventilated alveoli, through completely unventilated alveoli and by-passing the alveoli altogether (i.e. the bronchial and thebesian circulations). A combination of these effects produces the normal alveolar–arterial oxygen tension difference. The proportion of this difference which may be attributed to true shunt, i.e., blood passing through completely unventilated alveoli or normal anatomical vascular shunts, is revealed when the patient breathes a 100% oxygen; this manoeuvre readily corrects the hypoxaemia of ventilation/perfusion inequalities and is another useful measurement of gas exchange in shock. Such measurements have revealed that in the early stages of shock true shunt may fall although later, a substantial rise may occur as a result of pulmonary oedema or alveolar collapse. Pulmonary oedema may be produced by left heart failure or by the direct effects of poor perfusion on the integrity of the pulmonary capillaries; alveolar collapse may also result from poor perfusion leading to diminished production of surfactant, from medullary hypoxia or indirectly from the effects of various drugs which decrease compensatory hyperventilation.

As a result of diminished systemic blood flow during shock oxygen is extracted in large amounts from the blood returning to the heart with a consequent fall in mixed venous oxygen tension. Normally, the level of mixed venous oxygen tension does not significantly influence arterial oxygen tension but when a large shunt is present, as in the later stages of shock, the mixed venous oxygen tension becomes increasingly important as a cause of arterial oxygen desaturation.

The disturbances of gas exchange in the lung tend to disappear, or at least improve, on restoration of normal blood flow. In a few instances, however, gas exchange may further deteriorate giving rise to the condition commonly termed 'the shock lung'. It is likely that this condition, as commonly recognised, is multifactorial in origin and intravascular coagulation, infection, direct injury, intermittent positive pressure ventilation (IPPV) and excess oxygen have all been implicated.

The Kidney and Adrenal

Acute intrinsic renal failure is not an uncommon sequel to a period of shock although there is not necessarily a close relationship between the severity of shock and the incidence of renal failure. This is explained by the fact that although haemorrhage by itself will produce renal failure, a number of other factors modify the response e.g., sepsis, crush injury, pre-existing renal disease etc.

Urine formation ceases when the systemic arterial pressure falls to 50 mmHg. The autoregulatory control of renal blood flow is absent during haemorrhagic hypotension (Bell, 1972), and blood flow thus falls proportionately with blood pressure. This is particularly marked in the renal cortex and is not influenced by denervation (since the autotransplanted kidneys demonstrate the same phenomenon) or by the administration of mannitol before or during experimental haemorrhagic hypotension. The exact mechanism producing the changes in renal blood flow is uncertain although circulating catecholamines undoubtedly contribute. Glomerular filtration rate also falls in proportion to the fall in blood pressure, but the filtration fraction rises, presumably as a result of more marked vasoconstriction of the efferent glomerular arterioles. The changes produced by shock in the renal cortex may be patchy in character and although, in most cases, repletion of fluid deficit produces restoration of normal blood flow, in some, this patchy ischaemia may persist and may be related to the onset of acute intrinsic renal failure. Oxygen consumption in the kidney is closely related to sodium reabsorption in the tubules. Thus oxygen consumption falls pari passu with the fall in glomerular filtration rate and returns to normal on restoration of an adequate blood pressure.

The diagnosis of acute intrinsic renal failure is rarely a problem although the diagnosis should be established as quickly as possible if fluid overload in the shocked patient is to be avoided. The most important features in the diagnosis are a low urinary output and a high or rising blood urea; the urine urea is low and the urine sodium concentration exceeds 20 mEq/l.

In addition to these direct sequelae of shock on the kidney, other indirect effects succeed renal ischaemia, of which perhaps the most important is the release of aldosterone by the adrenal cortex. The juxta-glomerular apparatus in the renal cortex responds to blood volume depletion and sodium deficiency by producing renin which acts in the blood to form angiotensin II. This potent vasopressor stimulates the adrenal cortex to release aldosterone, the function of which is to conserve body sodium and thus blood volume.

Like aldosterone, both cortisol and corticosterone are produced in excess during shock and even when hypotension is severe and prolonged, adrenal cortical failure has been demonstrated only rarely. Thus the administration of hydrocortisone is not indicated on physiological grounds; nevertheless, large doses of steroids have been shown by some to exert a beneficial influence in experimental shock although only if given within a few minutes of the onset of shock. In the dose recommended (50 mg/kg of hydrocortisone), steroids exert a vasodilatory action, increase the production of adenosine triphosphate (ATP), increase the conversion of lactic acid to glycogen and stabilise lysosomal membranes. The adrenal medulla has already been shown to play an important role in the cardiovascular response to shock and it seems that low blood volume is more important than low blood pressure in initiating catecholamine release. In man, noradrenaline exceeds adrenaline production in the early stages of shock and the subsequent pattern of response appears to vary with the overall response of the patient to resuscitation (Griffiths, 1972).

Disturbances of Cell Metabolism

Disturbance of cell function is an early feature of the shock syndrome but, for obvious reasons, is less readily recognised than the haemodynamic and respiratory disturbances. Carbohydrate metabolism is impaired at an early stage with an accumulation within the cells of lactic acid resulting from an inability of pyruvate, in the absence of adequate oxygen, to pursue its normal pathway via co-enzyme A into the Kreb's citric acid cycle. This block in the normal glycolytic pathway leads to a tendency for glucose to leave the cell. The resultant hyperglycaemia is resistant to the administration of insulin; increased glycogenolysis occurs in an attempt to maintain normal levels of intracellular glucose. Associated mechanisms lead to elevated blood levels of amino acids and fats. The failure of carbohydrate metabolism to proceed to completion results in reduced formation of ATP. Consequently, there is a failure of the normal sodium pump mechanism and diminished formation of proteins including those contributing to the normal host defence mechanism e.g., immunoproteins (Schumer and Sperling, 1968). The inability of the cell to form ATP leads to an accumulation of phosphates within the cell and later in the blood. The failure of the sodium pump leads to extravasation of intracellular potassium and swelling of the cytoplasm and of the intracellular organelles as a result of sodium and water influx into the cell. These changes have been demonstrated using the electron microscope and are reversible with prompt correction of the defect in tissue perfusion.

The metabolic acidosis which begins within the cell, later becomes detectable as a fall in blood pH and is one of the commonest observations in shock. Lactic acidosis originates predominantly in ischaemic muscle but the liver itself may produce lactate in low flow states; these effects are thought to reflect the extent of vasoconstriction secondary to α-adrenoceptor stimulation. Recently it has been shown that circulating catecholamines, in the presence of α-blockade, can precipitate the production of lactate acidosis; β-adrenoceptor blocking agents effectively prevent this reaction. Failure of the ischaemic liver to metabolise the load of lactate presented to it during shock indicates a severe metabolic injury and sustained metabolic acidosis is a grave prognostic sign.

The secondary effect of a low blood pH on organ function is less certain than formerly. In isolated hearts Opie (1965) has shown that cardiac contractility only begins to be impaired below pH values of 7.10 units. Correction of profound metabolic acidosis during haemorrhagic hypotension and after retransfusion often has little influence on myocardial function and oxygen consumption (Ledingham et al., 1972). Nevertheless, there is good reason for restoration to normality of a disturbance in acid base balance in that it provides a reserve of buffer in the event of another shock episode and is stated to increase vascular responsiveness to vasoactive agents. Sodium bicarbonate is the usual solution administered and is given in a dose to correct extracellular acidosis. The use of so-called intracellular buffers, such as Tris-hydroxymethylaminomethane (THAM), has diminished in the past few years probably because of uncertainty as to the precise dosage required for an individual patient and because these substances can produce hypoventilation and a dangerous depression in serum potassium.

Septic Shock

Sepsis is an increasingly common feature of the shock state and septic shock is associated with a high mortality. This form of shock occurs most frequently in patients who have had operations on the genito-urinary system, the large bowel and the biliary system but any injury or major infection may permit bacteria to gain access to the bloodstream. The existence of other factors such as dehydration, hypoxia and debility increases the likelihood of bacteraemia being converted to bacteraemic shock. Although sharing many of the clinical features of shock in general, septic shock possesses characteristics which are sufficiently distinctive to justify separate appraisal in this chapter.

The causative organisms may be gram positive or gram negative but the latter are by far the more common. *Escherichia coli* bacteraemia occurs after biliary, colonic and urological surgery and *Pseudomonas aeruginosa* bacteraemia in burns. Recently the Bacteroides group of strictly anaerobic bacilli has become recognised as a particularly major problem in septic shock. The gram positive organisms include *Streptococcus, Staphylococcus* and *Cl. welchii.* The ultimate prognosis in patients with septic shock is influenced to a large extent by early diagnosis and the prompt administration of the appropriate antibiotic in adequate doses. A 'best guess' antibiotic regimen may have to be instituted initially and modified as soon as more specific bacteriological information becomes available.

Animal experiments have shown that the lethal nature of most forms of septic shock is related to the release into the blood stream of endotoxin, a large molecular weight lipopolysaccharide substance found in the O somatic antigen of the bacterial cell wall. Different bacteria produce endotoxins of different potency and chemical structure; the lipid fraction of the endotoxin produces its toxic effects while the polysaccharide fraction produces its antigenicity. Endotoxin, or similar substance, has been identified recently in patients with bacteraemia (Caridis et al., 1972) and its persistence in the blood is related to the presence of a septic focus or a depression in function of the reticulo-endothelial system. The precise mechanism of action of endotoxin is uncertain although it probably does not act directly on vessel walls. Its vasoactive properties may be attributable to an intermediary proteolytic substance formed in the blood causing the release from various cells of peptides e.g., bradykinin, amines, e.g., catecholamines, histamine and serotonin, and probably vasoactive lipid anions. Endotoxin has direct effects on certain intracellular enzymes and reduces oxygen consumption in rat liver mitochondria (Moss et al., 1969).

The clinical features of some patients with septic shock differ from the more usual pattern of shock. These patients have a hyperdynamic circulation with a raised cardiac output and low peripheral vascular resistance, and are often described as having warm hypotension. Only at a later stage do the more classical features of peripheral cyanosis and cardiovascular collapse emerge. In patients with sepsis combined with hypovolaemia, it is often possible to produce the hyperdynamic state with fluid repletion. Associated with these cardiovascular features is a low arterial-mixed venous oxygen content difference.

This distinctive clinical pattern may simply represent the response of the body to powerful circulating vasodilator substances (Hermreck and Thal, 1969) released from the septic region, with redistribution of blood flow towards the area of sepsis and a compensatory increase in cardiac output. Others have sought alternative additional explanations and these fall into two main categories. Some workers associate the haemodynamic changes and the low arteriovenous oxygen content difference with the opening up of arteriovenous shunts, particularly in the pulmonary and splanchnic regions (Berk et al., 1972). This mechanism is believed to involve the stimulation of β-adrenotropic receptors by catecholamines and has led to investigation of the use of β-blocking agents e.g., propranolol, in the treatment of advanced septic shock. The depressant effect of these agents on the myocardium has to be counteracted simultaneously with drugs having an inotropic action, e.g., digoxin and glucagon. The second mechanism is postulated by those who believe that the decrease in arteriovenous oxygen content difference is out of proportion to the increase in blood flow in septic shock. The demonstration by Wright et al. (1971) that muscle capillary blood flow is not defective in sepsis, has lent support to the concept that cell function is disturbed earlier in septic than in other forms of shock and that the hyperdynamic circulatory changes are purely secondary. Whatever the final explanation, it is clear that treatment of septic shock should be based not only on correction of fluid deficits but also on rapid elimination of the source of sepsis.

References

Bell, G. (1972): Renal blood flow during haemorrhagic shock. In: *Conference on 'Shock'*, p. 20. Editors: I.McA. Ledingham and T.A. McAllister. Henry Kimpton, London.

Berk, J.L., Hagen, J.F., Maly, G. and Koo, R. (1972): The treatment of shock with beta adrenergic blockade. *Arch. Surg. (Chicago)*, *104*, 46.

Caridis, D.T., Reinhold, R.B., Woodruff, P.W.H. and Fine, J. (1972): Endotoxaemia in man. *Lancet*, *1*, 1381.

Fisher, W.D., Heimbach, D.M., McArdle, C.S., Maddern, M., Hutchison, M.M. and Ledingham, I.McA. (1973): A circulating depressant effect following canine haemorrhagic shock. *Brit. J. Surg.*, *60*, 392.

Griffiths, J. (1972): The sequential assay of plasma catecholamines and whole blood histamine in early septic shock. In: *Conference on 'Shock'*, p. 76. Editors: I.McA. Ledingham and T.A. McAllister, Henry Kimpton, London.

Hackel, D.B., Ratliff, N.B. and Mikat, Eileen (1974): The heart in shock. *Circulat. Res.*, *35*, 805.

Hermreck, A.S. and Thal, A.P. (1969): Mechanisms for the high circulatory requirements in sepsis and septic shock. *Ann. Surg.*, *170*, 677.

Hinshaw, L.B., Greenfield, L.J., Owen, S.E., Black, M.R. and Guenter, C.A. (1972): Precipitation of cardiac failure in endotoxin shock. *Surg. Gynec. Obstet.*, *135*, 39.

Jakschik, B.A., Marshall, G.R., Kourik, J.L. and Needleman, P. (1974): Profile of circulating vasoactive substances in haemorrhagic shock and their pharmacologic manipulation. *J. clin. Invest.*, *54*, 842.

Ledingham, I.McA., Paratt, J.R. and Vance, J.P. (1972): Myocardial blood flow and metabolism in shock. In: *Conference on 'Shock'*, p. 13. Editors: I.McA. Ledingham and T.A. McAllister. Henry Kimpton, London.

Lefer, A.M. (1973): Blood-borne humoral factors in the pathophysiology of circulatory shock. *Circulat. Res.*, *32*, 129.

Mellander, S. and Lewis, D.H. (1963): Effect of haemorrhagic shock on the reactivity of resistance and capacitance vessels and on capillary filtration transfer in cat skeletal muscle. *Circulat. Res.*, *13*, 105.

Moss, G.S., Erve, P.P. and Schumer, W. (1969): Effect of endotoxin on mitochondrial respiration. *Surg. Forum*, *20*, 24.

Opie, L.H. (1965): Effect of extracellular pH on function and metabolism of isolated perfused rat heart. *Amer. J. Physiol., 209*, 1075.

Schumer, W. and Sperling, R. (1968): Shock and its effect on the cell. *J. Amer. med. Ass., 205*, 75.

Shoemaker, W.C., Brown, R.S., Mohr, P.A., Monson, D.O. and Carey, J.S. (1971): The cardiovascular system. In: *Cortico Steroids in the Treatment of Shock*, p. 16. Editors: W. Schumer and L.M. Nyhus. University of Illinois Press, Chicago, London.

Wiggers, C.J. (1950): *The Physiology of Shock*. Commonwealth Fund, New York.

Wright, C.J., Duff, J.H., McLean, A.P.H. and MacLean, L.D. (1971): Regional capillary blood flow and oxygen uptake in sepsis. *Surg. Gynec. Obstet.*, 637.

Ledingham (ed.). Shock

Pulmonary disturbances in shock

M.K. SYKES

There are relatively few reliable studies of lung function in patients with shock because such patients are usually in a very unsteady state. Furthermore it is often difficult to separate the direct effects of shock from those induced by trauma, therapy or pre-existing lung disease. Much of the information in this chapter is therefore derived from animal experiments. These should be interpreted with care, for there are often large variations in the response of different species. For example, the dog always develops splanchnic congestion in response to shock. This leads to a marked loss of fluid from the intravascular compartment and to bleeding into the intestines. The primate does not develop these changes and is, in many ways, more comparable with a human. However expense and difficulties in handling preclude the widespread use of the primate as an experimental animal.

Shock produces immediate effects on lung function which are closely related to the changes occurring in the pulmonary circulation. However, additional changes appear to be initiated during the hypotensive period. These may lead to the later development of the shock–lung syndrome. The manifestations of this syndrome usually appear 12–72 hours after the hypotensive period but the pathophysiological changes are extremely variable and the aetiology is, as yet, unknown.

Causes of Shock

The immediate effects of shock on lung function depend on the cause of the shock. For the purposes of this discussion three main types of shock are recognised.

1. *Hypovolaemic shock.* This includes all those conditions which result in a relative depletion of blood volume. The most obvious example is haemorrhage but similar effects are produced by peripheral vasodilatation and fluid loss in anaphylactic shock, or by plasma loss in patients with severe burns. The reduction in blood volume leads to a reduction in venous return and this leads to a decrease in pulmonary blood flow and pulmonary artery pressure.

2. *Cardiogenic shock.* This most commonly occurs after myocardial infarction or open-heart surgery. There is an acute increase in left atrial pressure which leads to pulmonary congestion and oedema.

3. *Septic shock.* Severe sepsis is associated initially with a high cardiac output, but later the cardiac output falls. There appears to be a marked increase in capillary permeability and pulmonary oedema is common.

These three types of shock have very different effects on pulmonary haemodynamics. In order to understand the effects of the haemodynamic changes on lung function it is necessary to consider the main factors governing the distribution of pulmonary blood flow.

Distribution of Pulmonary Blood Flow

The pulmonary circulation is a low pressure, low resistance system. As a result the distribution of pulmonary blood flow is primarily determined by the effects of gravity. The capillaries are believed to function rather like Starling resistors so that their blood flow is governed by the relationship between the alveolar gas pressure and the pressures in the arterial and venous ends of the capillary (Fig. 1). In the upper part of the lung (zone 1) the pressure in the pulmonary arteries is less than atmospheric throughout most of the cardiac cycle. Capillary blood flow is negligible so that no gas exchange can occur. Since the ventilation distributed to these alveoli is wasted, it is known as the alveolar dead space ventilation.

In the lower parts of the lung the pressure in the pulmonary arteries is

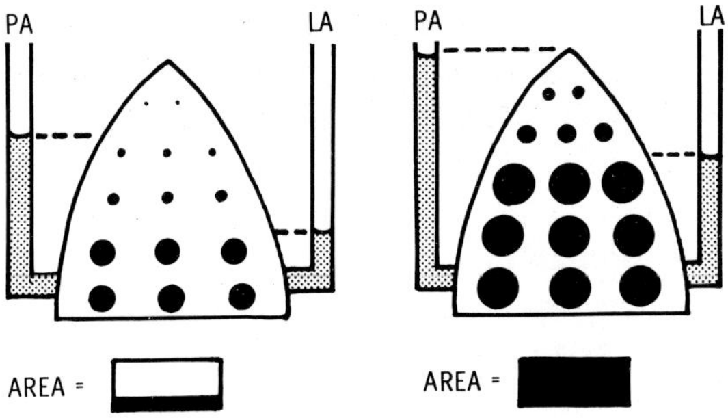

Fig. 1. Gravitational distribution of blood flow in the erect posture. Left: low flow. Right: high flow. The manometers indicate pulmonary artery (PA) and left atrial (LA) pressures. The black areas represent the cross sectional area of blood vessels in different zones of the lung. The total cross sectional area is increased at high blood flows because of the increase in zones 2 and 3 (see text).

greater than atmospheric. Blood is therefore forced along the pulmonary capillaries towards the venous end. Because of the resistance of the capillaries there is a lower pressure at the venous end than at the arterial end. Capillary flow is therefore determined by the relationship between the alveolar pressure and the pressure at the venous end of the capillary, the capillary collapsing when alveolar pressure exceeds that in the capillary. In the region where this mechanism is dominant (zone 2) there is a linear increase in flow from the top to the bottom of the zone (West, 1974).

The junction between zones 2 and 3 is determined by the left atrial pressure. In zone 3 the pulmonary venous pressure exceeds the pressure in the alveoli. The principle of the Starling resistor no longer applies and there is relatively little increase in flow down the zone. A fourth zone has been described at the base of the lung in patients with a high left atrial pressure. This is a zone of reduced blood flow which is believed to be produced by the presence of interstitial and alveolar oedema. This is thought to alter the tissue pressure, so narrowing the pulmonary arterioles and reducing blood flow.

Acute Effects of Hypovolaemic Shock on the Lung

Control of respiration

There is a marked increase in respiratory rate with variable alterations in tidal volume. Arterial PCO_2 is usually reduced to 20–30 mmHg. The increase in respiratory activity may be partly due to the metabolic acidosis which usually accompanies haemorrhage (Freeman and Nunn, 1963). However it appears that the main drive results directly from the reduction in blood flow which fails to wash anaerobic metabolites out of the glomus tissue in the peripheral chemoreceptors (Joels and Neil, 1963). In the later stages of shock the reduction in cerebral blood flow may depress the respiratory centre. A gasping or Cheyne–Stokes type of respiration may then be seen. This occurrence may be delayed by the administration of oxygen but is accelerated by the administration of respiratory depressant drugs.

Mechanics

Variable changes in lung compliance and airway resistance have been reported in animals. However in many of these experiments no precautions were taken to prevent progressive atelectasis. In primate experiments where such precautions were taken compliance increased during haemorrhage and returned to normal on reinfusion of the shed blood (Proctor et al., 1969). However Bø and Hauge (1973) observed biphasic changes in cats. In the earlier stages of haemorrhage dynamic compliance increased, but later dynamic compliance fell. These authors suggested that the late fall was due to narrowing or collapse of terminal airways secondary to the deposition of platelet aggregates in the pulmonary circulation (see page 25).

Pulmonary circulation and gas exchange

Carbon dioxide. When blood volume is reduced cardiac output falls and the arterio-venous difference for oxygen and carbon dioxide rises in order to maintain adequate transport of these gases. The lung is thus supplied with reduced quantities of blood with a low PO_2 and high PCO_2 but there is no reduction in the total volumes of oxygen and carbon dioxide which have to be exchanged. The reduction in pulmonary blood flow leads to a reduction in pulmonary artery and left atrial pressure, thus increasing the number of capillaries subject to zone 1 and 2 conditions. Since fewer capillaries are perfused, the cross-sectional area of the pulmonary vascular bed is effectively reduced and calculated pulmonary vascular resistance is increased (Fig. 1).

The increase in the number of non-perfused and relatively under-perfused alveoli increases alveolar dead space and dead space/tidal volume ratio. This has been clearly demonstrated in the isolated perfused lung by West and Jones (1965) and in the intact animal by Gerst et al. (1959) and Freeman and Nunn

(1963). Calculations made from the data of Cournand et al. (1943) and studies by Askrog (1966) reveal that similar changes are seen in man. The increase in dead space reduces alveolar ventilation so that CO_2 elimination becomes less efficient. However, it is uncommon to see much increase in arterial PCO_2 even when ventilation is maintained artificially at pre-haemorrhagic levels. The reason for this is that pulmonary artery pressure falls relatively less than systemic pressure because of the increase in pulmonary vascular resistance already noted. By the time that the fall in pulmonary artery pressure is of sufficient magnitude to cause a significant increase in dead space, cardiac output is grossly reduced. In order to maintain blood flow to the vital centres flow is redistributed away from non-essential areas (Rutherford et al., 1968). As a result there is a reduction in the volume of tissue perfused and, consequently, a reduction in the total CO_2 load imposed on the lung. When blood flow is restored the oxygen debt is made good, and the CO_2 load is increased above normal. An increase in the CO_2 load may also be imposed by the metabolism of citrate or bicarbonate or by shivering. When the blood loss is rapidly restored the pulmonary artery pressure usually returns to normal levels or above. However dead space may not return to normal for 15–30 minutes. This phenomenon is often seen after temporary total cessation of pulmonary blood flow during total cardiopulmonary bypass or cardiac arrest and is thought to be due to critical closure of vessels or to transient intravascular aggregation (Pauca and Sykes, 1966; Suwa et al., 1969).

Similar changes are seen when blood loss is not replaced and systemic hypotension persists. For example Kim and Shoemaker (1971) have noted elevations of pulmonary artery pressure in patients who have suffered trauma and haemorrhage, whilst in dogs bled to a constant low systemic pressure there is a gradual increase in pulmonary artery pressure and pulmonary vascular resistance though cardiac output remains at a low level. Furthermore, Naimark et al. (1968) have shown that the increase in pulmonary artery pressure is accompanied by a redistribution of blood flow from the base of the lung to the apex so that the blood flow becomes more evenly distributed throughout the lung. However, the enlarged alveolar dead space persists.

There are many possible explanations for these changes. Focal atelectasis and oedema were present in the dependent portions of the lungs and may have diverted flow by a mechanical effect or by inducing hypoxic vasoconstriction. A metabolic acidosis was pronounced at this time and might have produced preferential vasoconstriction in the lower zones. However the persistence of the increased alveolar dead space suggests that obstruction of portions of the pulmonary vascular bed may have occurred. Focal areas of reduced blood flow have been demonstrated in rabbit lungs by Allardyce et al. (1969). The obstruction may have been due to microaggregates in the blood taken up from the arterial reservoir, to vasoactive substances or to disseminated intravascular coagulation. Bø and Hognestad (1971) provided evidence that platelets were involved in hypovolaemic shock in cats. They showed that the increase in pulmonary vascular resistance was accompanied by a fall in platelet count and that the increase in pulmonary vascular resistance could be prevented by inducing thrombocytopenia before subjecting the cats to haemorrhage.

It was originally suggested that the increase in pulmonary vascular resistance was due to obstruction of the pulmonary circulation by microaggregates (Allardyce et al., 1969). However there is now a great deal of evidence to suggest that most of the increase in resistance is due to the release of vasoconstrictor substances from the platelet during the process of aggregation (Bø et al., 1972; Ljungqvist, 1973). The vasoconstrictor substances released by the platelet vary with the species but in the dog the evidence suggests that the vasoconstriction is mediated mainly by serotonin (Kusajima et al., 1974a; Swedenborg, 1971).

The reason for the deposition of platelet microaggregates in the lung is not clear. Ljungqvist (1970) showed that there was an increase in platelet adhesiveness, aggregability and aggregate formation within minutes of an acute massive haemorrhage in the dog and postulated that this reflected the activation of a homeostatic mechanism for control of haemorrhage. However it has been shown that tissue hypoxia or direct trauma can also result in the formation of platelet and fibrin microaggregates and that these may then migrate to the lung (Berman et al., 1971; Blaisdell et al., 1966, 1970). Furthermore, microaggregates are present in stored blood. These are often small enough to pass standard infusion filters and so may pass directly into the pulmonary circulation (Connell and Swank, 1973).

Whatever their origin, there seems to be no doubt that platelet microaggregates may modify the gross effects produced by a reduction in pulmonary blood flow. However, the importance of this mechanism in human shock remains to be determined.

Oxygen. Arterial hypoxaemia has been commonly recorded in patients with shock even though the arterial PCO_2 is normal or low. However hypoxaemia has not occurred in many carefully conducted animal studies. Thus West and Jones (1965) found no change in venous admixture when blood flow was reduced in the isolated lung whilst other workers have found that venous admixture is the same or reduced during haemorrhagic hypotension in intact animals (Gerst et al., 1959; Freeman and Nunn, 1963; Sykes et al., 1970).

Indeed in both animals and humans there seems to be a close positive correlation between shunt or total venous admixture and cardiac output (Hedley-Whyte et al., 1966; Yamamura et al., 1969). The discrepancy between the animal and human PO_2 data is therefore probably due to the presence of physiological or pathological changes in the lungs of humans. For example, it has been shown that the arterial PO_2 falls with age, a normal 70 year old patient having a PO_2 of between 70 and 80 mmHg (Sorbini et al., 1968). Furthermore, the arterial PO_2 of patients over the age of 40–45 years is usually lower in the supine position than in the erect position because the reduction in functional residual capacity in the former position causes dependent airways to close within the range of tidal breathing (Craig et al., 1971b). The assumption of a head-down tilt may further decrease functional residual capacity and so cause even more airways to close (Craig et al., 1971a). The closure of airways during part or all of the respiratory cycle will lead to underventilation and so will contribute to a venous admixture effect. This is one cause of arterial hypoxaemia in patients with apparently normal lungs.

However pathological changes in the lungs are quite common in patients with shock. These may be due to existing lung disease or to direct or indirect lung damage. Direct damage to the lung may result from trauma, aspiration or vomit, lung burns or smoke aspiration whilst indirect damage may be caused by the blast from an explosion. Head injuries are well known to cause pulmonary oedema whilst overtransfusion may produce a similar picture.

When venous admixture is increased, hypoxaemia may be accentuated by the reduction in mixed venous PO_2 resulting from the fall in cardiac output (Sykes et al., 1965). It has also been shown that, in dogs, shunt flow through an atelectatic lobe increases during shock. It is postulated that the redistribution of flow in this model is due either to impaired hypoxic vasoconstriction in the atelectatic lobe or to a disproportionate increase in pulmonary vascular resistance in the ventilated lung tissue (Wahrenbrook et al., 1970).

Another possible cause of hypoxaemia is terminal airway narrowing due to the release of serotonin, histamine or other substances from the platelet microaggregates in the lung. Stein et al. (1970) have shown that autologous thrombo-emboli increase airway resistance in dogs and that the changes can be prevented by pharmacological agents which decrease the number of platelets, inactivate thrombin, prevent platelet aggregation or antagonise serotonin. Arfors et al. (1972) showed that thrombin-induced disseminated intravascular coagulation produced a fall in PO_2 but further studies by Jastrzebski et al. (1975a) showed that the fall in PO_2 was mainly due to the reduction in cardiac output without much change in the proportion of venous admixture. However Jastrzebski et al. subjected the lungs to periodic hyperinflations throughout the period of study. This procedure appears to overcome terminal airway closure due to platelet aggregation and may therefore provide yet another cause for the great variation in results recorded in different studies.

A further possible cause of hypoxaemia is an increase in the pulmonary extravascular water volume. This is known to occur in dogs but has not yet been convincingly demonstrated in humans (Aarseth and Bø 1972; Wyche et al., 1971). It has been suggested that the increase in lung water is due to pulmonary venous constriction during and after the period of shock but it is also known that platelet amines can increase vascular permeability (Nachman et al., 1972). The increase in interstitial fluid appears to increase closing volume, thus producing dependent airway closure in the tidal volume range. When the lymphatic pathways become overloaded alveolar oedema may occur. However it is uncommon to see alveolar oedema after haemorrhagic shock unless the patient has been overtransfused.

Pulmonary Effects of Cardiogenic Shock

Respiratory control

Hyperventilation is characteristically present in patients with cardiogenic shock. Since the respiratory rate can be reduced by vagal blockade it has been postulated that the response is mediated by stimulation of the 'J' receptors. These are triggered by pulmonary congestion (Paintal, 1973). Hyperventilation gives way to hypoventilation when severe pulmonary oedema develops.

Lung mechanics

There is a marked reduction in lung compliance and an increase in airway resistance. Very high inflation pressures may be required when severe pulmonary oedema is present.

Pulmonary circulation and gas exchange

The increase in left atrial pressure alters the Starling equilibrium so that fluid passes out of the pulmonary capillaries into the interstitial space. The increased fluid transudation is at first drained away by the lymphatics but when these become overloaded interstitial oedema occurs. Initially the oedema is localised to the bases of the lungs where it appears to reduce pulmonary blood flow. It may also cause terminal airway closure (Hughes et al., 1968, 1970; Kazemi et al., 1970). Later the accumulation of fluid increases and alveolar filling occurs (Staub et al., 1967). Arterial hypoxaemia during air breathing is an early sign of pulmonary oedema and, in the absence of treatment, the arterial PO_2 usually falls rapidly to very low levels despite the low arterial PCO_2. The low arterial PO_2 is due to both ventilation perfusion inequalities and right-to-left intrapulmonary shunting and is accentuated by the effects of the lowered mixed venous PO_2 resulting from the reduced cardiac output. Some increase in alveolar dead space occurs as a result of the ventilation/perfusion inequalities but the increase in shunt is the dominant feature (McNicol et al., 1964; Al Bazzaz and Kazemi, 1972).

Pulmonary Disturbances Associated with Septic Shock

Respiratory control

Hyperventilation is the earliest sign of respiratory involvement both in animals and humans (Walt and Wilson, 1970). It has been suggested that the low arterial PCO_2 may be due to stimulation of the 'J' receptors or lung irritant receptors by congestion, oedema, serotonin or alterations in lung mechanics (Paintal, 1973). Respiratory stimulation may also be produced by the severe metabolic acidosis which is commonly found in septic shock.

Lung mechanics

Little is known about changes in mechanics in the early stages of septic shock in humans although there is an obvious increase in airway resistance and reduction in lung compliance when pulmonary oedema occurs. In experimental endotoxin or septic shock there is an early reduction in dynamic compliance and an increase in airway resistance. Stein and Thomas (1967) showed that the changes resulting from the injection of endotoxin in dogs could be diminished by the prior injection of heparin or serotonin antagonists or by the previous induction of thrombocytopenia. They therefore postulated that the changes were mediated by the release of serotonin during platelet aggregation. However in the later stages of endotoxin or septic shock there is a marked increase in interstitial and alveolar fluid. This produces similar but more pronounced changes in lung mechanics.

Gas exchange

The pattern of septic shock varies greatly. Some patients have a clearly defined hyperdynamic phase with a raised cardiac output, low perfusion pressure and hot extremities whilst others pass straight into the low output phase with constricted peripheral vessels and a diminished urine output. Since these gross changes in cardiac output have major effects on the pulmonary circulation, it is not surprising that there are wide variations in the reported changes in lung function. In experimental models there is an even greater variation in response, for not only are there differences in response between species, and differences between the response to endotoxin and to live organisms (Hinshaw, 1972), but there are also differences between the responses obtained in the conscious state and those obtained during anaesthesia or sedation (Herman et al., 1972).

In animals there is an early rise in the pulmonary artery pressure after the injection of endotoxin or live organisms but no change in left atrial pressure. It has been suggested that both pre- and postcapillary sphincters are affected and that capillary congestion could lead to subsequent transudation of fluid to the interstitial space (Kuida et al., 1958). It is not yet clear whether the changes in pulmonary artery pressure are due to a generalised rise in circulating vasoconstrictor substances or to the local release of vasoconstrictors during platelet aggregation in the lung. However Motsay et al. (1973) found that the previous administration of phenoxybenzamine or methylprednisolone prevented the rise in postcapillary resistance after injection of endotoxin and diminished the rate of water accumulation in the lung.

An increase in lung water is the dominant feature of septic shock. It has been shown that endotoxin increases capillary permeability to water and macromolecules (Chien et al., 1964; Coalson et al., 1970) and it is known that platelet aggregates may have a similar effect. Riordan and Walters (1968) recorded the results of autopsies on five patients who died from septic shock. These patients received no intravenous fluid and had no signs of cardiac disease but all had severe pulmonary oedema. McLean et al. (1968) recorded a high incidence of pulmonary oedema in patients with septic shock whilst McLaughlin (1971) noted that in a group of shocked patients the intrapulmonary shunt was greatest in those suffering from concomitant sepsis.

Patients with septic shock therefore develop a widening of the alveolar-arterial PO_2 difference at an early stage of the disease. However the arterial PO_2 is not greatly reduced because the arterial PCO_2 is low. As the disease progresses interstitial and alveolar oedema develops. This results in a marked increase in intrapulmonary shunt and severe hypoxaemia. In the terminal stages there is gross respiratory distress, cyanosis and an increase in arterial PCO_2.

Disseminated intravascular coagulation is a common complication of septic shock. Thus Milligan et al. (1974) reported that 19 out of 21 patients in septic shock had haematological changes which were indicative of disseminated intravascular coagulation, whilst Stoddart and Wardle (1974) documented a further case which ultimately died from the shock-lung syndrome. However there is still some doubt as to whether the lung damage is due to the endotoxin or to the accompanying disseminated intravascular coagulation (Jastrzebski, 1975b).

Delayed Effects of Trauma and Shock

Pulmonary complications have always been a major cause of death after both civilian and military trauma (Simeone, 1968). However improvements in the resuscitation and intensive care of casualties have led to an increased awareness of the problem of respiratory failure after injury. The syndrome occurs in a small proportion of seriously injured and shocked patients and has been variously termed the 'shock-lung syndrome', the 'acute respiratory distress syndrome of the adult', the 'wet-lung syndrome', 'Da Nang lung' and even the 'pushmi-pullyu syndrome' (Baue, 1972).

The clinical picture

It is usually possible to recognise four phases (Moore, 1968). The first is the phase of haemorrhagic hypotension. The patient hyperventilates, is severely shocked and lung function alters in the manner already described. Resuscitative measures are applied and surgery is carried out. The patient then enters the second or stable phase when both cardiac and respiratory systems appear to be performing normally. Usually this phase is indistinguishable from that following any major surgery, the respiratory changes being characterised by a raised respiratory rate, reduced tidal volume, normal or reduced PCO_2 and mild hypoxaemia. Such changes usually reach a peak on the first or second postoperative day and then regress. However when patients develop the shock lung syndrome there is a rapid increase in respiratory distress. This may occur at any time up to three or four days after the period of shock. The respiratory rate increases, respiration becomes laboured and there is a marked fall in arterial PO_2 despite a relatively normal PCO_2. The patient becomes restless and distressed and there may be diffuse opacities on the radiograph. This marks the third phase of the syndrome. If treatment is not actively pursued the patient passes into the fourth phase. This is characterised by increasing respiratory distress, a depressed level of consciousness and cardiovascular collapse. There is a progressive increase in intrapulmonary shunt, a marked increase in dead space/tidal volume ratio and an increase in arterial PCO_2. There is severe hypoxaemia, despite the administration of high concentrations of oxygen, and a severe metabolic acidosis develops. Gross opacities are present on the radiograph. Death results from the effects of the severe hypoxia.

Pathological changes

These have been well described by Blaisdell (1974). If death occurs during the early hypotensive phase there may be platelet or fibrin microemboli in the small pulmonary arterioles. By 16–18 hours after injury there is pulmonary vascular congestion and a number of periarteriolar haemorrhages are apparent. By 24 hours there is obvious intra-alveolar haemorrhage and interstitial and alveolar oedema and there are scattered areas of haemorrhage on macroscopic examination. These haemorrhages gradually become confluent until the lung has a liver-like appearance. On the third or fourth day after injury hyaline membranes become obvious and the haemorrhage and oedema is less marked. In patients dying more than 5 days after the original injury there are usually areas displaying a bronchopneumonic pattern of change. Wilson (1974) has pointed out that the pathological changes in the lung are common to many different types of injury. Oxygen toxicity, shock, cardiopulmonary bypass, circulatory overload, the inhalation of irritant gases and sepsis all produce similar reactions. Electron microscopy reveals that the tight junctions between endothelial cells are opened so that fluid, red cells, platelets and white cells leak out into the interstitial space. The endothelial cells frequently show damage to the pinocytotic vesicle system so that there is a drastic reduction in the lung's ability to control the movement of protein and alveolar type I pneumocytes (Shea et al., 1969). There is a proliferation of the connective tissue and the type II cells and mast cells also appear to be damaged.

Aetiology

The analysis of clinical data has contributed little to the elucidation of the aetiology of the condition, for most of the patients have been subjected to a number of different insults of varying severity. For example they have usually suffered major trauma, have been severely shocked and have undergone major surgery. Direct injury to the lungs and major sepsis are further complicating factors. Some of the possible aetiological factors can be isolated in experimental preparations but, again, the interpretation of results is hindered by the complex nature of the shock process. Furthermore there are large species variations which lead to contradictory conclusions. For these reasons it is only possible to indicate current lines of thought concerning possible aetiological mechanisms. Although many of the factors interact, an attempt has been made to simplify the discussion by grouping the possible aetiological factors under four headings:

Factors resulting in direct injury to the lung. One possible explanation for the syndrome is that it represents the delayed response to lung trauma sustained at the time of the original injury. This may arise in a number of ways. First, there may be obvious or concealed blunt trauma to the lungs. This leads to contusion with pulmonary congestion, interstitial and alveolar haemorrhages and localised oedema. However it has now been shown that contusion in one lung may lead to increased vascular permeability in the other (non-traumatised) lung. It is not clear why this occurs, but the implication is that generalised congestion and oedema may result from quite moderate volume replacement (Fulton and Peter, 1973, 1974). Trauma to the lung may also be caused by the blast from an explosion. This may not produce symptoms immediately but may lead to the later onset of severe respiratory distress (Falla, 1940; Zuckerman, 1940). Thermal or smoke injuries may also remain unrecognised at first but may later lead to severe respiratory embarrassment (Di Vincenti et al., 1971). Finally there is always the possibility that stomach contents may have been aspirated. This usually occurs during a transient period of unconsciousness or when the laryngeal reflexes are depressed by heavy sedation.

Factors associated with tissue injury elsewhere. Tissue injury results in the release of thromboplastins which induce local and generalised platelet aggregation with the production of platelet–fibrin microaggregates. Microaggregates from the traumatised area may enter the venous system and be filtered by the lung (Blaisdell et al., 1970).

Fat emboli are commonly associated with damage to the long bones but fat is often found in the lung after other types of trauma. It is not yet clear whether the fat damages the lung by obstructing the microcirculation or by liberating fatty acids (Sevitt, 1973) but the time of onset (12–48 hours after the injury) closely parallels the time at which the shock lung develops. Fat embolism leads to an increase in alveolar dead space and shunt and there is often severe pulmonary oedema.

A third factor which may be considered under this heading is sepsis. This may develop in the lung as a result of some postoperative pulmonary complication or may occur elsewhere. Sepsis increases capillary permeability and commonly results in pulmonary oedema. The association between sepsis and shock lung is very common and many authors believe that this is one of the most important aetiological factors (Wilson et al., 1969; Hirsch et al., 1971). Indeed it has recently been suggested that endotoxin may be released from the gut when massive burns are inflicted on animals and that this might account for the lung lesions commonly associated with severe burns (Cuevas et al., 1974) or haemorrhagic shock (Soma et al., 1974).

Factors associated with the period of shock. It was originally postulated that one of the causative factors was ischaemia of the lung during the period of shock. However this seems unlikely for the lesions can be prevented by excluding the lung from the circulation during the period of shock (Sykes et al., 1966; Willwerth et al., 1967). Henry et al. (1967) suggested that surfactant might be decreased and that the alteration in surface forces might lead to the later occurrence of lung lesions. Although the epithelial type II cells are undoubtedly damaged (Wilson, 1974) it is not yet clear whether the changes in surfactant are the cause or the result of the lung lesions.

A somewhat more likely cause of the lung lesions is prolonged pulmonary vasoconstriction. If this produced a greater increase in postcapillary than in precapillary resistance it could result in a increased pressure in the pulmonary capillary. The resulting congestion could then cause capillary leakage and rupture. The three most likely causes of pulmonary vasoconstriction are acidosis, circulating vasoconstrictor substances and autonomic activity (Cook and Webb, 1968; Berk et al., 1973). The correction of the acidosis in shock diminishes but does not eliminate the increase in pulmonary vascular resistance. This suggests that it is not an important factor.

Vasoconstrictor substances may originate from lung tissue, from platelet microaggregates or from other parts of the body. Thus histamine is probably released from mast cells in the lung during haemorrhage (Wilson, 1974) but in many species (including man) it is also released from the platelet during aggregation. Platelets release many other vasoactive substances during aggregation, but the substances most likely to cause pulmonary vasoconstriction and an increase in capillary permeability are serotonin and histamine. Circulating vasoactive substances known to be increased during shock include vasoactive peptides (Bayley et al., 1967) and kinins (Massion and Blümel, 1971).

Support for the possible role of the autonomic nervous system in the production of pulmonary venous constriction was provided by Sugg et al. (1969). These authors claimed that pulmonary venous constriction could be prevented if the lung was completely denervated by autotransplantation. Moss (1974) postulated that the increased autonomic activity was due to stagnant hypoxia of the brain resulting from the reduction in cerebral blood flow in severe shock. He demonstrated that typical lung lesions could be produced by perfusing the brain with mixed venous blood for 2 hours and that lesions did not develop in a lung which had been previously denervated by autotransplantation. Although this evidence, and the association between head injury and pulmonary oedema (Simmons et al., 1969), supports the centroneurogenic theory it is worth noting that Kusajima et al. (1974b) failed to produce lung lesions when they restricted the arterial inflow to the dog brain to such an extent that ischaemic changes occurred. Furthermore there is no firm evidence that pulmonary venous constriction occurs in man.

Factors associated with therapy. Early reports implicated oxygen toxicity as a possible cause of the syndrome. However, many patients developed the syndrome before oxygen was administered so it seems unlikely that this factor could have initiated the changes even though it may have been responsible for a deterioration in lung function after treatment was started.

Most of the patients have received massive fluid replacement and in the earlier series there were undoubtedly some cases where the condition was caused by the excessive infusion of crystalloid solutions (Mills, 1968). Such solutions diffuse rapidly throughout the extravascular space and pulmonary oedema may occur without any rise in central venous pressure. The increased likelihood of pulmonary oedema in the contused lung is a further factor to be considered.

Transfusions of blood have been known to cause pulmonary oedema by the induction of a hypersensitivity reaction to leuko-agglutinins (Thompson et al., 1971) or by the administration of incompatible blood (Halmagyi et al., 1963; Byrne and Dixon, 1971). Platelet–leucocyte microaggregates develop as blood is stored and these may be filtered out in the smaller vessels in the lung. Such aggregates pass through normal blood filters but can be removed by passing the blood through a special dacron wool filter. When this is done there is a marked reduction in the incidence of lung changes (Reul et al., 1973).

It is apparent that many authors feel that microaggregates play an important role in the development of the lung lesion. Intravascular aggregation may result from a generalised reduction in capillary flow, from peripheral tissue damage or from the infusion of stored blood. However, microaggregates are normally rapidly removed from the lung by the activation of the fibrinolytic system. If aggregates are to be implicated in the aetiology of the shock lung it is necessary to postulate that they initiate a series of changes which do not manifest themselves clinically until some time after the original injury. This hypothesis remains to be proved.

In summary, it appears likely that the so called shock-lung represents a non-specific reaction to a number of different stimuli. It is probable that many factors combine to cause the syndrome in any one patient and that prevention can only be accomplished by minimising the effects of different factors by meticulous attention to all aspects of resuscitation and subsequent patient care.

Treatment

Haemorrhagic shock

The first essential is the early and correct treatment of the shock with fluids and supplementary oxygen. This necessitates accurate and frequent measurements of arterial and central venous pressure and, if possible, pulmonary artery wedge pressure. Blood should be as fresh as possible, should be subjected to special filtration and should be warmed in the usual way. Colloids may be used to supplement blood but crystalloids must be administered with some care. If blood volume has been rapidly restored the excess lactate will be quickly metabolised. However if there is a severe and persistent metabolic acidosis, bicarbonate should be given.

When the acute phase is over the patient should be carefully observed and blood gases measured at least daily. If the shock-lung develops the treatment outlined below should be given.

Septic shock

The occurrence of hyperventilation and restlessness in a patient with sepsis should lead to an immediate arterial blood-gas analysis with calculation of the alveolar–arterial PO_2 difference. If a low output is suspected a central or mixed venous PO_2 should be obtained as well. The sepsis should be treated vigorously and supplementary oxygen should be provided if the arterial PO_2 is below about 70 mmHg. A reduced cardiac output should be treated by blood volume expansion and a close watch kept on the patient's condition and arterial PO_2. When this falls to 60–70 mmHg on 30% oxygen mechanical ventilation should be considered. It is important to start ventilation early rather than late and, once started, there should be no hesitation in applying an end-expiratory positive pressure. Particular care should be taken when attempting to wean the patient from the positive end-expiratory pressure for oedema quickly reaccumulates if the lung damage is incompletely resolved.

Cardiogenic shock

Similar considerations apply. However specific cardiac treatment will also be required.

Shock–lung

The mortality from this condition is high. The early application of mechanical ventilation with positive end-expiratory pressure is essential. Although it is desirable to restrict the inspired oxygen concentration to 50–60% this may have to be exceeded in the severe case. The circulation should be closely monitored and fluid or inotropic drugs administered as required. Diuretics may prove useful. Massive doses of steroids have been recommended but there is no evidence that they have any useful effect. It is possible that long-term extracorporeal oxygenation may prove helpful in the future.

Summary

Acute, severe haemorrhage leads to a fall in pulmonary artery and left atrial pressures and a reduction in pulmonary blood volume and flow. Alveolar dead space is increased but there is no increase in shunt or total venous admixture. The deposition of platelet microaggregates during prolonged haemorrhage leads to the release of amines which cause pulmonary vasoconstriction and may cause narrowing or closure of terminal airways. As a result there is an increase in pulmonary vascular resistance, a continued increase in dead space despite the increase in pulmonary artery pressure, and often arterial hypoxaemia. In patients arterial hypoxaemia is most likely to be due to preexisting lung disease, direct or indirect damage to the lung or overtransfusion. The effects of an increased venous admixture from any of these causes will always be accentuated by the reduction in mixed venous PO_2 resulting from the low cardiac output.

Both cardiogenic and septic shock lead to pulmonary oedema. This will usually be treated with mechanical ventilation and the application of end-expiratory pressure. Similar considerations apply to the treatment of the shock lung.

References

Aarseth, P. and Bø, G. (1972): Pulmonary blood- and extravascular water volumes during prolonged post-hemorrhagic hypotension. *Acta physiol. scand.*, *85*, 353.

Al Bazzaz, F.J. and Kazemi, H. (1972): Arterial hypoxemia and distribution of pulmonary perfusion after uncomplicated myocardial infarction. *Amer. Rev. resp. Dis.*, *106*, 721.

Allardyce, B., Hamit, H.F., Matsumoto, T. and Moseley, R.V. (1969): Pulmonary vascular changes in hypovolemic shock: radiography of the pulmonary microcirculation and the possible role of platelet embolism in increasing vascular resistance. *J. Trauma*, *9*, 403.

Arfors, K-E., Busch, C., Jakobson, S., Lindquist, O., Malmberg, P., Rammer, L. and Saldeen, T. (1972): Pulmonary insufficiency following intravenous infusion of thrombin and AMCA (tranexamic acid) in the dog. *Acta chir. scand.*, *138*, 445.

Askrog, V. (1966): Changes in (a–A) CO_2 difference and pulmonary artery pressure in anesthetized man. *J. appl. Physiol.*, *21*, 1299.

Baue, A.E. (1972): The pushmi–pullyu syndrome. *Surgery*, *72*, 655.

Bayley, T., Clements, J.A. and Osbahr, A.J. (1967): Pulmonary and circulatory effects of fibrinopeptides. *Circulat. Res.*, *21*, 469.

Berk J.L., Hagen, J.F., Koo, R., Beyer, W., Dochat, G.R., Rupright, M. and Nomoto, S. (1973): Pulmonary insufficiency caused by epinephrine. *Ann. Surg.*, *178*, 423.

Berman, I.R., Smulson, M.E., Pattengale, P. and Schoenbach, S.F. (1971). Pulmonary microembolism after soft tissue injury in primates. *Surgery*, *70*, 246.

Blaisdell, F.W. (1974): Pathophysiology of the respiratory distress syndrome. *Arch. Surg.*, *108*, 44.

Blaisdell, F.W., Lim, R.C., Amberg, J.R., Choy, S.H., Hall, A.D. and Thomas, A.N. (1966): Pulmonary microembolism. A cause of morbidity and death after major vascular surgery. *Arch. Surg. (Chicago)*, *93*, 776.

Blaisdell, F.W., Lim, R.C. and Stallone, R.J. (1970): The mechanism of pulmonary damage following traumatic shock. *Surg. Gynec. Obstet.*, *130*, 15.

Bø, G., Hauge, A. and Hognestad, J. (1972): Pulmonary hypertension during systemic hypotension. Effects of oxygen breathing and of vasodilators. *Acta physiol. scand.*, *86*, 466.

Bø, G. and Hognestad, J. (1971): Thrombocytes and pulmonary vascular resistance during hemorrhagic hypotension. *Acta physiol. scand.*, *82*, 218.

Bø, G. and Hauge, A. (1973): A two-phased change in dynamic lung compliance during hemorrhagic hypotension. *Acta physiol. scand.*, *87*, 448.

Byrne, J.P. and Dixon, J.A. (1971): Pulmonary edema following blood transfusion reaction. *Arch. Surg. (Chicago)*, *102*, 91.

Chien, S., Sinclair, D.G., Dellenback, R.J., Chang, C., Peric, B., Usami, S. and Gregersen, M.I. (1964): Effect of endotoxin on capillary permeability to macromolecules. *Amer. J. Physiol., 207*, 518.

Coalson, J.J., Hinshaw, L.B. and Guenter, C.A. (1970): The pulmonary ultrastructure in septic shock. *Exp. molec. Path., 12*, 84.

Connell, R.S. and Swank, R.L. (1973): Pulmonary microembolism after blood transfusions: an electron microscopic study. *Ann. Surg., 177*, 40.

Cook, W.A. and Webb, W.R. (1968): Pulmonary changes in hemorrhagic shock. *Surgery, 64*, 85.

Cournand, A., Riley, R.L., Bradley, S.E., Breed, E.S., Noble, R.P., Lauson, H.D., Gregersen, M.I. and Richards, D.W. (1943): Studies of the circulation in clinical shock. *Surgery, 13*, 964.

Craig, D.B., Wahba, W.M. and Don, H.F. (1971a): Airway closure and lung volumes in surgical positions. *Canad. Anaesth. Soc. J., 18*, 92.

Craig, D.B., Wahba, W.M., Don, H.F., Couture J.G. and Becklake, M.R. (1971b): 'Closing volume' and its relationship to gas exchange in seated and supine positions. *J. appl. Physiol., 31*, 717.

Cuevas, P., Ishiyama, M., Koizumi, S., Woodruff, P., Kaufman, A. and Fine, J. (1974): Role of endotoxemia of intestinal origin in early death from large burns. *Surg. Gynec. Obstet., 138*, 725.

Di Vincenti, F.C., Pruitt, B.A. and Peckler, J.M. (1971): Inhalation injuries. *J. Trauma, 11*, 109.

Falla, S.T. (1940): Effect of explosion-blast on the lungs. Report of a case. *Brit. med. J., 2*, 255.

Freeman, J. and Nunn, J.F. (1963): Ventilation–perfusion relationships after haemorrhage. *Clin. Sci., 24*, 135.

Fulton, R.L. and Peter, E.T. (1973): Physiologic effects of fluid therapy after pulmonary contusion. *Amer. J. Surg., 126*, 773.

Fulton, R.L. and Peter, E.D. (1974). Compositional and histologic effects of fluid therapy following pulmonary contusion. *J. Trauma, 14*, 783.

Gerst, P.H., Rattenborg, C. and Holaday, D.H. (1959): The effects of hemorrhage on pulmonary circulation and respiratory gas exchange. *J. clin. Invest., 38*, 524.

Halmagyi, D.F.J., Starzecki, B., McRae, J. and Horner, G.J. (1963): The lung as the main target organ in the acute phase of transfusion reaction in sheep. *J. surg. Res., 3*, 418.

Hedley-Whyte, J., Pontoppidan, H. and Morris, M.J. (1966): The response of patients with respiratory failure and cardiopulmonary disease to different levels of constant volume ventilation. *J. clin. Invest., 45*, 1543.

Henry, J.N., McArdle, A.H., Bounous, G., Hampson, L.G., Scott, H.J. and Gurd, F.N. (1967): The effect of experimental hemorrhagic shock on pulmonary alveolar surfactant. *J. Trauma, 7*, 691.

Herman, C.M., McKee, A.E., Schilling, P.W., Dickson, L.G., Horwitz, D.L., Coran, A.G., Cryer, P.E. and Kopriva, C.J. (1972): The baboon as a subhuman primate shock model. In: *Shock in Low and High Flow States*, p. 42. Editors: B.K. Forscher, R.C. Lillehei and S.S. Stubb. Excerpta Medica, Amsterdam.

Hinshaw, L.B. (1972): Comparison of responses of canine and primate species to bacteria and bacterial toxin. In: *Shock in Low and High Flow States*, p. 245. Editors: B.K. Forscher, R.C. Lillehei and S.S. Stubb. Excerpta Medica, Amsterdam.

Hirsch, E.F., Fletcher, R. and Lucas, S. (1971): Hemodynamics and respiratory changes associated with sepsis following combat trauma. *Ann. Surg., 174*, 211.

Hughes, J.M.B., Glazier, J.B., Maloney, J.B. and West, J.B. (1968): Effect of extra-alveolar vessels on distribution of blood flow in the dog lung. *J. appl. Physiol., 25*, 701.

Hughes, J.M.B. and Rosenweig, D.Y. (1970): Factors affecting trapped gas volume in perfused dog lungs. *J. appl. Physiol., 3*, 332.

Jastrzebski, J., Arnot, R.N., Hilgard, P. and Sykes, M.K. (1975a): Thrombin induced disseminated intravascular coagulation in the dog. II. Cardiorespiratory changes during spontaneous and controlled ventilation. *Brit. J. Anaesth., 47*, 658.

Jastrzebski, J., Hilgard, P., Henry, K. and Sykes, M.K. (1975b): Early cardiorespiratory effects of endotoxin shock in dogs. Effect of pretreatment with epsilon amino caproic acid (EACA). Submitted for publication.

Joels, N. and Neil, E. (1963): The excitation mechanism of the carotid body. *Brit. med. Bull., 19*, 21.

Kazemi, H., Parsons, E.F., Valenca, L.M. and Strieder, D.J. (1970): Distribution of pulmonary blood flow after myocardial ischemia and infarction. *Circulation, 41*, 1025.

Kim, S.I. and Shoemaker, W.C. (1971): Development of pulmonary, hemodynamic and functional changes after operative and accidental trauma. *Surg. Gynec. Obstet., 133*, 617.

Kuida, H., Hinshaw, L.B., Gilbert, R.P. and Visscher, M.B. (1958): Effect of gram-negative endotoxin on pulmonary circulation. *Amer. J. Physiol., 192*, 335.

Kusajima, K., Ozdemir, A. and Webb, W.R. (1974a): Role of serotonin and serotonin antagonist on pulmonary hemodynamics and microcirculation in hemorrhagic shock. *J. thorac. cardiovasc. Surg., 67*, 908.

Kusajima, K., Wax, S.D. and Webb, W.R. (1974b): Cerebral hypotension and shock lung syndrome. *J. thorac. cardiovasc. Surg., 67*, 970.

Ljungqvist, U. (1970): Platelet response to acute haemorrhage in the dog. *Acta chir. scand., Suppl.*, 411.

Ljungqvist, U. (1973): Platelets in shock and trauma. *J. surg. Res., 15*, 132.

Massion, W.H. and Blümel, G. (1971): Irreversibility of shock: role of vasoactive kinins. *Curr. Res. Anesth., 50*, 970.

McLaughlin, J.S. (1971): Physiologic consideration of hypoxaemia in shock and trauma. *Ann. Surg., 173*, 667.

McLean, A.P.H., Duff, J.H. and MacLean, L.D. (1968): Lung lesions associated with septic shock. *J. Trauma, 8*, 891.

McNicol, M.W., Kirby, B.J., Bhoola, K.D., Everest, M.E., Price, H.V. and Freedman, S.F. (1965): Pulmonary function in acute myocardial infarction. *Brit. med. J., 2*, 1270.

Milligan, G.F., MacDonald, J.A.E., Mellon, A. and Ledingham, I.McA. (1974): Pulmonary and haematological disturbances during septic shock. *Surg. Gynec. Obstet., 138*, 43.

Mills, M. (1968): The clinical syndrome. *J. Trauma, 8*, 651.

Moore, F.D. (1968): Discussion in 'pulmonary effects of nonthoracic trauma'. *J. Trauma, 8*, 666.

Moss, G. (1974): The role of the central nervous system in shock: the centroneurogenic etiology of the respiratory distress syndrome. *Crit. Care Med., 2*, 181.

Motsay, G.J., Alho, A.V., Romero, L.H. and Lillehei, R.C. (1973): The pulmonary microcirculation in endotoxin-shocked dogs: effect of phenoxybenzamine and methylprednisolone on the precapillary and postcapillary resistances. *J. surg. Res., 14*, 406.

Nachmann, R.L., Weksler, B. and Ferris, B. (1972): Characterization of human platelet vascular permeability – enhancing activity. *J. clin. Invest., 51*, 549.

Naimark, A., Dugard, A. and Rangno, R.E. (1968): Regional pulmonary blood flow and gas exchange in hemorrhagic shock. *J. appl. Physiol., 25*, 301.

Paintal, A.S. (1973): Vagal sensory receptors and their reflex effects. *Physiol. Rev., 53*, 159.

Pauca, A. and Sykes, M.K. (1966): Elimination of carbon dioxide after total body perfusion. *Brit. J. Anaesth., 38*, 39.

Proctor, H.J., Moss, G.S., Homer, L.D. and Litt, B.D. (1969): Changes in lung compliance in experimental hemorrhagic shock and resuscitation. *Ann. Surg., 169*, 82.

Reul, G.J., Greenburg, S.D., Lefrak, E.A., McCollum, W.B., Beall, A.C. and Jordan, G.L. (1973): Prevention of post-traumatic pulmonary insufficiency. *Arch. Surg. (Chicago), 106*, 386.

Riordan, J.F. and Walters, G. (1968): Pulmonary oedema in acterial shock. *Lancet, 1*, 719.

Rutherford, R.B., Kaihara, S., Schwentker, E.P. and Wagner, H.N. (1968): Regional blood flow in hemorrhagic shock by the distribution of labelled microspheres. *Surg. Forum, 19*, 14.

Sevitt, S. (1973): The significance of fat embolism. *Brit. J. Hosp. Med., 9*, 784.

Shea, S.M., Karnovsky, M.J. and Bossert, W.H. (1969): Vesicular transport across endothelium: simulation of a diffusion model. *J. theor. Biol., 24*, 30.

Simeone, F.A. (1968): Pulmonary complications of nonthoracic wounds: a historical perspective. *J. Trauma, 8*, 625.

Simmons, R.L., Martin, A.M., Heisterkamp, C.A. and Ducker, T.B. (1969): Respiratory insufficiency in combat casualities. II. Pulmonary edema following head injury. *Ann. Surg., 170*, 39.

Soma, L.R., Neufeld, G.R., Dodd, D.C. and Marshall, B.E. (1974): Pulmonary function in hemorrhagic shock. The effect of pancreatic ligation and blood filtration. *Ann. Sug., 179*, 395.

Sorbini, C.A., Grassi, V., Solinas, E. and Muiesan, G. (1968): Arterial oxygen tension in relation to age in healthy subjects. *Respiration, 25*, 3.

Staub, N.C., Nagano, H. and Pearce, M.L. (1967): Pulmonary edema in dogs, especially the sequence of fluid accumulation in the lungs. *J. appl. Physiol., 22*, 227.

Stein, M., Hirose, T., Yasutake, T. and Khan, M.A. (1970): The effects of platelet amines on airway function, p. 283. In: *Airway Dynamics*, p. 283. Editor: A. Bouhuys, C.C. Thomas, Springfield, Ill.

Stein, M. and Thomas, D.P. (1967): Role of platelets in the acute pulmonary responses to endotoxin. *J. appl. Physiol., 23*, 47.

Stoddart, J.C. and Wardle, E.N. (1974): Post-traumatic respiratory distress due to endotoxinaemia and intravascular coagulation. *Brit. J. Anaesth., 46*, 892.

Sugg, W.L., Craver, W.D., Webb, W.R. and Ecker, R.R. (1969): Pressure changes in the dog lung secondary to hemorrhagic shock: protective effect of pulmonary re-implantation. *Ann. Surg., 169*, 582.

Suwa, K., Yamaguchi, Y. and Yamamura, H. (1969): Arterial–alveolar CO_2 gradient after cardiac resuscitation in the dog. *Anesthesiology, 30*, 37.

Swedenborg, J. (1971): On the role of vasoactive substances in haemodynamic changes induced by thrombin. *Acta chir. scand., Suppl., 4*, 3.

Sykes, M.K., Adams, A.P., Finlay, W.E.I., Wightman, A.E. and Munroe, J.P. (1970): The cardiorespiratory effects of haemorrhage and overtransfusion in dogs. *Brit. J. Anaesth., 42*, 573.

Sykes, M.K., Robinson, B., Melrose, D.G. and Nahas, R. (1966): Pulmonary changes after extracorporeal circulation in dogs. *Brit. J. Anaesth., 38*, 432.

Sykes, M.K., Young, W.E. and Robinson, B.E. (1965): Oxygenation during anaesthesia with controlled ventilation. *Brit. J. Anaesth., 37*, 314.

Thompson, J.S., Severson, C.D., Parmely, M.J., Marmorstein, B.L. and Simmons, A. (1971): Pulmonary hypersensitivity reactions induced by transfusion of non-HL-A leukoagglutinins. *New Engl. J. Med., 284*, 1120.

Wahrenbrock, E., Carrico, C.J., Amundsen, D.A., Trummer, M.J. and Severinghaus, J.W. (1970): Increased atelectatic pulmonary shunt during hemorrhagic shock in dogs. *J. appl. Physiol., 29*, 615.

Walt, A.J. and Wilson, R.F. (1970): Clinical, haemodynamic and respiratory changes in sepsis due to peritonitis and methods of management. *Proc. roy. Soc. Med., 63*, 31.

West, J.B. (1974): *Respiratory Physiology – the Essentials*. Blackwell Scientific Publications, Oxford.

West, J.B. and Jones, N.L. (1965): Effects of changes in topographical distribution of lung blood flow on gas exchange. *J. appl. Physiol., 20*, 825.

Wilson, J.W. (1974): Pulmonary microcirculation. Cellular pathophysiology in acute respiratory failure. *Crit. Care Med., 2*, 186.

Wilson, R.F., Kafi, A., Asuncion, Z. and Walt, A.J. (1969): Clinical respiratory failure after shock or trauma. Prognosis and methods of diagnosis. *Arch. Surg. (Chicago), 98*, 539.

Willwerth, B.M., Crawford, F.A., Young, W.G. and Sealy, W.C. (1967): The role of functional demand on the development of pulmonary lesions during hemorrhagic shock. *J. thorac. cardiovasc. Surg., 54*, 658.

Wyche, M.Q., Marshall, B.E., Mehall, S.L. and Schuetze, M.M. (1971): Lung function, pulmonary extravascular water volume and hemodynamics in early hemorrhagic shock in anaesthetized dogs. *Ann. Surg. (Chicago), 174*, 296.

Yamamura, H., Kaito, K., Ikeda, K., Nakajima, M. and Okada, K. (1969): The relationships between physiologic shunt and cardiac output in dogs under general anaesthesia. *Anesthesiology, 30*, 406.

Zuckerman, S. (1940): Experimental study of blast injuries to the lungs. *Lancet,* 219.

Ledingham (ed.). Shock

Blood flow, oxygen transport and metabolic rate in experimental shock

D.F.J. HALMAGYI

Not hypotension but a gross discrepancy between supply and demand of oxygen is the principal abnormality in shock states.

Oxygen transport (= cardiac output × arterial oxygen content = Flux_{O_2}) and oxygen consumption ($\dot{V}_{O_2}$) are connected by the oxygen extraction ratio (= $\dot{V}_{O_2} \times 100/\text{Flux}_{O_2} = \text{Ex}_{O_2}$). Thus Ex_{O_2} is a determinant of $\dot{V}_{O_2}$ yet little is known of its function and control.

At rest (Reeves et al., 1961) and in hypothermia (Thauer, 1965) $\dot{V}_{O_2}$ was found to be linearly related to cardiac output, and Ex_{O_2} (measured as arteriovenous O_2 difference) remained virtually unchanged over a wide range of flow rates. In decapitated dogs (Granger and Guyton, 1969) $\dot{V}_{O_2}$ was found to be maintained chiefly by changes in Ex_{O_2}, and only when the venous reserves were depleted, i.e. when Ex_{O_2} reached its natural limit, did $\dot{V}_{O_2}$ again become flow-dependent.

In shock some investigators found $\dot{V}_{O_2}$ reduced and concluded that this 'oxygen deficit' is indicative of depressed cellular function and predicts fatal outcome (Crowell and Smith, 1964; Smith and Crowell, 1964; Rush et al., 1965; Neuhof et al., 1973). However, others found $\dot{V}_{O_2}$ normal in fatal shock (Post et al., 1958; Halmagyi and Gillett, 1966; Rothe, 1968) suggesting that this phenomenon may not be cellular in origin but could be due to the failure of Ex_{O_2} to increase sufficiently and compensate for the excessive reduction in Flux_{O_2}.

In addition to cellular metabolism, Ex_{O_2} is affected by the contact-time between blood and tissue: increased velocity of the circulation reduces Ex_{O_2} and vice versa, and this inverse relationship between $Flux_{O_2}$ and Ex_{O_2} has been suggested to cushion the dependence of $\dot{V}_{O_2}$ on $Flux_{O_2}$ yet its effectiveness has never been quantified. Functional capillary surface area is another determinant of Ex_{O_2} (Mellander and Johansson, 1968) and this is controlled by the contractile state of the precapillary sphincters which respond to physical and chemical stimuli. Thus when the distending pressure is reduced the microvasculature dilates ('Bayliss phenomenon') (Baez, 1968), resulting in an increase in femoral (Halmagyi et al., 1969), hepatic (Halmagyi et al., 1970) and systemic (Halmagyi and Kennedy, 1970) Ex_{O_2}. Accumulation of local metabolites may also dilate the precapillary sphincters (Mellander and Johansson, 1968) while the reduction in Ex_{O_2} observed in hypercapnia (Halmagyi et al., 1970) was related to the contraction of the precapillary sphincters.

In shock sudden fall in blood pressure and flow are accompanied by drastic changes in arterial P_{CO_2}, accumulation of tissue metabolites, sometimes even fever and it appeared logical to study this complex situation.

Methods

Ninety-one greyhounds weighing 20–35 kg were studied. The thiopentone-anesthetized and intubated animals were bled into a hydrostatic reservoir to 50 mmHg pressure and 3 hours later the shed blood was reinfused. Cardiac output, femoral arterial blood flow, total body and femoral $\dot{V}_{O_2}$, arterial, mixed venous and femoral venous blood O_2 contents, arterial blood gases, lactic acid plasma level, core temperature, systemic and pulmonary blood pressures were measured before, during and after blood loss as described in previous publications contained in the reference section of this paper. Variations in body temperature were induced by surface cooling as previously described (Halmagyi et al., 1973); in the normal animals shivering was prevented by anesthesia and in shocked animals shivering does not occur. Variations in $Flux_{O_2}$ were induced by bleeding and by the infusion of 5% dextran in saline (Macrodex, Pharmacia).

After reinfusion of the shed blood twenty dogs were submitted to combined (alpha + beta) adrenergic receptor blockade as previously described (Halmagyi et al., 1971) using phenoxybenzamine and propranolol.

Regression analysis was carried out using a standard IBM program. The logarithm of $\dot{V}_{O_2}$ was the dependent variable; logarithm $Flux_{O_2}$, blood temperature and arterial P_{CO_2} were the independent variables. The effect of hypotension was assessed by comparing the results obtained in the control animals with those in the bled (mean blood pressure 50 ± 4 Torr) and re-infused (mean blood pressure 80 ± 19 Torr) dogs.

The correlation matrices displayed in the Tables are composed of the correlation coefficients for each independent variable on the dependent variable and on all other independent variables. The partial regression coefficients indicating the regression of each independent variable on the dependent variable, after removing the effects of all other independent variables, were also calculated and when significant ($P < 0.02$) were incorporated into the regression equations which were written in the following form:

$$Y_r = \beta_1 X_1 + \beta_2 X_2 + \beta_3 X_3 + \ldots + \alpha$$

where Y_r = mean value of frequency distribution of Y for specified X_1, X_2, X_3, etc. The partial regression coefficient β_1 measures the average of expected changes in Y when X_1 changes 1 Unit, X_2, X_3, etc. remaining unchanged. A measure of the validity of the regression equation was obtained by calculating the F value. The regression lines were compared by a standard test of parallelism and equality.

Results

Intact dogs (Table I)

The logarithm of total body $\dot{V}_{O_2}$ was directly related to the logarithm of $Flux_{O_2}$, to body temperature (T) and, inversely, to arterial P_{CO_2}. The overall correlation coefficient (r) was highest for log. $Flux_{O_2}$ and was only marginally improved by the inclusion of other parameters. Log $Flux_{O_2}$ was also significantly related to T.

The logarithm of hind limb $\dot{V}_{O_2}$ was related only to log femoral $Flux_{O_2}$.

In this group arterial P_{O_2} was normal (86 ± 9 Torr) and there was no evidence of anaerobic metabolism (plasma lactic acid 0.90 ± 0.71 mEq/l).

Bled dogs (Table II)

The logarithm of total body $\dot{V}_{O_2}$ was directly related to the logarithm of $Flux_{O_2}$ and to T; again the principal correlation was with log. $Flux_{O_2}$ and inclusion

Table I
Correlation matrices and regression equations for oxygen consumption in normal dogs.

Total body (71 dogs, 89 observations)

	log $\dot{V}_{O_2}$	T	log $Flux_{O_2}$	Pa_{CO_2}	Mean	S.D.	F
log $\dot{V}_{O_2}$	1.0000				2.1993	0.1512	
T	0.6778*	1.0000			36.8	2.4	
log $Flux_{O_2}$	0.8165*	0.6201*	1.0000		2.8846	0.1869	
Pa_{CO_2}	−0.2264^{+}	0.1163	−0.2022	1.0000	41.8	8.7	
r	....	....	....	....	0.86*	0.08	
$\log \dot{V}_{O_2} = 0.0212T + 0.4671 \log Flux_{O_2} - 0.0025$							77.76*
$\log Flux_{O_2} = 0.0482T + 1.1121$							

Hind limb (42 dogs, 42 observations)

	log $\dot{V}_{O_2}$	T	log $Flux_{O_2}$	Pa_{CO_2}	Mean	S.D.	F
log $\dot{V}_{O_2}$	1.0000				1.0028	0.1453	
T	0.1222	1.0000			37.6	0.7	
log $Flux_{O_2}$	0.4820*	0.1027	1.0000		1.6768	0.1702	
Pa_{CO_2}	0.0899	−0.0333	−0.0512	1.0000	39.1	1.5	
r	....	....	....	....	0.48	0.13	
$\log \dot{V}_{O_2} = 0.4115 \log Flux_{O_2} + 0.3128$							12.11*

Table II
Correlation matrices and regression equations for oxygen consumption in bled dogs.

Total body (35 dogs, 105 observations)

	log $\dot{V}_{O_2}$	T	log $Flux_{O_2}$	Pa_{CO_2}	Mean	S.D.	F
log $\dot{V}_{O_2}$	1.0000				2.1809	0.1605	
T	0.5362*	1.0000			37.7	1.4	
log $Flux_{O_2}$	0.8995*	0.4422*	1.0000		2.3478	0.1690	
Pa_{CO_2}	−0.0277	0.1764	0.1264	1.0000	33.0	8.7	
r	....	....	....	....	0.93*	0.06	
$\log \dot{V}_{O_2} = 0.0225T + 0.7917 \log Flux_{O_2} - 0.0031\, Pa_{CO_2} - 0.4241$							207.9*
$\log Flux_{O_2} = 0.0532T + 0.3458$							25.04*

Hind limb (26 dogs, 72 observations)

	log $\dot{V}_{O_2}$	T	log $Flux_{O_2}$	Pa_{CO_2}	Mean	S.D.	F
log $\dot{V}_{O_2}$	1.0000				0.8875	0.3819	
T	0.4080*	1.0000			37.9	1.2	
log $Flux_{O_2}$	0.9750*	0.4430*	1.0000		1.0433	0.3564	
Pa_{CO_2}	0.1479	0.2482^{+}	0.1773	1.000	33.5	9.6	
r	....	....	....	....	0.97*	0.09	
$\log \dot{V}_{O_2} = 1.0448 \log Flux_{O_2} - 0.2025$							1346.79*
$\log Flux_{O_2} = 0.1322T - 3.9680$							16.90*

of T improved r only marginally. Log. $Flux_{O_2}$ was also significantly related to T. The logarithm of hind limb $\dot{V}_{O_2}$ was directly related to femoral log. $Flux_{O_2}$ and also to T but inclusion of the latter did not further improve r which was already very high for log $Flux_{O_2}$. Log $Flux_{O_2}$ was also related to T.

Arterial P_{O_2} was normal in this group (89 ± 12 Torr) and the presence of anaerobic metabolism was indicated by the elevated level of plasma lactic acid (5.65 ± 3.35 mEq/l).

Reinfused dogs (Table III)

The logarithm of total body $\dot{V}_{O_2}$ was directly related to log $Flux_{O_2}$, T, and inversely to Pa_{CO_2}. The principal correlation was on T and it was only marginally improved by the inclusion of the other parameters. Log $Flux_{O_2}$ was directly related to T. The logarithm of hind limb $\dot{V}_{O_2}$ was directly related to log. femoral $Flux_{O_2}$ and to T; femoral log $Flux_{O_2}$ was also related to T.

Arterial P_{O_2} was normal (86 ± 16 Torr) and plasma lactic acid level was 3.62 ± 3.03 mEq/l.

Table III
Correlation matrices and regression equations for oxygen consumption in reinfused dogs.

Total body (26 dogs, 98 observations)

	log $\dot{V}_{O_2}$	T	log $Flux_{O_2}$	Pa_{CO_2}	Mean	S.D.	F
log $\dot{V}_{O_2}$	1.0000				2.2039	0.2027	
T	0.8090*	1.0000			35.6	3.0	
log $Flux_{O_2}$	0.5415*	0.4295*	1.0000		2.7666	0.2020	
Pa_{CO_2}	−0.3795*	−0.2157^{+}	−0.0681	1.0000	36.7	10.3	
r	....	....	....	....	0.86*	0.10	
log $\dot{V}_{O_2} = 0.0441T + 0.2454$ log $Flux_{O_2} - 0.0043\ Pa_{CO_2} + 0.1144$							92.67*
log $Flux_{O_2} = 0.0287T + 1.7424$							

Hind limb (17 dogs, 46 observations)

	log $\dot{V}_{O_2}$	T	log $Flux_{O_2}$	Pa_{CO_2}	Mean	S.D.	F
log $\dot{V}_{O_2}$	1.0000				1.0238	0.2741	
T	0.7017*	1.0000			37.6	1.9	
log $Flux_{O_2}$	0.6675*	0.4055*	1.0000		1.4273	0.3494	
Pa_{CO_2}	0.1212	0.0180	0.1609	1.0000	32.2	8.7	
r	....	....	....	....	0.82*	0.16	
log $\dot{V}_{O_2} = 0.0739T + 0.3596$ log $Flux_{O_2} - 2.2741$							43.22*
log $Flux_{O_2} = 0.0740T - 1.3603$							8.66*

Blocked dogs (Table IV)

In these animals the logarithm of total body $\dot{V}_{O_2}$ was directly related to log $Flux_{O_2}$, T and Pa_{CO_2}. Log $Flux_{O_2}$ in this group was not related to T.

Table IV
Correlation matrices and regression equations for total body oxygen consumption in reinfused dogs subjected to combined adrenergic receptor blockade.

	log $\dot{V}_{O_2}$	T	log $Flux_{O_2}$	Pa_{CO_2}	Mean	S.D.
log $\dot{V}_{O_2}$	1.0000				2.0436	0.2027
T	0.5991*	1.0000			34.2	1.5
log $Flux_{O_2}$	0.3884*	−0.0360	1.0000		2.6256	0.1475
Pa_{CO_2}	−0.4691*	−0.5281*	0.1636	1.0000	37.9	6.1
r	. . . .	. . . .	. . . .	. . . .	0.77*	

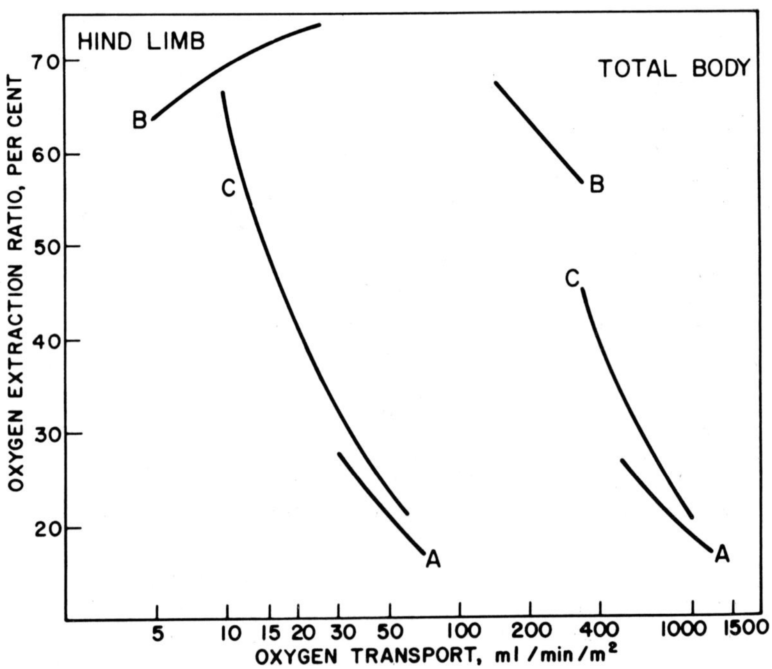

Fig. 1. Relationship of oxygen transport and oxygen extraction ratio in the hind limb and total body of normal (A), bled (B) and reinfused (C) greyhounds (body temperature 37°C, arterial P_{CO_2} = 40 Torr).

Discussion

Except in the hind limb of hypovolemic dogs Ex_{O_2} was inversely related to the logarithm of $Flux_{O_2}$ in both the total body and the hind limb circulations (Fig. 1). The $Flux_{O_2}$-related changes were not fully corrective but, as previously assumed, only cushioned the dependence of $\dot{V}_{O_2}$ on $Flux_{O_2}$. However, the degree of the cushioning was not fixed but variable.

In the reinfused dogs Ex_{O_2} was higher than in normals suggesting that, in the former group, $\dot{V}_{O_2}$ could be sustained by a lower cardiac output than in normals. However, in normal animals an increase in $\dot{V}_{O_2}$ from 156 to 192 ml (+23%) required a calculated increment in cardiac output from 3.5 to 5.5 l or +57% while in reinfused dogs a similar increase in $\dot{V}_{O_2}$ involved a calculated increment in cardiac output from 1.75 to 4.25 l, or +143% revealing one of the limitations of the post-shock circulation. In the blocked reinfused animals, whose $\dot{V}_{O_2}$ was generally lower, an increase in $\dot{V}_{O_2}$ from 125 to 153 ml (+23%) was associated with a calculated increment in cardiac output from 1.8 to 3.3 l, or +83%. It is mentioned here that while all non-medicated shocked dogs died within 6 hours after reinfusion, all blocked animals were alive next day.

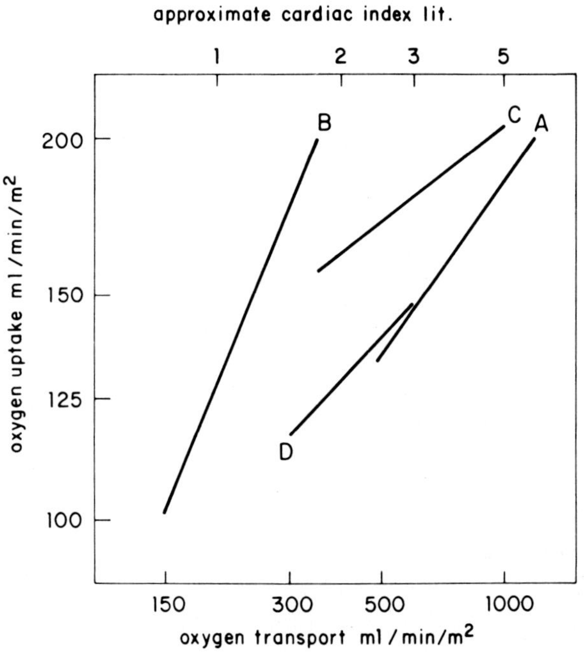

Fig. 2. Relationship of total body oxygen transport and oxygen uptake in normal (A), hypovolemic (B), reinfused (C) and blocked + reinfused (D) dogs.

The relationship between total body Flux_{O_2} and $\dot{V}_{O_2}$ is shown in Figure 2, that between hind limb Flux_{O_2} and $\dot{V}_{O_2}$ in Figure 3.

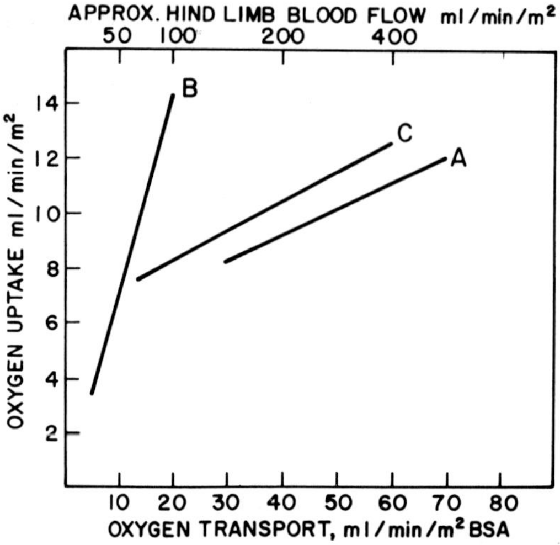

Fig. 3. Relationship of oxygen transport and oxygen uptake in the hind limb of normal (A), hypovolemic (B) and reinfused (C) greyhounds.

Had Flux_{O_2} been the singular determinant of Ex_{O_2} a fall in cardiac output from 2.8 to 1.4 l, as seen regularly in shocked animals, would have resulted in a drop in $\dot{V}_{O_2}$ from 140 to 110 ml but, instead, $\dot{V}_{O_2}$ averaged 160 ml in our shocked animals. The maintenance of $\dot{V}_{O_2}$ at pre-shock level was largely due to the Bayliss response which emerged here as the principal mechanism protecting the tissues against hypoxia. However, at this stage $\dot{V}_{O_2}$ was closely determined by blood flow since Ex_{O_2} could not further increase and a fall in cardiac output from 1.3 to 0.85 l (−35%) was associated with a calculated reduction in $\dot{V}_{O_2}$ from 158 to 120 ml, or −24%. This explain why $\dot{V}_{O_2}$ in shock can be both normal or reduced.

In the hind limb of shocked dogs Ex_{O_2} was found to increase with rising Flux_{O_2} as if the Bayliss response would have overruled the effect of Flux_{O_2} on Ex_{O_2} and, as a result, reducing femoral blood flow from 70 to 45 ml (−36%) produced an equal decrease in calculated femoral $\dot{V}_{O_2}$ from 10.0 to 6.4 ml (Fig. 3). With reinfusion of the shed blood the Flux_{O_2}–Ex_{O_2}–$\dot{V}_{O_2}$ relationship in the hind limb returned towards normal.

Body temperature and arterial P_{CO_2} are known to affect $\dot{V}_{O_2}$ and since $\dot{V}_{O_2}$ was shown here to be determined by the relationship of Flux_{O_2} and Ex_{O_2}, it appeared logical to study the effect of T and Pa_{CO_2} on the $\text{Flux}_{O_2}/\text{Ex}_{O_2}$ ratio, as shown in Figure 4.

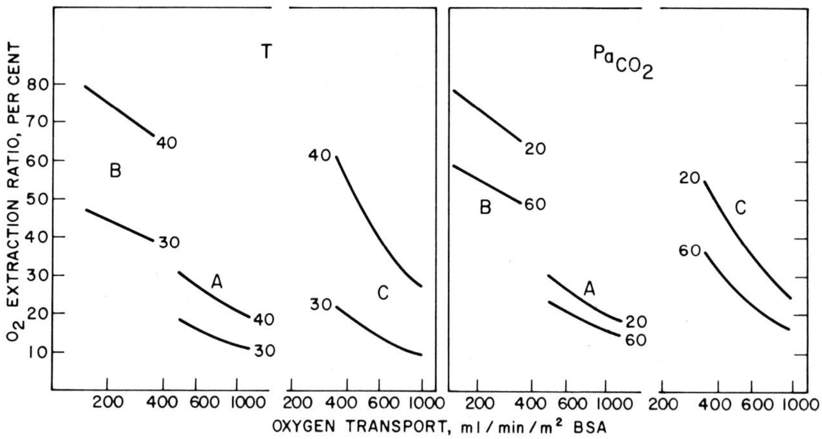

Fig. 4. Relationship of total body oxygen transport and extraction ratio in normal (A), bled (B) and reinfused (C) greyhounds. Effect of variations in body temperature (*T*, 30 and 40°C) and arterial P_{CO_2} (20 and 60 Torr).

The effect of body temperature was particularly marked in shocked and reinfused animals. However, the total effect was even more significant, since $Flux_{O_2}$ was significantly and positively related to *T* (Tables I–III).

In the hind limb the effect of *T* was different: it only affected $Flux_{O_2}$ but within the limits of these observations, did not appear to have any direct effect on $\dot{V}_{O_2}$.

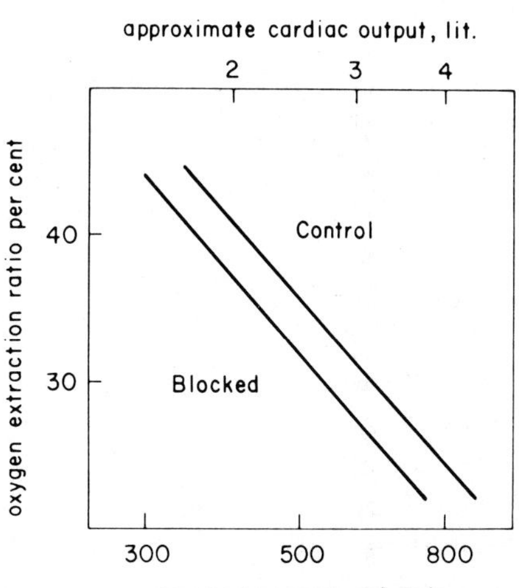

Fig. 5. Relationship of oxygen transport and oxygen extraction ratio following reinfusion in non-medicated dogs and in dogs subjected to combined adrenergic receptor blockade.

In combined adrenergic receptor blockade $\dot{V}_{O_2}$ was reduced via two mechanisms. First, for the same rate of $Flux_{O_2}$ Ex_{O_2} was significantly less, as shown in Figure 5. Secondly, in the blocked animals the dependence of $Flux_{O_2}$ on body temperature was abolished. As a consequence it was found that at any given temperature within the range of observations $\dot{V}_{O_2}$ was approximately 25% less than in the control dogs (Fig. 6). Reduced $\dot{V}_{O_2}$ in blocked dogs was not accompanied by signs of anaerobic metabolism or distress. On the contrary: combined adrenergic receptor blockade abolishes lactic acidosis (Halmagyi et al., 1968) and allows survival following an otherwise lethal insult (Halmagyi et al., 1971).

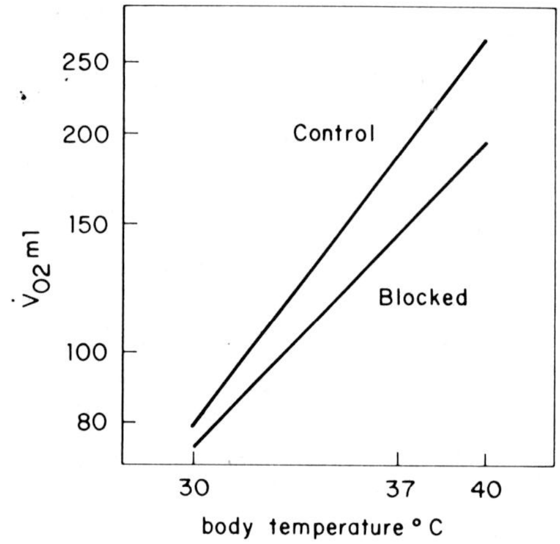

Fig. 6. Relationship of oxygen uptake and body temperature following reinfusion in normal dogs and in dogs subjected to combined adrenergic receptor blockade.

Ex_{O_2} was also profoundly affected by Pa_{CO_2}, as shown in Figure 4 but this effect was absent in the hind limb suggesting that the visceral circulation was the site of this action. For the same $Flux_{O_2}$, Ex_{O_2} (and thus $\dot{V}_{O_2}$) was higher in hypocapnia than in hypercapnia and this effect was more pronounced in the shocked and reinfused dogs than in the normal animals. In severe illness and circulatory failure Pa_{CO_2} was found reduced (Mazzara et al., 1974) and this may further increase O_2 demand. In febrile patients Pa_{CO_2} was found to be inversely related to body temperature (Chapot et al., 1974), and inspection of Tables I–IV reveals that a similar relationship was obtained in these dogs. Hypocapnia in fever is likely to accentuate the increased metabolic rate while hypercapnia by reducing O_2 demand may improve the tolerance to respiratory failure.

The assumption that O_2 supply follows O_2 demand is a time-honored axiom in physiology and suggestions that this relationship may also operate in reverse (Ziegler, 1965) have been rejected as heresy, yet at closer scrutiny this assumption does not appear totaly unfounded.

In the hind limb the majority of investigators found that variations in blood flow produce corresponding changes in $\dot{V}_{O_2}$ (Beer and Yonce, 1972; etc.) except Stainsby and Otis (1964) who, upon reducing blood flow through the resting muscle, found an increase in Ex_{O_2} and no change in $\dot{V}_{O_2}$. However, the latter authors reduced blood flow by lowering perfusion pressure and this probably triggered-off the Bayliss response creating a situation similar to what was described here for shock.

$\dot{V}_{O_2}$ of isolated muscle is reversibly depressed by reduced P_{O_2} without altering other measured cell functions suggesting that some oxidative processes simply generate heat if P_{O_2} exceeds a certain minimal level (Whalen, 1966). Indeed, when rats (Flueckiger, 1956), guinea pigs (Hill, 1959), kittens (Hill, 1959; Moore, 1959) and dogs (Blatteis and Lutherer, 1973) are exposed to cold environment and given 10% O_2 to breathe body temperature soon commences to fall and $\dot{V}_{O_2}$ gradually increases; and upon restoring air breathing, both body temperature and $\dot{V}_{O_2}$ return to the pre-hypoxic levels. These findings were interpreted to suggest that the thermoregulatory fraction of the resting $\dot{V}_{O_2}$ is negotiable and if $Flux_{O_2}$ decreases chemical thermogenesis is the first function to be sacrificed in order to protect and maintain other, more vital, mechanisms. In rats severe trauma causes impairment of the thermoregulatory mechanism ('Ebb phase'. Stoner, 1970) and this is likely to be related to the reduced $Flux_{O_2}$. On the other hand, in the resting muscle not all capillaries are perfused, mean tissue P_{O_2} is low and bound to rise steeply with increased perfusion. Once tissue P_{O_2} exceeds a certain minimal level more energy is produced and this additional 'luxury' $\dot{V}_{O_2}$ may be partly converted into heat (Whalen, 1966).

Substances such as thyroxin, dinitrophenol, and the catecholamines increase O_2 uptake in vitro and a similar effect observed in vivo is usually equated with their direct cellular action. However, in vivo these agents stimulate circulation, ventilation, and raise body temperature: their 'calorigenic' action is likely to represent a combination of metabolic and non-metabolic activities. Conversely, suppression of thyroid function, severe sedation, and hypothermia have an opposite effect on circulation and ventilation and the lowered metabolic rate may again represent a combination of metabolic and non-metabolic activities. The equations developed here may facilitate the in vivo assessment of interventions claimed to alter basal tissue metabolic rate.

Recognition of the urgency and the required magnitude of volume replacement, together with its ubiquitous availability account for the fact that, if bleeding can be controlled, today only laboratory animals die of post-hemorrhagic shock but not patients. Currently the singularly most important form of acute low flow state is cardiac shock which may well prove to be more difficult to solve than hemorrhagic shock. On the other hand, today the life of many patients is prolonged to reach more advanced, hitherto incompletely chartered, stages of their illness. At these stages blood pressure is normal and the numerical value of blood flow is correct but metabolic rate may be increased (Halmagyi et al., 1974). Increased metabolic rate, compounded with reduced arterial O_2 content secondary to pulmonary complications creates a less dramatic, but longer lasting, discrepancy between $Flux_{O_2}$ and $\dot{V}_{O_2}$. It is conceivable that the insight gained in post-hemorrhagic shock may prove to be useful in studying these more chronic conditions.

Acknowledgements

Part of the data shown here are based on an earlier paper: Halmagyi, D.F.J., Leigh, J., Goodman, A.H. and Varga, D. (1973): Factors determining total body and hind limb oxygen consumption in normal and shocked dogs. In: *Oxygen Transport to Tissues*, p. 491. Editors: Bicher, H.I. and Bruley, D.F. Plenum Press, New York.

The experiments described here were supported, over many years, by the National Heart Foundation of Australia, Imperial Chemical Industries Ltd., and Pharmacia Ltd., and were carried out in the Gordon Craig Research Laboratory, Department of Surgery, University of Sydney, Australia.

References

Baez, S. (1968): Bayliss response in the microcirculation. *Fed. Proc., 27*, 1410.

Beer, G. and Yonce, L.R. (1972): Blood flow, oxygen uptake and capillary filtration in resting skeletal muscle. *Amer. J. Physiol., 223*, 492.

Blatteis, C.M. and Lutherer, L.O. (1973): Cold-induced thermogenesis in dogs: its reduction by moderate hypoxia. *J. appl. Physiol., 35*, 608.

Chapot, G., Muller, M., Barrault, N., Dargnat, N. and Languillat, J.M. (1974): A correlation between Pa_{CO_2} and body temperature in febrile patients. *Thorax, 29*, 104.

Crowell, J.W. and Smith, E.E. (1964): Oxygen deficit and irreversible hemorrhagic shock. *Amer. J. Physiol., 206*, 313.

Flückiger, von E. (1956): Der Sauerstoffverbrauch der Ratte bei vermindertem Sauerstoff-Partialdruck. *Helvetica physiol. Acta, 14*, 369.

Granger, H.J. and Guyton, A.C. (1969): Autoregulation of the total systemic circulation following destruction of the central nervous system in the dog. *Circulat. Res., 25*, 379.

Halmagyi, D.F.J., Broell, J., Gump, F.E. and Kinney, J.M. (1974): Hypermetabolism in sepsis: correlation with fever and tachycardia. *Surgery, 75*, 763.

Halmagyi, D.F.J., Frazer, T.W. and Varga, D. (1973): Treatment of volume resistant experimental shock with hypervolemia and hypothermia. *Surgery, 74*, 370.

Halmagyi, D.F.J. and Gillett, D.J. (1966): Cardiorespiratory consequences of corrected gradual severe blood loss in unanesthetized sheep. *J. appl. Physiol., 21*, 589.

Halmagyi, D.F.J., Goodman, A.H., Little, M.J., Kennedy, M. and Varga, D. (1970): Portal blood flow and oxygen usage in hemorrhagic shock. *Ann. Surg., 172*, 284.

Halmagyi, D.F.J., Goodman, A.H. and Neering, I.R. (1969): Hind limb blood flow and oxygen usage in hemorrhagic shock. *J. appl. Physiol., 27*, 508.

Halmagyi, D.F.J., Irving, M.H. and Varga, D. (1968): The effect of adrenergic blockade on metabolic response to hemorrhagic shock. *J. appl. Physiol., 25*, 384.

Halmagyi, D.F.J. and Kennedy, M. (1970): Dependence of oxygen consumption on circulation in normovolemic and hypovolemic dogs. *J. appl. Physiol., 29*, 440.

Halmagyi, D.F.J., Kennedy, M. and Goodman, A.H. (1971): Response to dextran in post-hemorrhagic shock after combined adrenergic receptor blockade. *J. appl. Physiol., 30*, 186.

Halmagyi, D.F.J., Neering, I.R. and Varga, D. (1970): Response to hemorrhage during CO_2 breathing. *J. appl. Physiol., 28*, 465.

Hill, J.R. (1959): The O_2 consumption of newborn and adult mammals: its dependence on the O_2 tension in the inspired air and the environmental temperature. *J. Physiol. (Lond.), 149*, 346.

Mazzara, J.T., Ayres, S.M. and Grace, W.J. (1974): Extreme hypocapnia in the critically ill patient. *Amer. J. Med., 56*, 450.

Mellander, S. and Johansson, B. (1968): Control of resistance, exchange and capacitance functions in the peripheral circulation. *Physiol. Reviews, 20*, 117.

Moore, R.F. (1959): Oxygen consumption and temperature in newborn kittens subjected to hypoxia and reoxygenation. *J. Physiol. (Lond.), 149*, 500.

Neuhof, H., Hey, D., Glaser, E., Wolf, H. and Lasch, H.G. (1973): Schockueberwachung durch kontinuierliche Registrierung der Sauerstoffaufnahme und anderer Parameter. *Dtsch med. Wschr., 98*, 1227.

Post, R.S., Visscher, P.H. and Wiggers, J. (1948): Sequential changes in oxygen consumption during oligemic and normovolemic shock and their meaning. *Amer. J. Physiol., 152*, 71.

Reeves, J.T., Grover, R.F., Filley, G.F. and Blount, Jr.G. (1961): Cardiac output in normal resting man. *J. appl. Physiol., 16*, 276.

Rothe, C.F. (1968): Oxygen deficit in hemorrhagic shock in dogs. *Amer. J. Physiol., 214*, 436.

Rush, Jr., B.F., Rosenberg, J.C. and Spencer, F.C. (1965): Changes in oxygen consumption in shock. *J. surg. Res., 5*, 252.

Smith, E.E. and Crowell, J.W. (1964): Effect of hemorrhagic hypotension on oxygen consumption of dogs. *Amer. J. Physiol., 207*, 647.

Stainsby, W.N. and Otis, A.B. (1964): Blood flow, blood oxygen tension, oxygen uptake and oxygen transport in skeletal muscle. *Amer. J. Physiol., 206*, 858.

Stoner, H.B. (1970): The acute effects of trauma on heat production. In: *Ciba Foundation Symposium on Energy Metabolism in Trauma*, p. 1. Editors: Porter, R. and Knight, J. Churchill.

Thauer, R. (1965): The circulation in hypothermia of non-hibernating animals and man. In: *Handbook of Physiology, Circulation, Sect. II. Vol. III*, p. 1899. American Physiology Society, Washington.

Whalen, W.J. (1966): Intracellular pO_2: a limiting factor in cell respiration. *Amer. J. Physiol., 211*, 862.

Zierler, K.L. (1965): The skeletal muscle circulation. In: *Shock and Hypotension*, p. 170. Editors: Mills, L.C. and Moyer, J.H. Grune and Stratton, New York.

Ledingham (ed.). Shock

The early metabolic response to injury

A. FLECK

'... quand on trouble l'équilibre des fonctions vitales chez un animal, on voit généralement apparaître le sucre en beaucoup plus forte proportion.'

Claude Bernard (1877a)

About 100 years ago Claude Bernard (1877b) demonstrated that after 3 hours experimental haemorrhage in a dog the blood sugar rose from the initial level of 1.56 g/l to 3.30 g/l. He also confirmed as did Fischer (1862) that the insertion of a needle in a certain area in the floor of the IVth ventricle led to transient glycosuria.

The complexity of the response to injury is now apparent from recent comprehensive reviews (Sevitt and Stoner, 1970; Hunt, 1972). These have followed Cuthbertson's (1942) proposed stages of the metabolic response. After an acute injury, the first 'ebb' phase of depression of metabolism is followed by a longer period of increased metabolism – the 'flow' phase. Alternatively the 'ebb' phase may deteriorate into a terminal or necrobiosis stage associated with failing oxygen consumption (Stoner, 1961). This survey will be concerned mainly with the ebb phase which may last up to 24–48 hours in the experimental rat and man (Stoner, 1968) and which corresponds roughly with 'shock' (Stoner, 1958a, b).

Metabolism in the Ebb Phase

Carbohydrate metabolism

In his analytical studies referred to above, Claude Bernard (1877) measured the increase in blood glucose which occurred during experimental haemorrhage in dogs. This early observation has been confirmed subsequently by numerous investigators (Stoner and Heath, 1973) and in man the hyperglycaemic response seems to correlate with the degree of injury. This is not necessarily so in the rat (Heath and Corney, 1973) or in mice subjected to fatal doses of bacterial toxin. In the latter situation the blood glucose progressively falls until death after a few hours (Smith and Mukherjee, 1972).

Early in the 'ebb' phase increased glycogenolysis has been found both in skeletal muscle (Stoner 1958b) and liver (Heath, 1973) of animals subjected to hind limb ischaemia. Cardiac muscle glycogen increased marginally, except terminally when it decreased. The glycogen level of brain also fell terminally but was previously maintained near normal levels (Stoner, 1958b). After fatal septic shock in animals, liver glycogen is reduced to less than a quarter of that of normal animals and muscle glycogen is also significantly lower than normal (Smith and Mukherjee, 1972).

In contrast to the increased glycogenolysis, the rate of oxidation of carbohydrate is decreased soon after injury (Heath and Corney, 1973). This was demonstrated by using ^{14}C-labelled glucose to estimate the disposal rate (R) of glucose in injured rats. In these studies R was close to the carbohydrate oxidation rate and was reduced in the injured animals roughly in proportion to the decrease in oxygen consumption (Heath and Corney, 1973). In contrast, in the flow phase, Long et al. (1971b) have concluded that glucose oxidation is more than doubled and that glucose turnover is similarly increased.

It is widely assumed that glucose tolerance is decreased after injury (Stoner and Heath, 1973). In many studies, e.g. Allison et al. (1968), based on intravenous glucose tolerance tests, a K value determined from the semi-log plot of blood glucose against time is used as the index of glucose tolerance. This is obviously an oversimplification in the case of in vivo glucose metabolism as more detailed investigations have shown (Long et al., 1971a; Heath and Corney, 1973).

It is well known that circulating lactate and pyruvate may increase in 'shock' or hypoperfusion states (Huckabee 1961a, b; Peretz et al., 1965; Weil and Shubin, 1972), and greatly increased lactic acid has been correlated with reduced survival (Huckabee, 1961b; Peretz et al., 1965). During experimental haemorrhage the fall in arterial blood pH (e.g. to 7.06) is paralleled by falling bicarbonate and rising lactate (e.g. to 12 mmol/l) and pyruvate (Reivich et al., 1973). However, in the earlier stages, circulating lactate levels correlate better with organ surface pH than with arterial blood pH (Lemieux et al., 1969).

In a recent series of patients reported by Smith et al. (1975), all of whom had suffered accidental fracture, the highest level of lactate (2.1 mmol/l) was found in the initial sample taken 2 hours after injury. One group of the same series of patients had normal blood lactate and pyruvate levels although changes in other metabolites were found (see below). That the nature of the injury may influence the production or uptake of lactate is evident from the studies of Spitzer et al. (1972) who found that although arterial lactate was increased after both haemorrhage or endotoxic shock, the increase was very much greater after haemorrhagic hypotension.

Gump (1972) presented evidence that lactate may be increased after injury in the absence of hypoxia and questioned the assumption that decreased tissue perfusion is the explanation for lacticacidaemia after injury.

Gluconeogenesis, the synthesis of glucose from non-carbohydrate precursors the most important of which are lactate, glycerol and the amino acids (Newsholme and Start, 1973), may be an important aspect of carbohydrate metabolism after injury (Stoner and Heath, 1973). The comprehensive studies of Shoemaker et al. (1971) demonstrated increased hepatic output of glucose during the hypovolaemic period after injury, and it has been suggested that this indicates increased gluconeogenesis in the ebb phase (Stoner and Heath, 1973). This is certainly possible, although Ashby et al. (1965) had tentatively concluded from their studies of ^{14}C glucose and pyruvate metabolism that there was no great increase in gluconeogenesis; a block in pyruvate oxidation was more likely. From his studies in early shock, Kovách (1972) concluded that in the liver in early shock, gluconeogenesis was inhibited. In the later 'flow' phase, there is considerable indirect evidence for increased gluconeogenesis (Kinney et al., 1970). From consideration of the weight loss after injury, the loss of body protein, seen mainly as increased urine nitrogen, and indirect calorimetry, it is concluded that protein represents the only sizeable reserve for carbohydrate intermediates during the flow phase (Kinney et al., 1970). This conclusion is supported by the fact that total carbohydrate of the human body amounts to less than 1% of the body weight and can thus provide only a very small energy reserve.

A summary of some of the important reactions in carbohydrate metabolism is illustrated in Figure 1. From this the pathways of the main gluconeogenic substrates, glycerol (from fat), the amino acids, alanine and glutamine derived from protein, and lactic acid are evident. From the above description it will be

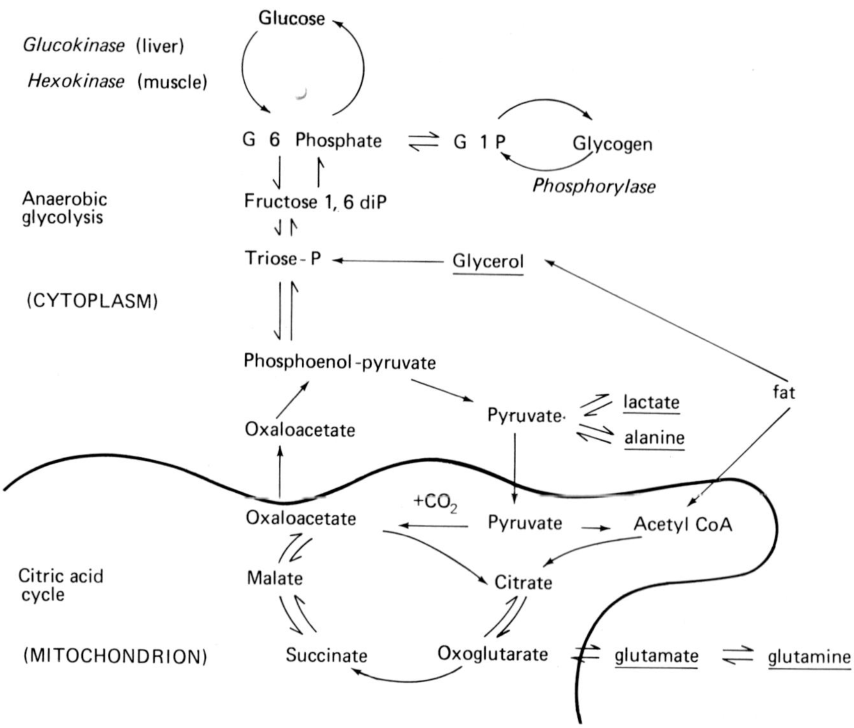

Fig. 1. Carbohydrate metabolism. *Note:* the substrates underlined, e.g. alanine are the main gluconeogenic substrates; enzymes are printed in italics, e.g. *phosphorylase*.

apparent that the hyperglycaemia of the ebb phase results from increased glycogenolysis, increased gluconeogenesis and decreased oxidation of glucose. Increases in the intermediate substrates such as pyruvate and lactate would also be expected to result from increased mobilisation of glucose accompanied by a reduction in its oxidation.

Fat metabolism

From their extensive studies in patients who had experienced a variety of injuries including burns, multiple injuries and extensive elective surgery, Kinney et al. (1970) concluded that although there was a net increase in protein catabolism, fat was the major source of energy in the post shock or flow phase of recovery. The proportion of the energy consumption contributed by fat could be as much as from 75–95% of the total energy requirement. The remaining energy was derived from protein.

Shoemaker et al. (1973) describe early, middle and late stages of the hypovolaemic response to haemorrhage. In the early stage there was a net increase in the release of triglycerides (TG) from the liver and increased uptake of free fatty acids (FFA), phospholipids and cholesterol. This effect was of short duration and the values returned to control levels in the middle stage of the response. In the late stage free fatty acids and phospholipids were released. The non-hepatic splanchnic tissue responded to haemorrhage with an increased output of FFA, TG and phospholipids which decreased in the late stage of hypovolaemia. Thirty minutes after injection of a fatal dose of *E. coli* endotoxin, the plasma FFA of baboons were significantly increased (Horwitz, 1972). The increase continued for more than 2 hours and during this time there was no change in total lipids.

Although Kovách (1972) found increased arterial glycerol concentrations during haemorrhage, he states that arterial free fatty acids do not rise during haemorrhage' and attributes this observation to a reduction in the blood flow in canine subcutaneous adipose tissue to 10% of the resting level (Rosell et al., 1973). Spitzer et al. (1973b) also report increased plasma glycerol to more than six times normal after haemorrhage but increased arterial FFA's were also found. The flux of FFA was increased but oxidation was variable.

However, other groups, including Spitzer and Kovách (1973a) studying the effects of endotoxin on adipose tissue metabolism, again found no change in plasma FFA but increased glycerol. Lipolysis in adipocytes was increased by endotoxin administration and by norepinephrine which also caused an additional stimulation and lipolysis in endotoxin affected animals.

In heart muscle the uptake of FFA is decreased during endotoxic shock (Scott et al., 1973) and lipoprotein lipase activity is increased after tourniquet stress (Borbola et al., 1973). The former group (Scott et al., 1973) also found that uptake and oxidation of FFA were reduced by endotoxin while lactate uptake was increased.

Despite the well-known concept of traumatic diabetes (Bernard, 1877; Kinney et al., 1970; Stoner and Heath, 1973) which leads one to suppose that ketosis would be a concomitant of the hyperglycaemia of injury, the occurrence of very high levels of ketones in injury uncomplicated by starvation is not common. For example, Smith et al. (1975) found one group (B) of their series of injured patients who had normal blood lactate levels to have ketones elevated to about 7 times normal. In contrast, a diabetic injured patient had blood ketone levels of about 80 times normal. The group (B) of patients with elevated ketones also tended to have elevated FFA's. In as yet unpublished observations, the author found small but significant increases in 3-hydroxybutyric acid excretion by humans and experimental rats after injury but the increases were almost negligible, approximately times two, in comparison with the massive increases seen in starvation (Cahill et al., 1966).

From a detailed study of ketone body metabolism in which ^{14}C-labelled β-hydroxybutyrate and acetoacetate were used, Barton (1973) concluded that if complete oxidation of ketones were assumed, the contribution of ketones to whole body oxygen consumption rose from 7 to 15% after injury. The increased disposal rate found reflected an increased rate of production by the liver.

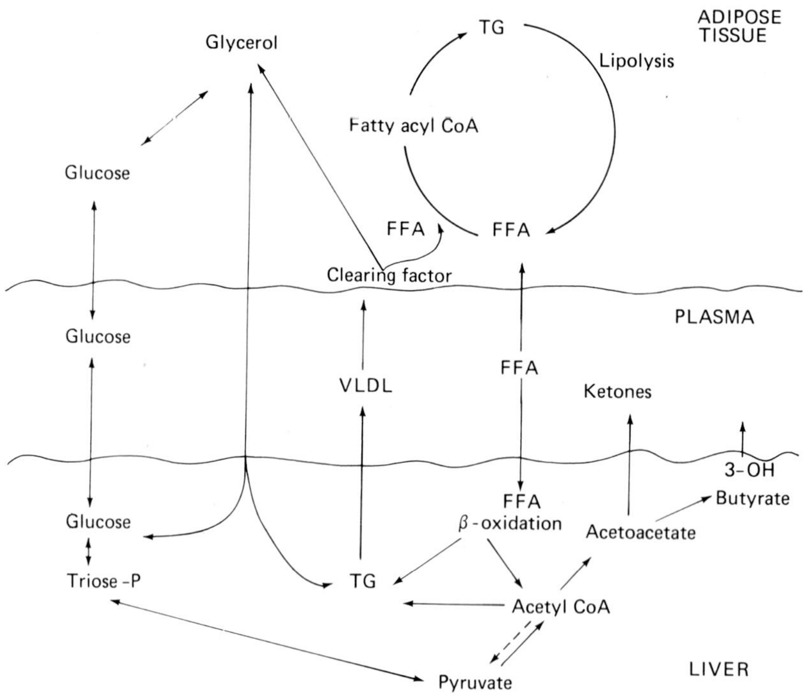

Fig. 2. Fat metabolism.

The main metabolic reactions of fat metabolism are summarised in outline in Figure 2. From this, the relation between carbohydrate and fat metabolism via pyruvate, acetyl CoA and glycerol can be seen. The fatty acid cycle of lipolysis and synthesis in adipose tissue may have an important regulatory function. The production of the ketones solely in the liver is also of note.

Protein metabolism

Most of the studies of the effects of injury on protein metabolism have been carried out on patients or experimental animals in the flow phase after recovery from shock or the ebb phase (Cuthbertson, 1964; Levenson et al., 1966; Davies, 1970; Gordon, 1970, 1973; Ballantyne et al., 1973; O'Keefe et al., 1974). However, there is evidence that in the rat the synthesis of α_1 AP globulin is increased within 5 hours after injury (Gordon, 1970). Wunnamacher (1972) has shown that liver protein synthesis is increased within 5 hours after injury. The response of the serum proteins known as the acute phase reactants to injury is complex because the synthesis rates of some may be increased, and that of others decreased, while the catabolic rates of others, e.g. transferrin, may be increased (Gordon, 1970).

Thus although the supply of amino acids influences protein synthesis in a complex fashion (Munro, 1970), the control of the response of the acute phase reactants is unlikely to be determined by tissue amino acid levels.

There have been few attempts to assess directly total body protein synthesis after injury. The general conclusion that protein catabolism is increased, at least in the 'flow' phase is mostly based on indirect evidence (Cuthbertson, 1964; Levenson et al., 1966; Kinney et al., 1970). However, recently, using a ^{14}C-leucine infusion technique, O'Keefe et al. (1974) concluded that protein synthesis in patients was reduced 48–60 hours after surgery. In in vivo studies in experimentally injured rats, Khan et al. (1974) found at 12 hours after injury increased liver polysome aggregation and increased incorporation of amino acids into polysome-protein. There was reduced incorporation at 24 hours and disaggregation 18–24 hours after injury. These observations are consistent with increased protein synthesis in liver in the ebb phase and a decrease in the late ebb or early flow phase.

As outlined above, gluconeogenesis from amino acids could be a significant aspect of the metabolic response, although whether there is a significant increase in the shock or ebb phase is dubious. After injury, glucose infusion did not depress gluconeogenesis as it did in control animals (Long et al., 1971b). However, these studies were carried out in the post-ebb phase.

It seems to be generally agreed that alanine (Felig et al., 1970; Felig and Wahren 1971 a, b) and glutamic acid or glutamine (Marliss et al., 1971) are key amino acids in gluconeogenesis (Kaplan and Pitot, 1970; Newsholme and Start, 1973) (see Fig. 1). It is therefore interesting to note that Smith et al. (1975) found plasma alanine and lactate and pyruvate to be raised in one group (A) of their small series of patients. In recent unpublished studies, Carlyle et al. (1975) have found plasma alanine to be raised for some days in rats after burning injury. Two of the amino acids of the urea cycle, ornithine and citrulline also showed increased plasma concentration in these injured animals.

Energy metabolism

There is widespread agreement that in the ebb phase both oxygen consumption and body temperature are reduced, hence heat production is reduced (Stoner, 1970).

With the knowledge of changes in oxygen consumption, transport and 2:3 diphosphoglycerate etc. (see Travis et al., 1971; Gump, 1972; this volume, chapters 3 and 12) it is not surprising that oxidative phosphorylation and mitochondrial function have received attention. More than 10 years ago Stoner (1961) reported his findings that in brain, phosphocreatine levels remained unchanged in shock and that liver ATP only decreased shortly before death. In muscle both phosphocreatine and ATP levels decline shortly before death. He did find, however, that in muscle both glucose-6-phosphate (G-6-P) and fructose-1:6-diphosphate (FDP) were increased while in liver only FDP was increased in shock. More recently, Rush (1972) referred to the depressed levels of cell ATP in haemorrhagic shock, to the well known increase in blood lactate and the increased output of lactate by the myocardium. Smith and Mukherjee (1972) concluded that oxidative phosphorylation was uncoupled because of the increase in inorganic phosphate and decrease in organic phosphates in the livers of animals in septic shock. Mela et al. (1973) found that the extent of the changes caused by pure tissue hypoxia were different from those caused by haemorrhage and endotoxaemia, and they suggested that release of lysosomal enzymes might be one possible cause of the mitochondrial damage they observed. Somogyi et al. (1973) have suggested that the decreased respiration capacity for rat brain mitochondria after injury might be related to the release of free fatty acids.

Summary of the metabolic changes in the ebb phase

1. Oxygen consumption and energy metabolism are decreased.
2. Glycogenolysis is increased and is accompanied by hyperglycaemia and lacticacidaemia which may be related to the degree of injury.
3. Gluconeogenesis may be increased in the ebb phase – there is good evidence for its increase in the flow phase. Plasma alanine may be increased.

4. FFA's may or may not be increased but there is a tendency for increased lipolysis in adipose tissue.
5. There may be increased production of ketones, but not to the levels seen in starvation.
6. The immediate effects on protein metabolism are complex. The synthesis of some of the acute phase reactants is increased.
7. These effects can be influenced by both the nature and severity of the injury.

Injury and Humoral Mechanisms

Endocrine changes

The endocrine response to trauma has been reviewed recently by Johnstone (1972, 1973) and more recently Allison (1974) has discussed some of the endocrine changes which influence energy and protein metabolism. Cuthbertson (1964) and Levenson et al. (1966) have also discussed in some detail the significance of the endocrine changes in injury. Most of the known changes in hormones after injury are summarised in Table I. This section will be restricted to a brief discussion of the endocrine changes of major significance in protein, carbohydrate, fat or energy metabolism.

Catecholamines (adrenaline and noradrenaline). Numerous observations have confirmed that both adrenaline and noradrenaline increase after injury

Table I
Changes in humoral factors or hormones after injury.

a) Increased plasma levels or urinary excretion			
Adrenaline[1,2]		Cortisol[1]	Antidiuretic hormone[1]
Noradrenaline[1,2]		Aldosterone[1]	Renin and angiotension[1]
ACTH[1]		Growth hormone (GH)[1]	
Insulin[1]	Glucagon[1]	Thyroxine[1]	
Histamine[1,2]			
b) Decreased plasma levels or urinary excretion			
Testosterone[2,3]		17 oxosteroids[2]	
c) Unchanged or dubious changes			
LH[1,3]	FSH[1]	TSH[1]	

[1] See Johnstone (1972); [2] See Birke et al. (1957); [3] see Cartensen et al. (1972).

(Cuthbertson, 1964; Hunt, 1972; Johnstone, 1972) that the rise is rapid, occurring immediately on injury, and in patients suffering from burns, may last at least 5 days (Birke et al., 1957). After stress the activity of several of the adrenal catecholamine producing enzymes is increased (Kvetnansky and Kopin, 1973). Adrenal medullectomy reduces both the hyperglycaemic, glycogenolytic response and survival time (Stoner, 1961).

Adrenal corticoids. These also show a rapid response to stress and injury. Peak plasma levels are usually attained in a few hours and return to normal within 24 hours (Birke et al., 1957; Johnstone, 1972). In injured patients the development of complications is associated with further increase in adrenocortical activity (Birke et al., 1957).

It has been recognised for many years that the adrenocortical response is 'permissive', in that the injury response occurs in adrenalectomised animals maintained on steroid replacement (Cuthbertson, 1964; Hunt, 1972; Johnstone, 1973).

The importance of the adrenal hormones in the acute response to stress can be judged from Stoner's (1961) observations on the considerable effects of adrenalectomy and adrenalmedullectomy on survival time in rats subjected to a 4 hour period of hind limb ischaemia. The average mortality of animals injured in this way was 85% and the mean survival time was 12.3 hours. Animals subjected to adrenal medullectomy before injury had 100% mortality and survived 5.8 hours on average whereas adrenalectomised animals also had 100% mortality but survived only 1.9 hours.

Anterior pituitary hormones. Apart from ACTH the role of which is in the feedback control of corticosteroid secretion, growth hormone (GH) would seem to have the most significant metabolic role in injury. There is a rapid rise, within the first hour or so, of GH after injury, including surgical operations (Johnstone, 1972; Oyama, 1973). Soldiers on combat patrol had increased levels of GH which further increased rapidly on injury; the levels gradually declined over a few days except in those who failed to survive in whom extremely high levels were maintained until death (Carey et al., 1971).

Very high levels of GH have been recorded during cardiac surgery and for up to 1 week afterwards (Salter et al., 1972).

Insulin. Reviewers (Johnstone, 1972, 1973; Allison, 1974) agree that the secretion of insulin in man is reduced early in shock but that within the first day high blood levels are found which may persist for up to one week. Recent observations by Russell et al. (1975) confirm this pattern during and after surgical operations. Experimental studies in baboons during haemorrhagic shock confirm that the fall in peripheral insulin reflects a decline in release of pancreatic insulin (Moss et al., 1973). However both Vigas et al. (1973) and Drucker et al. (1973) report that peripheral insulin and insulin secretion are increased early in experimental haemorrhagic shock in dogs. These apparent discrepancies may be related to factors such as adrenaline which inhibit insulin secretion (Johnstone, 1972; Jacobson, 1972).

In studies of lethal septicaemia in baboons, Cryer et al. (1972) found that during the rapid rise in blood glucose after injection of *E. coli* there was an equally rapid fall in insulin. Also the duration of survival correlated with the insulin levels but not with lactate, pH or blood pressure. Insulin secretion could be produced in hyperglycaemic shocked animals by α-adrenergic block. Insulin falls during surgical operation (Giddings et al., 1975; Russell et al., 1975) and in most cases during the shock phase after burning injury (Wilmore et al., 1974). It would seem safe to conclude that in man insulin secretion is depressed and plasma insulin is low in shock, but that the influence of catecholamines on insulin secretion may lead to a complex response.

Glucagon. Circulating glucagon as determined by radioimmunoassay (immunoreactive glucagon – IRG) increases after injury (Giddings et al., 1975; Russell et al., 1975) including burns (Wilmore et al., 1974). Wilmore et al. (1974) and Russell et al. (1975) found the increase to be early, during or immediately after the injury. In contrast Giddings et al. (1975) found no change in glucagon during operation, although they did find a low plasma insulin (immunoreactive insulin – IRI) at this time. It was not until the next morning that they found elevated IRG levels. All groups were in agreement that IRG remained elevated for several days or a week or more depending on the severity of the injury or complications. Wilmore et al. (1974) noted that in the early stages after a burning injury, the insulin/glucagon molar ratio was generally low and remained so for some days and that during convalescence the IRI/IRG ratio rose to higher than normal.

The thyroid response. From the changes in energy production and oxygen consumption after injury – the depressions in the shock phase and increases to above normal during recovery (Cuthbertson, 1964) – involvement of the thyroid and its hormones might be assumed. The role of the thyroid and its significance in the response remains however dubious (Johnstone, 1972). Harland et al. (1972) found no change in circulating blood levels of PBI (protein-bound iodine) although they did claim that thyroxine secretion was increased. Kirby and Johnstone (1973), in contrast, found no change in TSH (thyroid stimulating hormone) or circulating total thyroid hormone. They did find that free thyroxine was increased but this may have been due to a proportional fall in TBPA (thyroid binding pre-albumin) which was not accompanied by any change in TBG (thyroid binding globulin).

Histamine and other humoral agents. The release of histamine after tissue damage is well known, as is the stimulation of various proteolytic enzymes, the kinins etc. (see Hinshaw and Cox, 1972). The possible role of the proteases in the production of myocardial depressant factor (MDF) has been discussed by Lefer and Glen (1973). Resultant changes in cell membranes may lead to important sequelae in the maintenance of fluid and ion homeostasis (Flear, 1970) and also in mitochondrial energy metabolism (Mela et al., 1973). However the direct metabolic effects of these humoral agents is not clear and they will not be further discussed here.

Conclusions. Many hormones have been shown to have a clear response to injury. The duration of the changes and those of most metabolic significance are summarised in Figure 3. The response of the catecholamines (increased secretion of adrenaline and noradrenaline) is immediate and may last for several days depending on the severity of the injury. Cortisol also responds rapidly, considerable elevations being found within a few hours. The duration

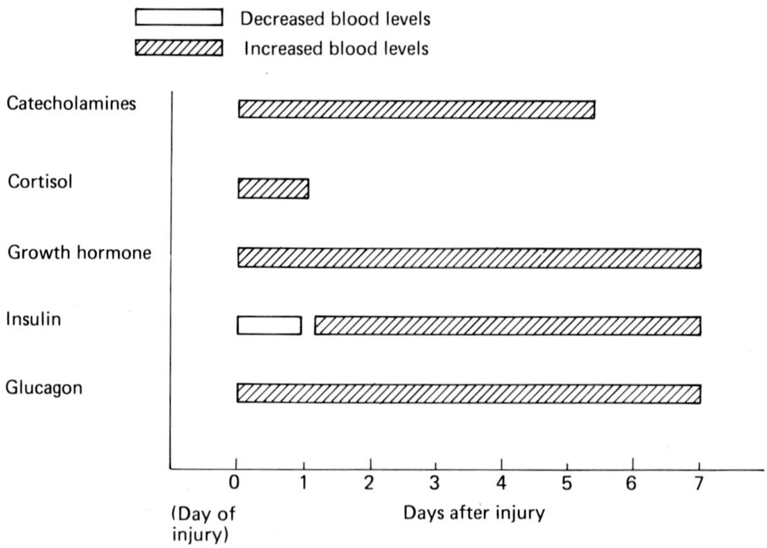

Fig. 3. Duration of endocrine response to injury.

of increased production is short and normal levels are usually found after the first day unless complications occur. Plasma growth hormone also increases very rapidly after injury, increased levels having been recorded during surgical operation. This response usually lasts about one week or more.

In man, insulin secretion seems initially to fall in the shock phase. This is followed on the first day after injury by increased secretion which may last for several days.

Glucagon levels rise rapidly after injury and slowly decline over the next seven or more days.

The normal metabolic roles of hormones

Each hormone may have several important effects on metabolism and the interactions may be very complex. In this section a brief and oversimplified summary of the main metabolic actions of the hormones mentioned above will be given as a preliminary to a discussion of their role in the injury response. Brief accounts are those of Jarrett (1971) and Allison (1974). For a more detailed discussion and an index of the metabolic effects of hormones Newsholme and Stuart (1973) should be consulted. There is, in addition, a recent definitive account of glucagon (Lefebvre and Unger, 1972).

Catecholamines. Adrenaline activates adenyl cyclase, hence leads to increased intracellular levels of cyclic AMP (cAMP). In the physiological range of concentrations adrenaline affects mainly muscle and adipose tissue. A principal effect of cAMP is to activate phosphorylase and so promote glycogenolysis (see Fig. 1). In both muscle and adipose tissue cAMP may activate triglyceride lipase and thus mobilise free fatty acids (FFA) (see Fig. 2). In muscle these will become available for metabolism and from adipose tissue will contribute to increased plasma FFA. Subsidiary but important effects of catecholamines are to inhibit pancreatic insulin secretion (Cryer et al., 1972) and stimulate glucagon secretion (Samols et al., 1972).

Cortisol. The roles and effects of steroid hormones in metabolism are very complex, possibly because of the variety of steroid hormones and also because their mode of action in general seems to be via nuclear protein binding to specific sites which results in a modification of specific messenger RNA synthesis. In the case of cortisol acting on the liver this leads to increased synthesis and activity of one or two gluconeogenic or amino acid degrading enzymes (Kenney, 1970). In general the glucocorticoids are agreed to have a predominantly catabolic role, mobilising amino acids from muscle (Munro, 1963; Manchester, 1970).

Growth hormone. An important action of GH is to mobilise fat from adipose tissue and thus increase plasma FFA's. The consequent inhibition of glucose utilisation probably potentiates ketone body production.

Growth hormone stimulates protein and RNA synthesis, and it may be that insulin aids or is necessary for this effect.

Insulin. It is probably best to outline the main functions of insulin on muscle, adipose tissue and liver, separately.

i. *Muscle.* Insulin stimulates directly the membrane transport of glucose into muscle cells. It also promotes glycolysis and glycogen synthesis from glucose. Muscle protein synthesis is also stimulated by insulin.

ii. *Adipose tissue.* In this tissue the increase in glycolysis stimulated by insulin leads to increased lipogenesis (see Figs. 1 and 2) (Denton, 1974). Lipolysis is also decreased.

iii. *Liver.* Glucokinase is stimulated, as is glycogen synthesis (see Fig. 1). Gluconeogenesis is inhibited but fatty acid and triglyceride synthesis are increased. Protein synthesis is also increased.

Glucagon. This hormone with insulin has a key role in glucose homeostasis (Lefebvre and Unger, 1972). Glucagon, like adrenaline, activates adenylate cyclase and increases cellular cAMP levels, although there are separate receptors for these hormones in liver. Glucagon has a very potent hyperglycaemic effect. In general, glucagon promotes glycogenolysis, gluconeogenesis, ureogenesis and ketogenesis and it is more effective in doing so than adrenaline. Lipolysis is also promoted by glucagon which therefore increases plasma FFA and ketones.

Table II
Hormones and metabolism.

	Glycogenolysis	Gluconeogenesis	Lipolysis	Protein synthesis
Catecholamines	+	+	+	
Cortisol		+		
Growth hormone			+	+
Insulin	−	−	−	+
Glucagon	+	+	+	

+ = Stimulation; − = inhibition.

A brief summary of the physiological actions of these 5 hormones is given in Table II. It is essential to note that the potency of the effects of each hormone and duration of action differ and that there are many mechanisms which may influence interactions (e.g. see Fig. 4).

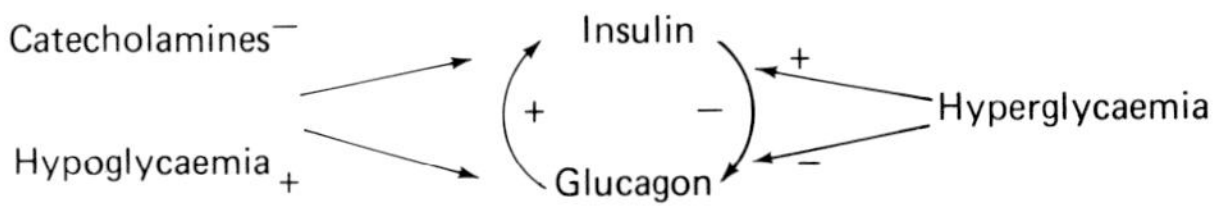

Fig. 4. Control of blood glucose levels.

An important interaction is that of insulin and glucagon in the maintenance of normal fasting blood sugar levels (Alford et al., 1974). The ratio of glucagon to insulin also controls glucose turnover. For example, maintaining normal glucagon levels while increasing insulin can lead to a considerable increase in glucose turnover without a significant change in blood glucose concentration (Cherrington and Vranic, 1971). This relationship may be important in determining glucose utilisation both in the ebb and flow phases (see under Glucagon, p. 67; and Wilmore et al., 1974). It is also of interest that glucagon can stimulate catecholamine secretion very rapidly (see Lefebvre and Unger, 1972) and that glucagon stimulates insulin secretion while insulin inhibits glucagon secretion (see Fig. 4).

The endocrine response and metabolism after injury

Reference to Figure 3 and Table II confirms Allison's (1974) conclusion that the change in the endocrine pattern after injury may explain, in part, at least some of the metabolic sequelae.

The rapid rise in catecholamines and glucagon during or immediately after injury with the early inhibition of insulin secretion presumably accounts for the now historic observation of hyperglycaemia during shock. This endocrine pattern can also account for glycogenolysis and with the increased growth hormone secretion, increased lipolysis and the rise in FFA and glycerol. The danger of oversimplification is illustrated when it is recalled that FFA is a potent inhibitor of glucagon secretion (Unger and Lefebvre, 1972), and this emphasises the importance of taking account of the relative effectiveness of the various interacting substances. The decreased insulin levels seen in shock are possibly due to the inhibitory effect of the catecholamines. Presumably their subsequent fall releases this inhibition and allows glucagon to stimulate insulin secretion with the resultant increase in glucose turnover seen in the flow phase. This, with the continuing stimulation of lipolysis may account for the increased oxygen consumption and heat production in the early flow phase. The change in body fuel consumption (increased fat and protein catabolism) observed by Kinney et al. (1970) are compatible with this argument.

An early reduction in protein synthesis followed by later stimulation by the combined effects of GH and insulin would also be predicted from the endocrine pattern and although the evidence for this is somewhat indecisive, it tends in that direction (Ballantyne et al., 1973; O'Keefe et al., 1974).

Hypoxia in the ebb phase would promote glycogenolysis but reduce gluconeogenesis (Park and Exton, 1972). This might explain the variable observations of inhibition of (Kovách, 1972) or increased (Stoner and Heath, 1973) gluconeogenesis in the ebb phase.

It is of interest to note that glucocorticoids are essential for the stimulation of gluconeogenesis by glucagon (Park and Exton, 1972) and that this is a permissive role related to the intracellular action of cAMP.

Stimulation of gluconeogenesis is not necessarily incompatible with the observed accumulations of lactate, pyruvate and alanine (Smith et al., 1975). It is merely necessary that the rates of production of these substrates exceed utilisation and, in the presence of decreased oxygen consumption, this is likely.

The problems of lacticacidaemia and ketonaemia remain to be rationalised. Although there must be some reduction in glycolysis in the ebb phase it might be assumed that the inhibition of pyruvate oxidation by FFA's, citrate, and acetyl CoA and CoA, all of which accumulate when lipolysis is stimulated, would lead to the accumulation of pyruvate and subsequently lactate (see Figs. 1 and 2).

The ratio of the adenine nucleotides $NAD^+/NADH$ in the cytoplasmic compartment falls to 60% and 20% of normal in starved and alloxan diabetes respectively (Newsholme and Start, 1973). This might explain the tendency to accumulation of lactate in the absence of hypoxia, in these conditions.

The degree of ketosis found in injury is much less than that in starvation or diabetes. However the duration of the ebb phase with its relative insulin lack and hypometabolism is short, whereas the massive ketosis of starvation takes several days to develop (Cahill et al., 1966).

Finally in considering the metabolic changes in the ebb phase some of the consequences of acidaemia should be noted. These have been discussed in some detail by Nahas (1970).

Firstly, although acidosis inhibits the metabolic effects of catecholamine activity such as increased lipolysis and the increase in plasma FFA, acidosis also stimulates catecholamine production so that an unstable equilibrium results.

Secondly, acidosis also reduces the glycogenolytic effects of catecholamines and thus the accumulation of pyruvate and lactate is reduced. Thus the presence or absence of acidosis might explain the contradictory observations of Kovách et al. (1973) and Spitzer et al. (1973b) on the effects of haemorrhage on plasma FFA's.

It will be apparent as demonstrated experimentally by Nahas (1970) that acidaemia could account for the failure to mobilise energy stores and hence the reduced oxygen consumption seen in the ebb phase.

Conclusions

By discussing the metabolic and endocrine changes which occur after injury in general terms, it is possible to arrive at a preliminary understanding of some of the mechanisms of the response. The changes in metabolites can be related to the known main endocrine changes and the important effects of acidosis.

Detailed understanding of the mechanism however still requires further investigation. For example, the reason for the duration of the response is not clear, nor is the initial 'trigger mechanism' which probably involves the hypothalamus (Stoner, 1970).

Acknowledgements

Stimulating and helpful discussion with Sir David Cuthbertson and Dr. K. Queen is gratefully acknowledged.

References

Alford, F.P., Bloom, S.R., Nabarro, J.D.N., Hall, R., Besser, G.M., Coy, D.H., Kastin, A.J. and Shally, A.V. (1974): Glucagon control of fasting glucose in man. *Lancet, 2*, 974.

Allison, S.P. (1974): Metabolic aspects of intensive care. *Brit. J. Hosp. Med., 11*, 860.

Allison, S.P., Hinton, P. and Chamberlain, M.J. (1968): Intravenous glucose tolerance, insulin and free fatty acid levels in burned patients. *Lancet, 2*, 1113.

Ashby, M.M., Heath, D.F. and Stoner, H.B. (1965): A quantitative study of carbohydrate metabolism in the normal and injured rat. *J. Physiol. (Lond.), 179*, 193.

Ballantyne, F.C., Tilstone, W.J. and Fleck, A. (1973): Effect of injury on albumin synthesis in the rabbit. *Brit. J. exp. Path., 54*, 409.

Barton, R.N. (1973): The interconversion and disposal of ketone bodies in untreated and injured post-absorptive rats. *Biochem. J., 136*, 531.

Bernard, C. (1877a): *Leçons sur le Diabète*, p. 408. Librairie J.B. Baillière et fils, Paris.
Bernard, C. (1877b): *Leçons sur le Diabète*, p. 410. Librairie J.B. Baillière et fils, Paris.
Birke, G., Duner, H., Liljedahl, S.O., Pernow, B., Plantin, L.O. and Troell, L. (1957): Histamine, catecholamines and adrenocortical steroids in burns. *Acta chir. scand., 114*, 87.
Borbola, J., Gesce, A. and Karady, S. (1973): The activity of lipoprotein in rat heart after tourniquet stress. *Advanc. exp. Med. Biol., 33*, 387.
Cahill, G.F. Jr., Herrara, M.G., Morgan, A.P., Soeldner, J.S., Steinke, J., Levy, P.L. and Reichard, G.A. Jr. (1966): Hormone–fuel interrelationships during fasting. *J. clin. Invest., 45*, 1751.
Carey, L.C., Cloutier, C.T. and Lowery, B.D. (1971): Growth hormone and adrenal cortical response to shock and trauma in the human. *Ann. Surg., 174*, 451.
Carlyle, J.E., Fleck, A., Drury, J.T. and Richards, J. (1975): Amino acids in plasma and tissues after injury. In preparation.
Cartensen, H., Terner, N., Thorén, L. and Wide, L. (1972): Testosterone, luteinizing hormone and growth hormone in blood following surgical trauma. *Acta chir. scand., 138*, 1.
Cherrington, A. and Vranic, M. (1971): Role of glucagon and insulin in control of glucose turnover. *Metabolism, 20*, 625.
Cryer, P.E., Herman, C.M., Sode, J., Coran, A.G. and Horwitz, D. (1972): Immunochemical and physiologic insulin lack during lethal scepticaemia in the subhuman primate. *Advanc. exp. Med. Biol., 23*, 155.
Cuthbertson, D.P. (1942): Post-shock metabolic response. *Lancet, 1*, 433.
Cuthbertson, D.P. (1964): Physical injury and its effects on protein metabolism. In: *Mammalian Protein Metabolism, Vol. 2*, Ch. 19, pp. 373–414. Editors: Munro, H.N. and Allison, J.B., Academic Press, New York, London.
Davies, J.W.L. (1970): Protein metabolism following injury. *J. clin. Path., 23, Suppl.* (Roy. Coll. Path.) *4*, 56.
Denton, R.M. (1974): Acute hormonal regulation of fatty acid synthesis in rat epidymal fat pads. *Biochem. Soc. Trans., 2*, 1208.
Drucker, W.R., Gallie, B.L., Lau, T.S., Farago, G., Levene, R.A. and Haist, R.E. (1973): The effect of persisting hypovolaemic shock on pancreatic output of insulin. *Advanc. exp. Med. Biol., 33*, 187.
Felig, P., Pozetsky, T., Marliss, E. and Cahill, G.F. Jr. (1970): Alanine: key role in gluconeogenesis. *Science, 167*, 1003.
Felig, P. and Wahren, J. (1971a): Influence of endogenous insulin secretion on splanchnic glucose and amino acid metabolism in man. *J. clin. Invest., 50*, 1702.
Felig, P. and Wahren, J. (1971b): Amino acid metabolism in exercising man. *J. clin. Invest., 50*, 2703.
Fischer, P. (1862): Du Diabète consécutif aux traumatismes. *Arch. gén. Méd., 5th Serie, 20*, 257.
Flear, C.T.G. (1970): Electrolyte and body water changes after trauma. *J. Clin. Path., 23, Suppl.* (Roy. Coll. Path.) *4*, 16.
Giddings, A., O'Connor, K.J., Rowlands, B.J., Mangnall, D. and Clark, R.G. (1975). Hyperglucogonaemia in the surgical patient. *Lancet, 1*, 570.
Gordon, A.H. (1970): The effects of trauma and partial hepatectomy on the rates of synthesis of plasma protein by the liver. In: *Plasma Protein Metabolism*, pp. 351–368. Editors: Rothschild, M.A. and Waldmann, T. Academic Press, New York, London.
Gordon, A.H. (1973): Acute phase plasma proteins in wound healing. In: *Protein Turnover. Ciba Foundation Symposium 9* (new series), pp. 73–85. Associated Scientific Publishers, Amsterdam.
Gump, F.E. (1972): What mechanisms influence oxygen transport and oxygen tissue delivery in endotoxic and haemorrhagic shock. *Advanc. exp. Biol. Med., 23*, 167.
Harland, W.A., Orr, J.S. and Richards, J.R. (1972): Increased thyroxine secretion following surgical operation. *Scot. med. J., 17*, 92.
Heath, D.F. (1971): Liver metabolism after injury. *Advanc. exp. Biol. Med., 33*, 271.

Heath, D.F. and Corney, P.L. (1973): The effects of starvation, environmental temperature and injury on the rate of disposal of glucose by the rat. *Biochem. J., 136*, 519.
Hinshaw, L.B. and Cox, B.G. (1972). The fundamental mechanisms of shock. *Advanc. exp. Med. Biol., 23.*
Horwitz, D.L. (1972): Effects of endotoxin and E. coli shock on the metabolism of lipids and carbohydrate. *Advanc. exp. Med. Biol., 23*, 195.
Huckabee, W.E. (1961a): Abnormal resting blood lactate. I. The significance of hyperlactataemia in hospitalised patients. *Amer. J. Med., 30*, 833.
Huckabee, W.E. (1961b): Abnormal resting blood lactate. II. Lactic acidosis. *Amer. J. Med., 30*, 840.
Hunt, A.G. (1972): *Pathology of Injury – Current Knowledge and Future Development.* Editor: Hunt, A.C. The report of a working party of the Royal College of Pathologists. Published for the Royal College of Pathologists by Harvey Miller and Medcalf Ltd., London.
Jacobson, E.D. (1972): Are adrenergic overactivity and splanchnic vasoconstriction the prime pathophysiological events in shock? *Advanc. exp. Med. Biol., 33*, 109.
Jarrett, R.J. (1971): Blood glucose homeostasis and its disorders. *Brit. J. Hosp. Med., 6*, 499.
Johnstone, I.D.H. (1972): The endocrine response to trauma. *Advanc. clin. Chem., 15*, 255.
Johnstone, I.D.H. (1973): The metabolic and endocrine response to injury: a review. *Brit. J. Anaesth., 45*, 252.
Kaplan, J.H. and Pitot, H.C. (1970): The regulation of intermediary amino acid metabolism in animal tissues. In: *Mammalian Protein Metabolism, Vol. 4*, Ch. 33, pp. 388–443. Editor: Munro, H.N. Academic Press, London.
Kenney, F.T. (1970): Hormonal regulation of synthesis of liver enzymes. In: *Mammalian Protein Metabolism, Vol. 4*, Ch. 31, pp. 131–176. Editor: Munro, H.N. Academic Press, London.
Khan, S.N., Tilstone, W.J., Fleck, A. and Broom, I. (1974): Protein synthesis in the rat liver after fracture of the femur. *Proc. Nutr. Soc., 33*, 93A.
Kinney, J.M., Duke, J.H. Jr., Long, C.L. and Gump, F.E. (1970): Tissue fuel and weight loss after injury. *J. clin. Path., 23, Suppl.* (Roy. Coll. Path.) *4*, 65.
Kirby, R. and Johnstone, I.D.H. (1973): Thyroid function after injury. *Advanc. exp. Med. Biol., 33*, 165.
Kovach, A.G.B. (1972): Metabolic changes in haemorrhagic shock. *Advanc. exp. Biol. Med., 23*, 275.
Kvetvansky, R. and Kopin, I.J. (1973): Activity of adrenal catechol producing enzymes and their regulation after stress. *Advanc. exp. Med. Biol., 33*, 517.
Lefebvre, P.J. and Unger, R.H. (1972): *Glucagon – Molecular Physiology, Clinical and Therapeutic Implications.* Pergamon Press, Oxford.
Lefer, A.M. and Glen, T.M. (1973): The lysosomal protease – myocardial depressant factor system in circulatory shock. *Advanc. exp. Med. Biol., 33*, 367.
Lemieux, M.D., Smith, R.N. and Couch, N.P. (1969): Surface pH and redox potential of skeletal muscle in graded haemorrhage. *Surgery, 65*, 457.
Levenson, S.M., Pulaski, E.J. and Del Guercia, L.R.M. (1966): Metabolic changes associated with injury. In: *Physiologic Principles of Surgery.* Saunders, Philadelphia, Penn.
Long, C.L., Spencer, J.L., Kinney, J.M. and Geiger, J.W. (1971a): Carbohydrate metabolism in normal man and effect of glucose infusion. *J. appl. Physiol., 31*, 102.
Long, C.L., Spencer, J.L., Kinney, J.M. and Geiger, J.W. (1971b): Carbohydrate metabolism in man: effects of elective operations and major injury. *J. appl. Physiol., 31*, 110.
Manchester, K.L. (1970): Sites of hormonal regulation of protein metabolism. In: *Mammalian Protein Metabolism, Vol. 4,* Ch. 33, pp. 229–298. Editor: Munro H.N. Academic Press, New York.
Marliss, E.B., Aoki, T.T., Pozefsky, T., Most, A.S. and Cahill, G.F. Jr. (1971): Muscle and splanchnic glutamine and glutamate metabolism in postabsorptive and starved man. *J. clin. Invest., 50*, 814.

Mela, L.M., Miller, L.D., Bacalzo, L.V. Jr., Olofsson, K. and White, R.R. (1973): Alterations of mitochondrial structure and energy linked functions in haemorrhagic shock and endotoxaemia. *Advanc. exp. Med. Biol., 33*, 231.

Moss, G.S., Cerchio, G.M., Siegel, D.C., Popovich, P.A. and Butler, E. (1970): Serum insulin response in haemorrhagic shock in baboons. *Surgery, 68*, 34.

Moss, G.S., Cerchio, G., Siegel, D.C., Reed, P.C., Cochin, A. and Fresquez, V. (1973): The decline in pancreatic insulin release during haemorrhagic shock in the baboon. *Advanc. exp. Med. Biol., 33*, 199.

Munro, H.N. (1964): General aspects of the regulation of protein metabolism by diet and by hormones. In: *Mammalian Protein Metabolism, Vol. 1*, Ch. 10, pp. 381–481. Editors: Munro, H.N., Allison, J.B. Academic Press, London.

Munro, H.N. (1970): A general survey of mechanisms regulating protein metabolism in mammals. In: *Mammalian Protein Metabolism, Vol. 4*, pp. 3–130. Editor: Munro, H.N. Academic Press, New York.

Nahas, G.G. (1970): The problems of acidosis. *J. clin. Path. 23, Suppl.* (Roy. Coll. Path.) *4*, 73.

Newsholme, E.H. and Start, C. (1973): *Regulation in Metabolism*. John Wiley & Sons, London.

O'Keefe, S.J.D., Sender, P.M. and James, W.P.T. (1974): The 'catabolic' loss of body nitrogen in response to surgery: a problem of protein synthesis. *Lancet, 2*, 1035.

Oyama, T. (1973): Endocrine responses to anesthetic agents. *Brit. J. Anaesth., 45*, 276.

Park, C.R. and Exton, J.H. (1972): Glucagon and the metabolism of glucose. In: *Glucagon – Molecular Physiology, Clinical and Therapeutic Implications*. Ch. 6, pp. 77–108. Editors: Lefebvre, P.J. and Unger, R.H., Pergamon Press, Oxford.

Peretz, D.I., Scott, H.M., Duff, J., Dosseter, J.B., MacLean, L.D. and McGregor, M. (1965): The significance of lacticacidaemia in the shock syndrome. *Ann. N.Y. Acad. Sci., 119*, 1133.

Reivich, M., Kovách, A.G.B., Spitzer, J.J. and Sandor, P. (1973): Cerebral blood flow and metabolism in haemorrhagic shock in baboons. *Advanc. exp. Med. Biol., 33*, 19.

Rosell, S., Sandor, P. and Kovách, A.G.B. (1973): Adipose tissue and haemorrhagic shock. *Advanc. exp. Med. Biol., 33*, 323.

Rush, B.F. Jr. (1972): Irreversibility in the post-transfusion phase of haemorrhagic shock. *Advanc. exp. Med. Biol., 23*, 215.

Russell, R.I.G., Walker, C.J. and Bloom, S.R. (1975): Hyperglucagonaemia in the surgical patient. *Brit. med. J., I*, 10.

Salter, C.P., Fluck, D.C. and Stimmler, L. (1972): Effect of open-heart surgery on growth-hormone levels in man. *Lancet, 2*, 853.

Samols, E., Tyler, J. and Marks, V. (1972): Glucagon–insulin interrelationships. In: *Glucagon*, pp. 151–173. Editors: Lefebvre, P.J. and Unger, R.H. Pergamon Press, Oxford.

Scott, J.C., Weng, J.T. and Spitzer, J.J. (1973): Myocardial metabolism during endotoxic shock. In: *Neurohumoral and Metabolic Aspects of Injury*. Editors: Kovach, A.G.B., Stoner, H.B., Spitzer, J.J. Plenum Press, London.

Sevitts and Stoner, H.B. (eds.) (1970): The pathology of trauma. *J. clin. Path., 23, Suppl.* (Roy. Coll. Path.) *4*.

Shoemaker, W.C., Stahr, L.J., Kim, S.I. and Elwyn, D.H. (1973): Sequential circulatory and metabolic changes in the liver and whole body during haemorrhagic shock. *Advanc. exp. Med. Biol., 33*, 293.

Smith, R., Fuller, D.J., Wedge, J.H., Williamson, D.H. and Alberti, K.G.G.M. (1975): Initial effect of injury on ketone bodies and other blood metabolites. *Lancet, 1*, 1.

Smith, I.M. and Mukherjee, K.L. (1972): Liver metabolism and energy in Staphylococcus aureus septic shock in mice. *Advanc. exp. Med. Biol., 23*, 253.

Somogyi, J., Cremer, J.E. and Ikrényi, K. (1973): Characterisation of rat brain mitochondria, the effect of injury. *Advanc. exp. Med. Biol., 33*, 345.

Spitzer, J.A., Kovách, A.G.B., Rosell, S., Sandor, P., Spitzer, J.J. and Storck, R. (1973a): Influence of endotoxin on adipose tissue metabolism. *Advanc. exp. Med. Biol.*, *33*, 337.
Spitzer, J.J., Spitzer, J.A., Weng, J.T. and Scott, J.C. (1972): Myocardial metabolism during acute haemorrhagic or endotoxic shock. *Advanc. exp. Med. Biol.*, *23*, 267.
Spitzer, J.J., Wiener, R. and Wolf, E.H. (1973b): Non-esterified fatty acid (FFA) metabolism following severe haemorrhage in the conscious dog. *Advanc. exp. Med. Biol.*, *33*, 221.
Stoner, H.B. (1958a): Studies on the mechanism of shock. The influence of environment on the changes in oxygen consumption, tissue temperature and blood flow produced by limb ischaemia. *Brit. J. exp. Path.*, *39*, 251.
Stoner, H.B. (1958b): Studies on the mechanism of shock. The quantitative aspects of glycogen metabolism after limb ischaemia in the rat. *Brit. J. exp. Path.*, *39*, 635.
Stoner, H.B. (1961): The biochemical response to injury. *The Scientific Basis of Medicine, Annual Review*, pp. 172–199. University of London, Athlone Press, London.
Stoner, H.B. (1968): Mechanism of body temperature changes after burns and other injuries. *Ann. N.Y. Acad. Sci.*, *150*, 722.
Stoner, H.B. (1970): Energy metabolism after injury. *J. clin. Path.*, *23, Suppl.* (Roy. Coll. Path.) *4*, 47.
Stoner, H.B. and Heath, D.F. (1973): The effects of trauma on carbohydrate metabolism. *Brit. J. Anaesth.*, *45*, 244.
Travis, S.F., Sugerman, H.J., Ruberg, R.L., Dudrick, S.J., Delivoria-Papadopoulos, M., Miller, L.D. and Oski, F.A. (1971): Alterations of red-cell glycolytic intermediates and oxygen transport as a consequence of hypophosphataemia in patients receiving intravenous hyperalimentation. *New Engl. J. Med.*, *285*, 763.
Unger, R.H. and Lefebvre, P.J. (1972): Glucagon physiology. In: *Glucagon*, Ch. 15, pp. 213–244. Editors: Lefebvre, P.J. and Unger, R.H. Pergamon Press, London.
Vigas, M., Haist, R.E., Bauer, F. and Drucker, W.R. (1973): Insulin secretion during haemorrhagic shock. *Advanc. exp. Med. Biol.*, *33*, 179.
Weil, M.H. and Shubin, H. (1972): Proposed reclassification of shock states with special reference to distributive defects. *Advanc. exp. Med. Biol.*, *23*, 13.
Wilmore, D.W., Lindsay, C.A., Moylan, J.A., Faloona, G.R., Pruitt, B.A. and Unger, R.H. (1974): Hyperglucagonaemia after burns. *Lancet*, *1*, 73.
Woods, H.F. (1974): Lactic acidosis. In: *Tenth Symposium on Advanced Medicine*, pp. 53–67. Editor: Ledingham, J.G.G. Pitman Medical in association with the Journal of the Royal College of Physicians of London.
Wunnamacher, R.W. Jr. (1972): Ribosomal RNA synthesis and function as influenced by amino acid supply and stress. *Proc. Nutr. Soc.*, *31*, 281.

Ledingham (ed.). Shock

*The role of humoral factors in shock**

A.L. NAGLER and Rita McCONN

Although the history of shock, especially hemorrhagic shock, is one of antiquity, dating prehistoria, when it was observed that there existed a quantitative relationship between blood loss, weakness and death, most of our present day knowledge has been derived over the last 50 years. Such accumulation of knowledge began with the recognition that the state of shock was a focal common point terminus of several convergent processes that could be induced by a variety of causes.

For the purpose of this chapter, shock will be considered a syndrome in which there is a sustained reduction in tissue perfusion resulting in various alterations in tissue metabolism, structure and function at the organic, cellular and systemic levels. Shock in the normovolemic and hypovolemic state has the common characteristic of circulatory failure, and a widely held shock theory is that the production of a humoral factor or factors is the cause of this hemodynamic state. With the identification throughout the years of various vasoactive compounds, investigators have attempted to define whether they have any role in the production of the shock state. The relationship of these

* Supported in part by Grants 1RO1 GM17423 and 1RO1 HL17479 from the National Institutes of Health, National Institutes of General Medical Sciences, Bethesda, Md., to the Albert Einstein College of Medicine, Yeshiva University, Bronx, N.Y., by gifts from The Prudential Insurance Company of America to the Albert Einstein College of Medicine, Yeshiva University, Bronx, N.Y.

various factors to tissue perfusion and metabolism in shock will be critically reviewed in this paper.

Prior to this discussion, however, let us consider the pathogenesis of the shock state resulting from blood loss. Upon initial blood loss the body's intrinsic hemostatic regulatory mechanisms attempt to compensate for the hemorrhage-induced initial fall in central venous and arterial pressures by vasoconstrictive reflex mechanisms. This is accomplished by reflexly increasing the tone of the vascular tree, thereby reducing its capacity; at the same time the heart rate is increased to improve perfusion. As hemorrhage progresses and less perfusion fluid is available for circulation, additional vascular reflex compensatory mechanisms are called upon to, in effect, diminish or 'cut-off' circulation to 'non-vital' areas such as the visceral circulation; this maintains the highest venous return to the heart permitting the lesser volumes available to circulate through the vital areas such as the heart and brain. Such a compensatory phase of shock is hallmarked by an alternating (as seen in the microcirculation) compensatory ischemia, permitting minimal intermittent non-vital tissue perfusion to occur, while maintaining venous return and systemic pressure by such selective perfusion; if the initial cause of bleeding is corrected at this time and the patient or animal given volume replacement therapy, resuscitation is possible, the patient or animal survives and the shock state is 'reversible'.

If however the loss of blood is not corrected and resuscitation therapy not instituted, an 'irreversible' period is entered which is proclaimed by the opening of the previously reflexly constricted vascular beds; there is a resultant pooling of the already decreased circulating volumes exaggerating the already decreased venous return to the heart, the forerunner to a decreased cardiac output. This decreased perfusion volume is subsequently pooled in other newly dilated beds, so on and till the patient dies in an ever diminishing systemic pressure state. Thus, shock is cyclic in nature, in that once initiated a sequence of hemodynamic events occurs, each adversely affecting the next. The cause and effect relationship of this syndrome (blood loss → vasoconstriction → vasodilation → decreased venous return → decreased cardiac output → vasoconstriction → vasodilation → decreased venous return) constitutes the vicious cycle contributing to its self-perpetuation.

Since these vascular phenomena are under the control of local and circulating humoral agents and are affected by anesthetics, a great deal of effort has been expended to elucidate their role in the pathogenesis of shock and its treatment.

Catecholamines

It is well documented that the release of catecholamines is a major aspect of the attempted compensatory life-sustaining reaction to injury enabling the animal to maintain blood flow to the heart and brain, yet investigations in this area have created one of the greatest controversies. Evidence has been accumulated both for and against this hormonal system being responsible for irreversibility in shock.

Through the media of electron microscopy and radioisotopic analysis the storage and release of such catecholamines is known to be associated with the granulated vesicles in post-ganglionic sympathetic nerve endings and the adrenal medulla (Egdahl, 1959; Nykeil and Glaviano, 1961). Their release is undoubtedly neurogenically mediated in part via: 1) moderator reflexes (Nakano and Schryver, 1963) 2) reduced blood flow and hypoxia of the adrenal medulla, and 3) secondarily by drugs (notably reserpine, tyramine, amphetamine, cocaine) and the humor histamine.

The best known hemodynamic effects of the catecholamines are inotropic and chronotropic stimulation of the heart, constriction of arterioles in skin, kidney and viscera, dilation of arteries in striated muscle and myocardium, and constriction in most veins. These effects vary considerably depending upon the metabolic state of the experimental animal, blood volume, anesthesia and the dose and type of adrenergic drug used.

Increased levels of catecholamines have been regularly measured in the plasma of animals and patients in shock resulting from all etiologies (Egdahl, 1959; Hall and Hodge, 1971; Jacobson et al., 1964; Nykeil and Glaviano, 1961) causing all investigators and clinicians to agree that such catecholamines play a significant role in the reaction to shock. Furthermore the facts that: 1) the effects of bacterial endotoxins are enhanced locally and systemically by catecholamines and vice versa (Hinshaw et al., 1962; Jacobson et al., 1964; Weiner and Zweifach, 1966; Zweifach et al., 1956), 2) such states can be mimicked physiologically, pathophysiologically and pathologically by the slow intravenous infusion of such catecholamines (Erlanger and Gasser, 1919; Lillehei et al., 1964b) and 3) blockade of adrenergic receptor sites almost invariably exerts protective actions in various types of experimental shock (Lillehei et al., 1964a; Motsay et al., 1970), have significantly contributed to the concept that catecholamines play an important role in the pathogenesis of shock state.

In Lillehei's schema (Lillehei et al., 1969a, b) the shock-initiating injury induces sympathetic nervous system and adrenal medullary activity culminating in the release of catecholamines. There is a resultant intense vasoconstriction of primarily skin and visceral precapillary arterioles and postcapillary venules with ischemia and hypoxia of the beds they perfuse. There is a lowering of the hydrostatic pressure in the capillary beds to cause tissue fluids to enter the circulatory system and produce a beneficial overall compensatory increase in circulating blood volume. The state of ischemia and hypoxia causes the local production and accumulation of metabolic acids, which in turn lower the responsiveness of the contracted vessels to catecholamines; at the same time there occurs an increase in the activity of histidine decarboxylase (which results in the production of vasodilation via histamine), both these events synergistically producing vasodilation. Such progress causes the tissue status to change from pale ischemic hypoxia to one of congested stagnant hypoxia. In an effort to reinstitute and maintain the original state of vasoconstriction, greater concentrations of catecholamines are liberated. This cyclical series of events proceeds until the arterioles lose their tone (possibly because of local acidosis and histamine endothelial damage) and blood enters the capillary beds – the venules maintain their tone and the microcirculation becomes engorged. The resultant elevation in hydrostatic pressure within the capillary bed causes a further loss of circulating blood volume; subsequent stagnation and hypoxia in the presence of the toxic metabolites therefrom, destroy the integrity of the capillary bed permitting the suffusion of whole blood into the tissues. This further reduces circulating blood volumes, all these events leading to irreversibility of the shock state, which, according to Lillehei, is due to failure of the microcirculation based upon overactivity of catecholamine attempts at compensation.

On the other hand, there is considerable evidence to indicate that over-activity of the sympathoadrenal system, presumably causing extensive fluid efflux into the skin and skeletal muscle, is not primarily involved in the genesis of irreversibility. Firstly, to the contrary, a number of earlier papers discussing the genesis of shock describe fluid loss from skin and muscle of a shocked dog forelimb, even during perfusion of the forelimb with a constant flow (Emerson et al., 1965, 1966; Hinshaw et al., 1965). Secondly, Grega and Haddy (1971), while measuring transcapillary fluid flux in the dog forelimb during catecholamine infusion shock, found that fluid efflux was minimal as shock progressed, and with further progression, fluid resorption into the vasculature was increased. Thirdly, little success has been reported with the use of adrenergic blockade, using phenoxybenzamine given before and after endotoxemia, in an attempt to prevent acidosis, hemoconcentration, the intravascular blood pooling, reduction in venous return or cardiac output, systemic hypotension and death (Brake et al., 1964; Hinshaw et al., 1965). It has been suggested that the lack of success of adrenergic blockade could be due to the 'too generalized catecholamine antagonistic effect'. It is thought that if specific organ blockade could be achieved beneficial results would occur. Fourthly, it was determined that neither sympathetic denervation of the splanchnic viscera nor adrenalectomy prevented the portal hypertension, systemic hypotension or intestinal hemorrhagic necrosis associated with endotoxic shock. Similarly, splanchnic sympathectomy was also without effect on survival rates (Emerson et al., 1965a, 1966).

Thus, in the light of conflicting data, we can only state that while we know these amines to play a role in shock, their role in the genesis of irreversibility remains uncertain. The possibility exists that while they may not play an overt role early in shock leading to irreversibility, they may exert their negative role late in shock. It should be borne in mind that in vivo studies of the microcirculation yield a biphasic response, initially a hyperreactive phase followed by hyporeactivity, depression and even reversal of epinephrine responsiveness. Perhaps it is in this latter phase, during hyporeactivity or reversal of reactivity, that the breakdown of compensatory vasoconstrictor mechanisms comes into play.

Histamine

A biochemical rationale was provided for the vasodilatory microvascular changes pathognomonic of the shock state with the discovery of histamine. Further investigations into this hypothesis provided data to buttress the theory since histamine also increased tissue permeability and produced severe hypotension upon intravenous administration to cats. The significance of histamine in this regard diminished when investigators were unable to demonstrate increased levels of circulating histamine during shock and that shock was not obviated by the use of antihistamines.

Interest in this material has since been rekindled by Schayer (1962) when the hypothesis was formulated that the balance between histamine and catecholamines *locally* exerts the major control over circulatory homeostasis with histamine being the chief regulator of the microcirculation. His work, showing increased levels of histidine decarboxylase in shock tissues (specifically during endotoxin shock), implies that the local synthesis of histamine ('induced histamine'), rather than 'preformed histamine' in mast cells, is the important physiologic mechanism controlling the microcirculation. This increased synthesis of histamine during shock may then produce small vessel damage, with the local histamine causing gradual alleviation of the reflex compensatory vasoconstriction (alternating opening and closing of the vessels) terminating in the hypothesized histamine-induced vasodilation which leads to intravascular pooling, etc. According to Zweifach, however, the primary actions of histamine, namely widespread vasodilation and endothelial damage, are not observed in most forms of shock (Zweifach, 1962) and therefore do not corroborate the role of histamine as stated by Schayer (1962) in shock (other than in endotoxin shock). Furthermore, Haddy and Visscher (1971) provided evidence that the increased capillary permeability brought about by histamine results from postcapillary venular spasm rather than from a direct toxic effect on endothelial cells. More recent evidence from Altura's (Altura and Zweifach, 1966) laboratory, however, has also cast serious doubt on this Schayer theory on the mechanism of microcirculatory control by histamine. These workers, using other procedures known to activate histidine decarboxylase, were not regularly able to achieve vasodilation of affected areas, or alter the vascular reactivity of these areas in the terminal microcirculatory beds.

With regard to the role of histamine in endotoxin shock, there is considerable evidence that the initial fall in blood pressure upon endotoxemia is due to the trapping or pooling of blood within the hepatic portal system and the splanchnic bed (Weil et al., 1956) apparently as a result of transient venous constriction (Haddy and Fisscher, 1971) due to histamine release (Hinshaw et al., 1961a, b, 1962; Vick, 1964). During endotoxin shock the initial histamine response triggers the release of epinephrine from the adrenal medulla (Jacobson et al., 1964). Such adrenal medullary secretion in turn stimulates an increase in blood histamine (Baur and Staub, 1949) providing evidence for a mutual secretory action of the humors (Went and Varga, 1952). Thus, the initial vascular histamine-mediated effect is manifest shortly thereafter by a decreased venous return to the heart and a decreased cardiac output resulting in the creation of the vicious cycle; the cycle secondarily involves the local tissues with their attempt to compensatorily vasoconstrict in order to maintain higher cardiac return and elevation of systemic pressure. Such local vasoconstriction gives way in the cycle to local histamine–hypoxia-initiated vasodilation and vascular collapse (the initial endotoxin-induced histamine response having started the cycle going in endotoxin shock). This local increase in histamine is evidenced by a marked increase of histidine decarboxylase locally (Schayer, 1960) during endotoxemia.

There are some key experiments aimed at corroborating this thesis, that have failed to do so. It has been demonstrated on several occasions that amelioration of the early vascular effects of histamine (Haddy and Fisscher, 1971; Hinshaw et al., 1961a, b, 1962a, b; Vick, 1964; Weil et al., 1956) does little if anything to prevent the mortality of endotoxemia (Hinshaw et al., 1965). Furthermore, Emerson (1972) found that bolus injections of endotoxin led to a decrease in blood pressure, supposedly histamine-induced, while a slow infusion had no hypotensive effect, yet death occurred in both groups of animals with no difference in survival time.

It therefore appears from all available evidence that while histamine release is no doubt harmful, there is little to support the hypothesis that endogenous histamine is responsible directly or indirectly for the irreversibility of endotoxin shock.

Serotonin

A vasoactive amine also thought by some to be involved in the pathogenesis of shock states is serotonin or 5-hydroxy-tryptamine. This humor, although present in several tissues of the body, has been found in largest concentrations in the brain, gastrointestinal tract, platelets and mast cells. In non-shock related experiments serotonin causes contraction of skin vessels. Its effects on other vascular smooth muscle are quite variable depending upon the physiologic state of the animal at the time of its administration; it may either raise or lower systemic blood pressure, the action on vascular tone often being opposite to that already present (Daugherty et al., 1968; Emerson et al., 1971). In vitro using vessel strips, serotonin increases smooth muscle tension regardless of the state of initial resistance (Ituri and Emerson, 1971). As a rule serotonin has little effect on venous return or cardiac output (Emerson, 1968) and has negligible effects on capillary filtration (Daugherty et al., 1968). The most notable effect of the humor has been shown to be on the pulmonary vessels (Hinshaw et al., 1957). Serotonin has been found to constrict the pulmonary vasculature in the perfused canine lung and increase pulmonary vascular resistance.

The role of serotonin in shock is undetermined. Kobald et al. (1964) have demonstrated such release from platelets and splanchnic visceral organs in endotoxin shock, while Baez and his associates (Janoff et al., 1961) have demonstrated such release in superior mesenteric artery occlusion (SMAO) and hemorrhagic shock. Endotoxin-induced serotonin release has also been demonstrated to occur from blood and splanchnic visceral organs in vitro (Kobald et al., 1964), and as a result of continued trauma to the formed elements of the blood during prolonged pump oxygenation. Davis et al. (1960,

1961) have shown in vivo that endotoxemia causes an initial short-lived plasma increase in serotonin peaking at about 30 seconds, with return to normal within 5 minutes, and thereafter falling to below normal levels (Jacobson et al., 1964; Rosenberg et al., 1959, 1961). It has been postulated that such serotonin release and circulation may be involved in the transiently increased pulmonary vascular resistance seen in the dog after intravenous endotoxin adminstration.

Investigations have shown the administration of the humor to be somewhat protective in shock. In fact, the data show that many procedures which enhance resistance to endotoxin shock (including neomycin pretreatment) also increase the serotonin content of the gut wall. A great deal of investigation is required before the role of this humor in shock can be determined.

Vasopressin and Angiotensin

Vasopressin is a peptide released from the neurohypophysis. It is vasoactive by virtue of its direct action on vascular contractile elements of the capillaries and arterioles and as such may elevate blood pressure. Vasopressin also causes decreases in coronary blood flow via coronary constriction and as such depresses myocardial function which, in conjunction with its pressor effects on capillaries and arterioles, may result in the appearance of no net response in particular in vivo experimental situations.

Several groups of investigators have reported a significant increase in circulating levels of blood vasopressin after hemorrhage. The pathway for such a response is thought to be via pressor receptors lying in the aortic arch, stretch receptors in the left atrium and carotid artery baroreceptors (Chien et al., 1962; Share and Levy, 1962). Other pathways must be present since bilateral vagotomy and carotid sinus denervation did not completely abolish the secretion of vasopressin in response to hemorrhage. Furthermore, a role for vasopressin in hemorrhage has been supported by the fact that animals with diabetes insipidus have an increased susceptibility to hemorrhage which can be reversed by the administration of vasopressin.

Angiotensin II is a vasoactive octapeptide formed by the action of renin on the plasma substrate, angiotensinogen. It is a potent vasoconstrictor of peripheral beds (Daugherty et al., 1968; Emerson et al., 1965b) causing a decrease in venous return and cardiac output and an increase in systemic blood pressure upon infusion into normal dogs (Emerson, 1966). During hemorrhage, renin is released secondary to renal ischemia (compensatory ischemia) with the consequent formation of angiotensin II (Davis et al., 1962).

The plasma concentration of angiotensin II rises early in shock, remaining elevated for at least 60–90 minutes (Hall and Hodge, 1971; White et al., 1966).

McNeil (1972) concluded from his data that angiotensin formation and vasopressin secretion play a major role in the intestinal and splenic vasoconstrictor reaction-response to hemorrhage, especially the former. The responses he observed with infusions of vasopressin and angiotensin on these circulatory beds were consistant with his postulated roles for the peptides in hemorrhage, the postulate being that the initial compensatory response of splanchnic vasoconstriction is due to these peptides. Although the evidence is limited, the fact that blood pressure of dogs in hypovolemic shock is markedly improved by subcutaneous or intramuscular injections of angiotensin provides a good indication that more research is required in this area (Derrick et al., 1962).

Lysosomal Enzymes

Lysosomal enzymes have been implicated in the production of the irreversible shock state though at the present time their exact role has not yet been clearly defined.

The name lysosome was first proposed by DeDuve in 1959, when it was found that in rat liver as many as five distinct acid-hydrolases, with widely differing specificities, appeared to be associated together with a special group of cytoplasmic particles. An important property of lysosomes is the structure linked latency of their enzymes which is attributed to the presence of a membrane-like barrier restricting the accessibility of their internal hydrolases to external substrate. Two possible roles were proposed for lysosomes, one of intracellular digestion, heterolysis, and the other, self-digestion, autolysis, of the cell which may result as a normal or pathological process in the life of a cell. The cytological identity of lysosomes has been fairly well established by electron microscopy studies and localization of acid phosphatase by cytochemical techniques. Studies in recent years have modified the concept of the lysosome into a dynamic intracellular entity, in which the activity of acid hydrolases depends on the metabolic state of the cell, the need for controlled degradation of macromolecules or the promotion of endocytosis or exocytosis. These lysosomal particles show an extraordinary intracellular mobility of an order that places them beyond Brownian movement (Verrity et al., 1973).

Lysosomes are widely distributed in mammalian tissues including brain, spleen, thyroid and lymph nodes. The highest concentrations are found in the liver, kidney, and spleen. While as many as twelve different acid hydrolases have been identified, their distribution and absolute concentration varies. One of the most important sites of lysosomes is in the phagocytic cells of the blood, namely, the polymorphonuclear leukocytes and the mononuclear elements which comprise the reticulo-endothelial system, in particular the alveolar macrophages. There is a fair amount of evidence to support Janoff's (1964) suggestion that lysosomal enzymes are released not only in dead cells undergoing autolysis, but also prior to cell death as a result of cellular anoxia or injury; hypoxia, ischemia and acidosis are well known to be effective stimuli for the disruption of lysosomes (Slater, 1969). The enzymes which are regarded as specific markers for lysosomes are β-glucuronidase and D-cathepsin; in the plasma acid phosphatase is not an enzyme specific only to lysosomes since it also occurs in the red cell. Lefer and Glenn (1972) found that the total tissue activity of pancreas and liver is markedly reduced in post-oligemia and splanchnic ischemia shock whereas the spleen and intestine are moderately influenced and the heart is not significantly involved. Furthermore, an increase in free lysosomal enzymes, i.e., unbound enzymes, has been found in the splanchnic viscera in shock as well as in the circulating plasma. Significant increases in the plasma levels of these enzymes have been reported in hemorrhagic, endotoxic and cardiogenic shock, splanchnic ischemia and burn trauma (Alexander, 1967; Berman et al., 1969; Glenn and Lefer, 1970; Glenn et al., 1971). However, the release of measurable quantities of lysosomal enzymes in shock has been questioned by Schumer et al. (1969). Several investigators did studies designed specifically to answer this question and were able to confirm the original observations and furthermore show that it is a time-related phenomenon (Clermont and Williams, 1962; Fredlund et al., 1972).

Plasma lysosomal enzymes may arise not only from tissues but also from the polymorphonuclear leukocytes (PMNL). Cohn (Cohn and Hirsch, 1960), in his studies of the cytoplasmic granules of the PMNL noted their sensitivity to the hydrogen ion concentration of the medium. Thus, the acidosis of shock may also be a contributing factor to the leakage of enzymes from the leukocytes. Further it is known that whenever cells engage in phagocytosis they release a portion of their lysosomal hydrolases into the surrounding medium unaccompanied by seepage of the cytoplasm marker enzyme; this occurs not only following uptake of immune complexes, but also accompanies ingestion of inert particles (Weissman et al., 1972). Stored blood may have significant concentrations of lysosomal enzymes resulting from leakage or disintegration of the PMNL (McConn and Nagler, 1974), thus transfusion of whole blood in the shock patient may further contribute to the circulating levels of lysosomal enzymes.

There is some evidence from animal studies to support the suggestion that high circulating levels of lysosomal enzymes produce cardiac depression and splanchnic vasoconstriction (Glenn et al., 1972). Studies in the isolated cat heart (Langendorf preparation) showed that the presence of these enzymes in the wash fluid reduced both coronary flow and contractile force. Additional studies in cat papillary muscle showed that the negative inotropic effect was not due solely to coronary vasoconstriction but also to a direct cardiodepressant effect. In the intact animal lysosomal enzymes were not found to exert any significant hemodynamic effect if there was normal functioning reticulo-endothelial system. The depression of the reticulo-endothelial system has been documented to occur in a variety of shock states (Altura and Hershey, 1972; Blattberg and Levy, 1963). In animals in whom the reticulo-endothelial system was excluded by surgical removal of the spleen and circulatory by-pass of the liver, infusion of lysosomal enzymes was associated with significant myocardial depression (Glenn et al., 1972).

Lysosomal enzymes have been implicated by a number of investigators in the production of a 'shock' factor by action on a modified tissue or plasma protein. This factor appears to have vasoactive and/or cardiodepressant effects. In discussion of the lysosomal enzymes it is generally understood that this term refers to the acid hydrolases and these have activity in the range pH 2–6 with maximum activity usually occurring around pH 4. The hydrogen ion concentration may well fall to this level in some tissues in shock. Thus, it is possible that there could be local production of a shock factor which could then enter the circulation. Alternatively the shock factor may be produced by the action of lysosomal enzymes on a modified plasma protein. It is doubtful that an acid hydrolase would have any significant activity at plasma pH values which are regarded as acidotic with respect to the patient. Movat, however, recently demonstrated the presence of neutral proteases in human PMNL (Movat et al., 1973). They reported that cells interacted with immune precipitates released β-glucuronidase, a neutral protease (hemoglobinase), and an enzyme capable of liberating kinin from kininogen at neutral pH. Ultrastructural studies showed that the leukocytes had undergone degranulation, and cell fractionation studies showed that hydrolase and kinin activity was present in the granule or lysosomal pellet. Thus the action of the lysosomal enzymes on a plasma substrate could result in the production of a kinin-type of compound.

If the release of proteolytic enzymes from lysosomes plays an important role in the development of shock, then pharmacological agents which either prevent the release of these enzymes or inhibit the activity of the 'free' enzymes should have a protective effect in experimental shock. Several groups have reported that protease inhibitors give some protection in endotoxic, thermal, pancreatitis, traumatic, tourniquet and hemorrhagic shock (Back et al., 1968; Berrelli and Donati, 1970; Haberland, 1970; Stock and Eigler, 1969). Furthermore the proteinase inhibitor, Trasylol, when given to a septic donor animal is capable of blocking pneumonitis in the perfused pulmonary lobe (Clowes, 1973).

Supra-physiologic doses of glucocorticoids bestow a protective action in shock. Several hypotheses have been proposed for the mechanism of action of steroids and this subject has been the topic of much investigative work and is discussed in detail later. However, one possible mode of action suggested is that these compounds stabilize lysosomal membranes. Methylprednisolone has been shown to stabilize lysosomal membranes and markedly retard the release of lysosomal hydrolases particularly in the pancreas, both in vivo in the control and shock state (Glenn and Lefer, 1970; Lefer and Glenn, 1972b) and in vitro (Jefferson et al., 1971). Glucocorticoids do not however inhibit lysosomal enzymes once they are released from lysosomes (Glenn and Lefer, 1971). Wilson (1974) gave tritiated labelled methylprednisolone sodium succinate in animals and then induced hemorrhagic shock and studied the distribution of the steroid by autoradiography in tissue sections taken after the animal was retransfused. Large numbers of labelled cells were found in almost every organ of the body. Lung biopsies showed heavy labelling of alveolar type II cells and nuclei of PMNL and granules of mast cells. Lysosomes within lung cells as well as free lysosomes in pulmonary circulation were also labelled. These pathological findings lend support to the hypothesis that steroids can interfere with the release of lysosomal enzymes in shock from tissues and blood elements as well as the reticulo-endothelial system.

The chemical identity of the compound(s) produced by the action of the proteolytic lysosomal enzymes is far from complete. Those which have been implicated are presented below.

Kinins

The interaction of proteolytic enzymes with plasma proteins results in the formation of polypeptides called kinins, with smooth muscle stimulating properties. Bradykinin, the prototype of this group of polypeptides is a nonapeptide derived from the kininogen in the alpha-2-globulin fraction of plasma. It has been implicated in shock because of its vasodilator activity and its action on capillary permeability. In hemorrhagic shock bradykininogen levels rise and then decline below normal (Dimiz and Carvalho, 1963).

A possible relationship between vasoactive peptides such as bradykinin and endotoxin was investigated by Siegel et al. (1965) using the isolated perfused limb of a dog. They reported that bradykinin decreased the arteriovenous oxygen differential associated with decreased vascular tone; in contrast, endotoxin did not show these effects. Siegel (1965) postulated that endotoxin effects may be mediated through the release of such a humoral product (i.e., kinins) and in this way produce the previously mentioned myocardial depression and other manifestations of endotoxin shock. Kobald et al. (1964) have demonstrated the in vitro release of such materials upon incubation of blood, blood fractions or homogenates of abdominal viscera with endotoxin. The substances produced as a result of such incubation are similar to those found in the circulation after shock induced by endotoxemia. The authors feel that these vasoactive mediators play an important role in the pathogenesis of endotoxin shock since the removal of the abdominal viscera (the prime source of such peptides upon in vitro incubation with endotoxin) delayed the onset of shock.

The decapeptide kalliden, with properties similar to those of bradykinin has been reported (upon injection) to cause shock like states. Subsequent investigations however have shown that purified preparations of kalliden (kallikrein) are less toxic and therefore attribute the earlier demonstrated toxicity to contaminating materials – especially since injections of kallikrein in concentrations 9 times that concentration reported to be lethal was not lethal in dogs (Webster and Clark, 1959).

More recently there has been a revival of the significance of such kinins in endotoxin shock (Erdos and Mina, 1968; Nies et al., 1968). Reichgott et al. (1971) concluded from their studies that bradykinin infusions reproduce the circulatory events, including regional blood flow distributions of early endotoxemia. Much of the other evidence is indirect, but implies that kallikrein substrate disappears during endotoxemia (Erdos and Mina, 1968) while kinin activity in blood increases (Shah et al., 1970; Wlodzimierz, 1972). These changes correlate well with the fall in total peripheral resistance in the early phases of shock.

It is conceivable that there are many compounds which could be classified as kinins although only a few have been specifically named and whose chemical structure has been elucidated. The initial identification of a kinin-type of compound is usually by means of bioassay using a smooth muscle preparation, and differentiation by dose/response in various preparations such as rat uterus, guinea pig ileum. While the results from several investigators would indicate the presence of a circulating toxic factor in shock it is conceivable that these entities could be related to kinins as yet not characterized.

Various theories have been postulated to explain possible mechanisms of such release, activation and activity of kinins in shock. They are: 1) direct activation of plasma kallikrein by endotoxin; 2) interaction of endotoxin with specific immunoglobulins (with or without complement or other enzymes (lysosomes and lysosomal enzymes) to convert kininogens to kinins (Nies et al., 1968); 3) activation of clotting system to activate kinins, perhaps via Hageman factor activation or plasmin activation (and serotonin); 4) interaction of endotoxin with PMNL to release activators to produce kinin (Greenbaum et al., 1969); or 5) interference with liver kinin inactivation or kininase systems (Abrams et al., 1969), and thus cause prolongation of kinin response.

In recent years a great deal of attention has focussed on the lung in shock and a concentrated effort has been made to determine the etiology of the progressive respiratory insufficiency which can occur in the shock patient who has no known history of chronic lung disease nor who has sustained any chest injury. Investigators have sought a circulating agent as the cause of the pulmonary lesion in a like fashion to the search for the shock factor which causes the failure in the hemodynamic system. It seems reasonable to postulate that the loss of integrity of the pulmonary circulation and the systemic circulation in shock could occur by the same mechanism. There is a fair amount of evidence to suggest that production of both proteolytic enzymes and vasoactive peptides occur in situ in the lung in shock. It is generally thought that the pulmonary circulation plays a prominent role in inactivating kinins (Erdos, 1971); however recent work by Greenbaum et al. (1969) indicates that a kinin compound is produced by alveolar macrophages acting on purified human plasma. This supports the concept of the production of a vasoactive peptide within the lung itself.

Passively transferable lethal factor (PTLF) and cardiovascular toxic factor (CVTF)

Over the last thirty years a number of investigators (Janoff et al., 1961; Nagler and Levenson, 1974; Ravin et al., 1958) have demonstrated the presence of a passively transferable lethal factor in the plasma of animals in experimental irreversible shock.

Nagler and Levenson (1974) using various techniques have been able to demonstrate that the toxicity of plasma resides in the gamma globulin fraction. Electrophoretic and ultracentrifugation studies indicate that it is an aggregated gamma globulin and is non-dialyzable. Incubation of this plasma fraction with a white cell lysate or with the first few ml of the effluent splenic blood following retransfusion of hemorrhaged rats produces a factor which has a marked ventricular depressant effect on the frog heart forming the basis of a bioassay for the material. Using this technique, significant amounts have been found of both the precursor and the cardiovascular toxin in the plasma of a variety of acutely-ill patients; the concentrations of these materials correlated well with severity of their shock clinically and with death. In addition, Frater et al. (1974) have found significant amounts of both factors in patients undergoing cardiopulmonary bypass, once again with good correlation between the amounts bioassayed and the clinical status of the patient. McConn and Nagler (1974) recently demonstrated that these factors were also produced during liquid preservation of whole blood at 4°C. Furthermore, they were able to demonstrate a significant depression of the isolated rabbit and dog heart by the material resulting from incubation of the stored plasma with white cell lysates and the decrease in ventricular function could not be attributed to a fall in coronary flow (McConn et al., unpublished observations).

This work suggests that the components which react to produce the humoral shock factor are contained within the blood and/or reticulo-endothelial system and it is the conditions to which it is exposed which precipitates the formation of such a compound. The work also indicates that the factor has a direct myocardial depressant effect.

Myocardial depressant factor (MDF)

Complementary to this work is the myocardial depressant first described by Brand and Lefer in 1966; their data indicate that this factor is produced by the action of lysosomal hydrolases upon a protein derived from the pancreas which then passes into the circulation (Ferguson et al., 1972). The presence of MDF is determined by bioassay in the cat papillary muscle (Lefer and Rovetto, 1970) and this factor has been demonstrated in the plasma of animals and man in various types of shock including hemorrhagic (Brand and Lefer, 1966; Lefer and Glenn, 1972b; Fisher et al., 1973), endotoxic (Wangensteen et al., 1971), cardiogenic (Glenn et al., 1971; Lefer et al., 1967), splanchnic ischemia (Glenn and Lefer, 1970), pancreatitis and burn shock (Lefer et al., 1971). MDF has now been identified as a peptide with a molecular weight of 500–1000 and its plasma activity is inversely related to survival in shock. The pancreas has been sited as the primary source of both the cardiotoxic peptide MDF, and the activating enzymes and co-factors (Lefer and Glenn, 1973).

MDF has been shown to have a direct depressant action on the myocardium, moderately to vasoconstrict the splanchnic vessels and there is some suggestion that it may depress the reticulo-endothelial system (Lefer and Glenn, 1973). These latter properties would form part of a positive feed-back system to further increase MDF concentration. Furthermore it appears that lysosomal enzymes sensitize the heart to the action of MDF.

The validity of MDF has been questioned by several investigators and it has been suggested that MDF is sodium chloride (Wangensteen et al., 1973), pentobarbital (Wilson and Ebert, 1972) or an artefact of freezing plasma (Urschel et al., 1972). Lefer and Glenn (1974) recently answered their critics in detail pointing out incorrect experimental technique and a poorly designed study respectively as the origin of the first two suggestions and showed new experimental work which indicated that MDF is not produced in shock plasma as a result of freezing nor is it due to inactivation of catecholamines by freezing and thawing.

The presence of a myocardial factor in hemorrhagic shock has been substantiated by the work of Fisher and colleagues (1973) in Scotland and furthermore they were also able to confirm the fact that the effects demonstrated were not due to changes in electrolyte composition.

Hemochromogens

Nemir et al. (1973) postulated that hemoglobin or the plasma proteins are enzymatically denatured in shock and at some stage in the proteolytic process a toxic factor is produced. In dogs subjected to low flow states in the gut for some 4–7 hours, Nemir and co-workers (1963) noted an extravasation of blood into the mucosa and submucosa, a dissolution of the mucosal integrity and a change in the spectra of the portal vein blood indicating the presence of abnormal hemin pigment resulting from the combination of hemin with a denatured globin or other peptides. These investigators stress that the lethal component is probably in the globin fraction and not the pigment itself; they simply regard the pigment as an indicator for the presence of a denatured protein. The actual toxic protein may merely be derived from a plasma protein rather than hemoglobin. Indeed this is more likely since the presence of hemochromogen has not been widely reported in man in shock.

A substance with a similar spectroscopic pattern to that found clinically has been produced by alkali denaturation of hemoglobin with 1 N sodium hydroxide. This synthetic hemochromogen produced is lethal on injection into animals. Intravenous injection in dogs resulted in a decrease in systemic pressure, cardiac output, arterial pH and a significant increase in pulmonary vascular resistance. This latter fact could not be accounted for by the passive effect of associated hemodynamic variables. This work indicates the lethality of a degraded globulin. Nemir et al. (1963) suggests that the lung may also serve as a site for production of this factor where blood extravasated into the interstitial tissue may be degraded by enzymes. Congestion of pulmonary capillaries and extravasation of blood into the parenchyma has been shown both in animals and man in shock.

Clowes pulmonary factor

It is a well known fact in shock that the coagulation equilibrium is shifted in the direction of hypercoagulability. The result is that blood coagulates intravascularly in the capillaries (diffuse intravascular coagulation (DIC)). Together with the intravascular clots, cellular aggregates and agglomerations of thrombocytes, erythrocytes and leukocytes obstruct the capillaries. The role of DIC in the lung in shock has been the subject of debate. There is evidence, however, to suggest that the increase in pulmonary vascular resistance in shock does not result from the mechanical plugging of the pulmonary vessels, but rather from a pulmonary vascular constriction which could occur as a result of vasoactive compounds released from the elements of the blood itself (Clowes, 1974). There are both experimental and clinical studies however which indicate that Trasylol, a proteolytic enzyme inhibitor, also interferes with the intravascular coagulation process. One study suggests that this compound also counteracts platelet aggregation and platelet trapping in the lung following soft tissue injury. While this would suggest that an increase in lysosomal enzymes is related to the hypercoagulability of the blood in shock, no mechanism has been found for this phenomenon (Clowes, 1974).

Clowes found that non-protein fractions of plasma from septic patients and animals prepared by cold vacuum filtration contain substances with molecular weights from 1000–10,000 which when added to blood perfusing the lobe of a dog lung in situ produced the histologic picture of pneumonitis and increase in pulmonary vascular resistance. His studies imply that proteolytic lysosomal enzymes are among the co-factors necessary for the production of this factor. Recently he has been able to develop a radio-immune assay for this factor which opens up the possibility of more detailed investigation (Clowes, 1974).

Endotoxin

There is a large amount of evidence which implicates bacterial endotoxin in the formation of the humoral shock factor. In 1967 it became possible to determine quantitatively the presence of biologically active endotoxin using a simple in vitro test, namely, the Limulus lysate technique of Levein and Bang (1968). This test is sensitive enough to detect 10^{-3} μg/ml endotoxin. False positives have never been observed in normal patients and/or experimental animals. Several groups have reported finding significant levels of endotoxin in patients with sepsis or with disorders in which the antibacterial defenses were depleted (Fine et al., 1972). Furthermore the levels were comparable to those found in experimental shock animals. Fine found endotoxin (Levein et al., 1970) to be present in the plasma of both animals in septic and non-septic but not hemorrhagic refractory shock. Prophylactic use of kanamycin was only effective in lowering mortality when placed in the gut; intramuscular administration of the antibiotic was ineffective. This indicated the gut as the source of circulating endotoxin in shock in which there is no septic focus. The route of entry of endotoxin into the circulation from the gut is transmural and thence via the peritoneal cavity. It is thought that a variety of stimuli such as ischemia, hypoxia, acidosis, vasoactive compounds, etc., affect the integrity of the gut wall and induce movement of endotoxin into the peritoneal cavity. Fine suggests that not only is the gut the route of endotoxin in non-septic shock, but also the major source in gram-negative shock. In burns both the skin and the gut appear to be the sources of circulating endotoxin (Fine et al., 1972).

It is widely accepted experimentally that circulating endotoxin can produce the pulmonary and hemodynamic response associated with shock, though recent work would indicate that endotoxin itself has no direct myocardial depressant action (Hinshaw et al., 1974; Nagler and Levenson, 1974) nor does it directly effect vasomotor tone (Hinshaw et al., 1974). Endotoxin apparently only becomes physiologically active after combination with complement or leukocytes. Several studies have shown that in experimental studies with endotoxin, plasma and buffy coat are necessary to produce pulmonary vasopressor responses (Hinshaw et al., 1957), the systemic hypotensive response (Vick, 1964) and the hepatic arterial constrictor response (Filkins, 1969). Cuevas et al. (1972) recently observed that endotoxin infusion caused rabbits to develop pneumonitis but animals made resistant to endotoxin did not develop this syndrome (Cuevas and Fine, 1973). Direct infusion of endotoxin into the dog lung perfused with heparinized blood caused a rise in perfusion pressure which was abolished by the use of citrated blood. The vascular response to endotoxin could be restored by the addition of calcium and heparin to ACD perfusate (Kux et al., 1972). This implicates the clotting system and the possible role of calcium ions in the production of a pulmonary toxic factor by endotoxin. It is generally now thought that many of the harmful effects of endotoxin are mediated through its release of catecholamines and kinins, white cell lysosomes and other vasoactive peptides (Cuevas and Fine, 1973; Hyman et al., 1974). Endotoxin shock itself may be caused by the action of endotoxin on such kinin systems [via white blood cell lysosomes and their production of cardiovascular depressant(s)]; the initial histamine–endotoxin induced hypotension starts the cycle which is propagated and advanced in its cyclic nature to a continuous self propagating CVTF productive state (Nagler and Levenson, 1974).

Steroids in Shock

Extracts of adrenal cortex were found to be effective in correcting the circulatory failure of both adrenalectomized animals and Addison's disease. This was interpreted to indicate that cortical hormones had a regulatory effect on peripheral vascular tone (Swingle et al., 1938). With the subsequent isolation and purification of the various adrenal steroids, studies began on the effectiveness of these compounds as therapeutic agents in experimental and clinical shock.

Spink (1960) first proposed the use of hydrocortisone in large doses for the treatment of shock. Pretreatment with corticosteroid was found to be effective in preventing the lethal course of endotoxin shock in a variety of animals (Lillehei and MacLean, 1958; Spink and Anderson, 1954; Thomas and Smith, 1954). Lillehei and MacLean postulated that the protective action of the corticosteroids lay in the fact that they protect the animal from the pernicious effects of prolonged vasoconstriction or perhaps decrease the intensity of the duration of vasospasm. This hypothesis was supported by their experiments in which pretreatment with hydrocortisone protected dogs against the lethal effect of high concentrations of epinephrine given intravenously. Lillehei subsequently advocated the use of high doses of corticosteroids in septic (Dietzman et al., 1971) and cardiogenic shock (Schutz et al., 1972) since he postulated that the common factor in these shock states which ultimately caused the detrimental hemodynamic changes was the microcirculatory changes in the visceral circulation resulting from catecholamine release.

His suggestion to use massive doses of corticosteroids to decrease the adverse effects of catecholamines came under severe criticism. There has been a great deal of work in recent years to determine the mechanism whereby these steroids exert a protective effect in shock and also to evaluate these compounds as therapeutic agents in the clinical treatment of shock.

Altura's group, using their sophisticated model for studying the microcirculation in vivo attempted to determine if hydrocortisone sodium succinate and methylprednisolone sodium succinate had a direct effect on the diameter of the microvasculature or acted through their ability to alter the arteriolar response to catecholamines and vasopressin (Altura et al., 1974). Their data suggested that pharmacological doses of glucocorticoids prevent the intense peripheral vasoconstrictor action of constrictor substances released in shock. This would result in an apparent vasodilator action thus restoring the vasomotor tone of the microcirculation toward normal. These studies support Lillehei's concept of steroid action.

It is conceivable that corticosteroids exert their beneficial effect on shock by virtue of a positive inotropic effect on the heart. Hinshaw et al. (1974) have designed an isolated heart preparation, in which the left ventricle from a donor dog receives a constant input of blood from a donor animal and pumps it out against a known resistance, to study whether a compound has a direct inotropic effect on the heart; complicating variables of venous return, changing afterload and varying degrees of adrenergic neural influences are not present. Using this approach he showed that methylprednisolone sodium succinate had a positive inotropic action on the left ventricle, lowered left ventricular pressure, increased coronary blood flow, decreased vascular resistance and increased oxygen delivery to myocardial tissue. These favorable effects were observed in normal hearts and in some endotoxin heart failure preparations. However, there were some endotoxin heart preparations in which the steroid had no beneficial effect, and in some instances ventricular failure increased. In this group, digoxin was found to be effective in improving ventricular function and coronary flow.

Vyden et al. (1974) recently reported on the use of massive doses of corticosteroids early in the treatment of experimental acute myocardial infarction in dogs. His data showed that while methylprednisolone sodium succinate reduced the systemic vascular resistance, the major region to experience a drop in resistance was the coronary circulation. Furthermore it diminished heart rate, afterload and preload in the first 15 minutes after its administration. These effects all contributed favorably to improving the demand between myocardial oxygen demand and supply – a critical balance in infarcted hearts.

In contrast to these studies, Lefer (1974) using papillary muscles and isolated heart preparations from cats and guinea pigs was unable to demonstrate positive inotropic action of glucocorticoids in normal or shock preparations, nor did these compounds potentiate or antagonize the inotropic effects of catecholamines, angiotensin or cardiac glycosides. Furthermore, Kadowitz and his colleagues (1974) found that hydrocortisone in protective doses for endotoxin shock was neither a positive inotropic agent nor an alpha adrenergic blocking agent in the cat. These workers also demonstrated in a perfused dog lung preparation in a control animal that the steroid did not alter resistance across the lung nor change venous pulmonary tone nor alter the response of the lobar arteries and veins to epinephrine or norepinephrine.

It is difficult to evaluate critically the significance of experimental data on the hemodynamic effects of steroids in shock because of the differences in animal preparations and the use of natural and synthetic steroids in varying doses. Frankel (1974) at a recent meeting on steroids noted that in the course of the papers, 635 cats, 290 dogs, 12 baboons and over 174 humans had been saved from a variety of shock states by these compounds. He made the point that to a clinician it is difficult "to lump all of these very different shock states into one...The problem of cardiogenic shock is different from hemorrhagic shock", but in this condition also it is difficult to evaluate the circulatory effects of steroids from the heterogenous collection of experimental work. It may well be that these compounds are effective through a multiplicity of actions. There is a growing amount of work which indicates that these compounds may act at the cellular level. One theory for the anti-shock action of glucocorticoids is the membrane stabilizing effect. There is work which indicates that these compounds stabilize capillary endothelium (Motsay et al., 1974), prevent platelet adhesiveness (Pierce et al., 1972) and prevent disruption of lysosomes as discussed earlier. An additional benefit from the stabilization of lysosomal membranes is the prevention of the production of toxic factors which appear to be catalyzed by lysosomal enzymes, such as the myocardial depressant factor (MDF) of Lefer and Glenn. However, glucocorticoids have been shown not to interfere with the formation of MDF once lysosomal enzymes have been liberated. Furthermore, glucocorticoids do not appear to interfere with any other action of lysosomal hydrolases. This would indicate that the time to give these steroids in shock is prior to lysosomal disruption.

This brings up the question of when and how the corticosteroids should be used clinically in the treatment of shock. It is now generally known that glucocorticoids, not mineralocorticoids are the effective agents in shock and should be given early in shock. This latter admonition is a difficult one to qualify because no one has drawn up any critical index which can be used to determine the point to begin therapy.

The relationship between the Humors and Metabolism in Shock

During the induction and progression of shock several investigators have reported a host of metabolic alterations in almost every metabolic system studied, these changes being characteristic of but not specific to the shock syndrome.

The blood, being so readily accessible, has been the major source of such studies and as such, has revealed a progressive shock-induced accumulation of many metabolites indicative of failing anabolic circuits during a hypercatabolic state. Notably, an early hyperglycemia (and late hypoglycemia) in conjunction with a hyperlipidemia and a hyperaminoacidemia and azotemia occurs producing an acidosis that is buttressed by a lactacidemia and a pyruvicacidemia. As intracellular fluid and contents enter the circulation, the ions of potassium and magnesium rise, as do such hydrolytic enzymes including cathepsins, phosphatases, proteases, glucuronidases, lysosomal and cytoplasmic enzymes; there is a coincident decrease in serum sodium, chloride and ascorbic acid.

Such biochemical alterations are associated with decreases in body temperature reflecting a reduction in total energy metabolism, oxygen consumption and heat production. Tissue levels of adenosine triphosphate are markedly reduced, supposedly due to an uncoupling of mitochondrial oxidative phosphorylation.

For the most part, the biochemical and metabolic alterations that have been observed during shock have been ascribed to: 1) the specific humors released to produce compensatory reflex activities, 2) the hypoxia resulting from the characteristic reduction in blood flow (due to blood loss or reflexly), and 3) the tissue toxic materials (intracellular contents and or metabolites) initially released and their subsequent secondary effects on such metabolic and biochemical systems.

With regard to (1) above, the relationship to specific humors released, it is well recognized that the early compensatory release of catecholamines induces via the increase in heart rate and myocardial contractility, a greater need for glucose and energy metabolism. In addition, such catecholamines increase lipolysis to produce a lipidemia, a hyperglycemia and cause a hypoinsulinemia, secondarily decreasing glucose uptake and fatty acid synthesis. Such metabolic alterations are apparently mediated via the catecholamine-induced acceleration of cyclic AMP via catecholamine stimulation of adenyl cyclase. The overall effects are to breakdown glycogen to glucose-6-phosphate, which in muscle (because of a lack of the appropriate phosphatase) is metabolized to lactic acid and produces the lactacidemia; in the liver the presence of the phosphorylase and the appropriate phosphatase causes the split in the molecule to form glucose and thus the hyperglycemia. The specific lipase in adipose tissue is also apparently activated by cyclic AMP and adenyl cyclase via catecholamines and thus the lipidemia.

The shock-induced release of glucosteroids results in glycogenolysis augmenting the catecholamine-induced hyperglycemia and in addition causes the release of intracellular potassium and acceleration of proteolysis. Little is known of the effects of other humors on such metabolic systems except as catecholamines and other humors effect the hypoxia secondary to their vasoconstrictive effects (Alexander, 1967). In this regard it is well known that hypoxia will potentiate a change from aerobic glycogenolysis to anaerobic glycogenolysis and enhance the production of lactacidemia and pyruvicacidemia and acidosis, a less efficient production of ATP, a decrease in the liver's ability to synthesize urea and to metabolize deaminated amino acids and/or to remove amino acids from the blood because of a decreased hepatic circulation (the amino acids coming from a protein hypercatabolism as well as directly from the products of tissue injury). As a result, under such circumstances of hypoperfusion and disturbed metabolism (with or without direct tissue injury), organs, tissues and cells are irreparably damaged, their contents are extruded locally and systemically to cause a cluster of reactions specifically related to their release.

With the body in a constant state of flux and with an ever constant attempt at maintenance of dynamic equilibrium, it is not surprising to note that each of the effects on metabolism in turn are reflected by feed-back responses in the microcirculatory beds. For example, the local increase in lactic acid lowers the pH, rendering the vascular bed less responsive to vasoconstrictor amines and thus a tendency toward less constriction or relative vasodilation; these tissue metabolites, and cellular 'toxins' as well, increase the permeability of the vessels. All these adjustments aimed at facilitating the removal of local metabolites and tissue toxins tend to increase oxygen locally and to restore a normal vasculature. Yet, at the 'whole organism level' such improvement in local perfusion would defeat the body's purposeful attempt at compensation and thus, with higher levels not permitting the local changes to occur, a greater order from the hierarchy is once again brought forth to constrict the local vascular areas. These influences tend to increase the local state of anoxia, local lactacidosis, histamine synthesis, etc., reflexly to trigger vasodilation. Thus, in the interrelationships, there is the creation of a feed-back mechanism in which ischemia provokes metabolic derangements which then provoke capillary membrane permeability, which leads to further loss of function of organs, including the myocardium which creates further ischemia. The excursions of this inherently unstable state escalate until failure of the systems, collapse and death occurs.

Summary 1

It is perhaps a little unfortunate for the reader, who has had sufficient patience to stay with this work up to the finale, that there is no resolution to the problem raised in the introduction, namely, is there a specific humor responsible for the initiation of irreversible shock states. Inevitably, there are fashions in science, and clinical science is no exception to this rule. Current thinking in the shock field is strongly leaning toward the thesis that the shock factor is a vasoactive compound produced by the action of proteolytic enzymes, of tissue or blood origin, on some as yet unknown precursor material. Concentrated efforts are being made in this direction in a number of laboratories to resolve the problem. Only time and labor will tell if this is the winning horse in the field.

Summary 2

All that's left is to summate
The information we've tried to relate.
The literature is replete, with attempts at this feat,
So, in brief, we want to restate:
  While histamine, vasopressin and catechols
  No doubt play significant roles,
  What now learn-ed reader, would seem to be the leader
  Are the lysosomes, with the *hearts* paying the tolls.
With cardiotoxia produced by hypoxia,
The cycle goes on 'till St. Peter's.
What is best to prevent, is the initial event
And stop these iambic pentameters.

Acknowledgement

We wish to acknowledge the expert assistance of Mrs. Rosalie Nagler in several phases of the writing of this chapter.

References

Abrams, J.S., Hopkins, R.W., Perlman, R. and Simeone, F.A. (1969): Effect of phenoxybenzamine on endotoxic shock in dogs: metabolic changes. *J. Trauma, 9*, 614.

Alexander, J.W. (1967): Serum and leukocyte lysosomal enzymes – derangements following severe thermal injury. *Arch. Surg. (Chicago), 95*, 482.

Altura, B.M., Altura, B.T. and Hershey, S.G. (1974): Pharmacodynamic actions of corticosteroids on the microcirculation and vascular smooth muscle. In: *Steroids and Shock*, p. 67. Editor: T. Glenn. University Park Press, Baltimore, Md.

Altura, B.M. and Hershey, S.G. (1972): Sequential changes in reticulo-endothelial function after acute hemorrhage. *Proc. Soc. exp. Biol. (N.Y.), 139*, 935.

Altura, B.M. and Zweifach, B.W. (1966): Microvascular effects of endogenous histamine formation. 4th European Conference on Microcirculation, Cambridge. England, 1966. *Bibl. Anat. (Basel), 9*, 22.

Back, N., Wilkens, H. and Steger, R. (1960): Proteinases and proteinase inhibitors in experimental shock states. *Ann. N.Y. Acad. Sci., 146*, 491.

Baur, H. and Staub, H. (1949): Histamin und peripher Leukocytose nach Sympathomimetica. *Helv. physiol. pharmacol. Acta, 7*, 482.

Berman, I.R., Mosley, R.V., Lamborn, P.P. and Sleeman, H.K. (1969): Thoracic duct lymph in shock: gas exchange, acid base balance and lysosomal enzymes in hemorrhagic and endotoxic shock. *Ann. Surg., 169*, 202.

Berrelli, A. and Donati, L. (1970): The influence of some enzymes and enzyme inhibitors. In: *Shock: Biochemical Pharmacological and Clinical Aspects*. Editors: A. Berrelli and N. Back, Plenum Publ. Co., New York.

Blattberg, B. and Levy, M.N. (1963): Mechanism of depression of the reticulo-endothelial system in shock. *Amer. J. Physiol., 204*, 899.

Brake, C.M., Emerson, Jr., T.E., Wittmers, L.E. and Hinshaw, L.B. (1964): Alteration of vascular responses to endotoxin by adrenergic blockade. *Amer. J. Physiol., 207*, 149.

Brand, G.C. and Lefer, A.M. (1966): Myocardial depressant factor in plasma from cats in irreversible post oligemic shock. *Proc. Soc. exp. Biol. (N.Y.), 122*, 200.

Chien, S., Peric, B. and Usami, S. (1962): The reflex nature of release of antidiuretic hormone upon common carotid occlusion in vagotomized dogs. *Proc. Soc. exp. Biol. (N.Y.), 111*, 193.

Clermont, H.G. and Williams, J.S. (1962): Lymph lysosomal enzyme acid phosphatase in hemorrhagic shock. *Ann. Surg., 155*, 90.

Clowes, G.H.A. (1973): The pulmonary response to circulating agents in post traumatic and septic states. In: *6. New aspects of Trasylol Therapy. The Lung in Shock*, p. 71. Editors: G.L. Haberland and D.H. Lewis, F.K. Schattauer Verlag, Stuttgart.

Clowes, G.H.A. (1974): Pulmonary abnormalities in sepsis. *Surg. Clin. N. Amer., 54*, 993.

Cohn, Z.A. and Hirsch, J.G. (1960): The isolation and properties of the specific cytoplasmic granules of rabbit polymorphonuclear leukocytes. *J. exp. Med., 112*, 983.

Cuevas, P., De la Maza, M., Gilbert, J. and Fine, J. (1972): The lung lesion in four different types of rabbits. *Arch. Surg. (Chicago), 104*, 319.

Cuevas, P. and Fine, J. (1973): Production of fatal endotoxin shock by vasoactive substances. *Gastroenterology (Basel), 64*, 285.

Daugherty, R.M. Jr., Scott, J.B., Emerson, T.E. Jr. and Haddy, F.J. (1968): Comparison of intravenous and intraarterial infusion of vasoactive agents on dog forelimb blood flow. *Amer. J. Physiol., 214*, 611.

Davis, J.O., Carpenter, C.C.J. and Ayers, C.R. (1962): Relation of renin and angiotensin II to the control of aldosterone secretion. *Circulat. Res., 11*, 171.

Davis, R.B., Meeker, W.R. and Bailey, W.L. (1961): Serotonin release by bacterial endotoxin. *Proc. Soc. exp. Biol. (N.Y.), 108*, 774.

Davis, R.B., Meeker, W.R. and McQuarrie, D.G. (1960): Immediate effects of intravenous endotoxin on serotonin concentrations and blood platelets. *Circulat. Res., 8*, 234.

De Duve, C. (1959): Lysosomes, a new group of cytoplasmic particles. In: *Subcellular Particles*, p. 128. Editor: T. Hayashi. Ronald Press Co., New York.

Derrick, J.R., Roland, B. and Anderson, J. (1962): Angiotensin – a new pressor agent. *Ann. Surg. (Chicago), 156*, 214.

Dietzman, R.H., Motsay, G. and Lillehei, R.C. (1971): The use of corticosteroids in the treatment of septic shock. In: *Septic Shock and Man*, p. 231. Editors: S.G. Hershey and L.R.M. Delguercio and R. McConn. Little and Brown Co., Boston.

Dimiz, C. and Carvalho, I. (1963): A micro method for determination of bradykininogen under several conditions. *Ann. N.Y. Acad. Sci., 104*, 77.

Egdahl, R.H. (1959): The differential response of the adrenal cortex and medulla to bacterial endotoxin. *J. clin. Invest., 38*, 1120.

Emerson, T.E. Jr. (1966): Effect of angiotensin, norepinephrine, epinephrine and vasopressin on venous return. *Amer. J. Physiol., 210*, 933.

Emerson, T.E. Jr. (1968): Effects of acetylcholine, histamine and serotonin infusion on venous return in dogs. *Amer. J. Physiol., 215*, 41.

Emerson, T.E. Jr. (1972): Participation of endogenous vasoactive agents in the pathogenesis of endotoxin shock. *Advanc. exp. Med. Biol., 23*, 25.

Emerson, T.E. Jr., Brake, C.M. and Hinshaw, L.B. (1965a): Endotoxin shock in splanchnic denervated dogs. *J. Trauma, 5*, 737.

Emerson, T.E. Jr., Brake, C.M. and Hinshaw, L.B. (1966): Splanchnic sympathetic and adrenal participation in endotoxin shock. *J. Okla. med. Ass., 59*, 425.

Emerson, T.E. Jr., Hinshaw, L.B. and Brake, C.M. (1965b): Vascular effects of angiotensin and norepinephrine in the dog, cat and monkey. *Amer. J. Physiol., 208*, 260.

Emerson, T.E. Jr., Meir, P.D. and Daugherty, E.R.M. (1971): Local vascular responses to serotonin in dog skeletal muscle at different levels of resistance. *Fed. Proc., 30*, 212.

Erdos, E.G. (1971): Enzymes that inactivate vasoactive peptides. In: *Concepts in Biochemical Pharmacology, Part 2*, p. 620. Springer Verlag, Publ. New York.

Erdos, E. and Mina, I. (1968): Effect of endotoxin on the plasma kallikrein-kinin system in the rabbit. *Fed. Proc., 27*, 92.

Erlanger, J. and Gasser, H.S. (1919): Studies in secondary traumatic shock. II. Shock due to mechanical limitation of blood flow. III. Circulatory failure due to adrenalin. *Amer. J. Physiol., 49*, 151; 345.

Ferguson, W.W., Glenn, T.M. and Lefer, A.M. (1972): Mechanisms of production of circulatory shock factors in isolated perfused pancreas. *Amer. J. Physiol., 222*, 450.

Filkins, J.R. (1969): Hepatic vascular response to endotoxin. *Proc. Soc. exp. Biol. (N.Y.), 131*, 1235.

Fine, J., Caridis, D.T., Cuevas, P., Ishiyama, R. and Reinhold, R. (1972): Therapeutic implication of new developments in the study of refractory non-septic shock. In: *Shock in Low and High Flow States*, p. 1. Editors: B.K. Forscher, R.C. Lillehei and S.S. Stubbs. Excerpta Medica, Amsterdam.

Fisher, W.D., Heimbach, D.M., McArdle, C.S., Maddern, M., Hutcheson, M.M. and

Ledingham, I.McA. (1973): Circulating depressant effect following canine hemorrhagic shock. *Brit. J. Surg., 60*, 392.

Fredlund, P.E., Ockerman, P.A. and Vang, J.O. (1972): Plasma activities of acid hydrolases in experimental oligemic shock in the pig. *Amer. J. Surg., 124*, 300.

Frankl, E. (1974): Discussion. In: *Steroids and Shock*, p. 433. Editor: T. Glenn, University Park Press, Baltimore, Md.

Frater, R.W.M., McConn, R., Oka, Y., Yellin, E. and Nagler, A.L. (1974): *Cardiovascular Toxic Factor (CVT) in Patients Undergoing Cardiopulmonary Bypass. Proc. Texas Heart Institute*, Appelton-Century-Crofts.

Glenn, T.M. and Lefer, A.M. (1970): Role of lysosomes in the pathogenesis of splanchnic ischemia shock. *Circulat. Res., 27*, 783.

Glenn, T.M. and Lefer, A.M. (1971): Significance of splanchnic proteases in production of a toxic factor in hemorrhagic shock. *Circulat. Res., 29*, 338.

Glenn, T.M., Lefer, A.M., Beardsley, A.C., Ferguson, W.W., Lopez-Rasi, A.M., Serate, T.S., Morris, J.R. and Wangensteen, S.L. (1972): Circulatory responses to splanchnic lysosomal hydrolases in the dog. *Ann. Surg., 176*, 120.

Glenn, T.M., Lefer, A.M., Martin, J.B., Lovett, W.L., Morris, J.N. Jr. and Wangensteen, S.L. (1971): Production of a myocardial depressant factor in cardiogenic shock. *Amer. Heart J., 82*, 78.

Greenbaum, L.M., Freer, R., Chang, J., Semente, E. and Yamafuji, K. (1969): PMN-kinin and kinin metabolizing enzymes in normal and malignant leukocytes. *Brit. J. Pharmacol., 36*, 623.

Grega, G.J. and Haddy, F.J. (1971): Forelimb transcapillary fluid fluxes and vascular resistance in catecholamine shock. *Amer. J. Physiol., 220*, 1448.

Haberland, G.L. (1970): The effect of Trasylol in shock. In: *Shock: Biochemical, Pharmacological and Clinical Aspects*. Editors: A. Berrelli and N. Back. Plenum Publ. Co., New York.

Haddy, F.J. and Visscher, M. (1971): In: *Shock – A Physiologic Basis for Treatment*, Chapter 2, Editors: Thal, Brown, Hermreck and Bill, Yearbook Med. Publ. Inc., Chicago, Ill.

Hall, R.C. and Hodge, R.L. (1971): Vasoactive hormones in endotoxin shock: a comparative study in cats and dogs. *J. Physiol. (Lond.), 213*, 69.

Hinshaw, L.B., Archer, L.T., Black, M.R., Elkins, R.C. and Brown, P.B. (1974): Myocardial function in shock. *Amer. J. Physiol., 226*, 357.

Hinshaw, L.B., Archer, L.T., Black, M.R. and Greenfield, L.J. (1974): Effects of methyl prednisolone sodium succinate on myocardial performance, hemodynamics and metabolism in normal and failing hearts. In: *Steroids and Shock*, p. 253. Editor: T.M. Glenn. University Park Press, Baltimore, Md.

Hinshaw, L.B., Brake, C.M. and Emerson, T.E. Jr. (1965): Biochemical and pathological alterations in endotoxin shock. In: *Shock and Hypotension, Pathogenesis and Treatment*. Grune and Stratton, New York.

Hinshaw, L.B., Emerson, T.E. Jr., Iampietro, P.F. and Brake, C.M. (1962a): A comparative study of the hemodynamic actions of histamine and endotoxin. *Amer. J. Physiol., 203*, 600.

Hinshaw, L.B., Jordan, M.M. and Vick, J.A. (1961a): Mechanism of histamine release in endotoxin shock. *Amer. J. Physiol., 200*, 987.

Hinshaw, L.B., Kuida, H., Gilbert, R.P. and Visscher, M.B. (1957): Influence of perfusate characteristics on pulmonary vascular response to endotoxin. *Amer. J. Physiol., 191*, 293.

Hinshaw, L.B., Vick, J.A., Jordan, M.M. and Wittmers, L.E. (1962b): Vascular changes associated with development of irreversible endotoxin shock. *Amer. J. Physiol., 202*, 103.

Hinshaw, L.B., Vick, J.A., Wittmers, L.E., Worthen, D.M., Nelson, D.L. and Swenson, O.P. (1961b): Changes in total peripheral resistance in endotoxin shock. *Proc. Soc. exp. Biol. (N.Y.), 108*, 24.

Hyman, A.L., Pennington, D.G., Kadowitz, P.J. and Jaques, W.E. (1974): Studies of the mechanisms of the pulmonary vasopressor response to endotoxin. Effects of corticosteroids and catecholamines. In: *Steroids and Shock*, p. 129. Editor: T.M. Glenn. University Park Press, Baltimore, Md.

Ituri, S. and Emerson, T.E. Jr. (1971): Responses of arterial vessel strips from skin and muscle to serotonin. *Proc. Soc. exp. Biol. Med. (N.Y.), 137*, 416.

Jacobson, E.D., Mehlman, B. and Kalas, J.P. (1964): Vasoactive mediators as the 'trigger mechanism' in endotoxin shock. *J. clin. Invest., 43*, 1000.

Janoff, A. (1964): Alterations in lysosomes (intracellular enzymes) during shock: effects of preconditioning (tolerance) and protective drugs. In: *Shock*. Editor: S.G. Hershey. Little, Brown, Co., Boston, Mass.

Janoff, A., Nagler, A.L., Baez, S. and Zweifach, B.W. (1961): Pathogenesis of experimental shock. III. A lethal factor in the blood of rabbits following occlusion of the superior mesenteric artery. *J. exp. Med., 114*, 205.

Jefferson, T., Glenn, T.M. and Lefer, A.M. (1971): Cardiovascular and lysosomal actions of corticosteroids in the intact dog. *Proc. Soc. exp. Biol. (N.Y.), 136*, 276.

Kadowitz, P.J., Yard, A.C., Greenberg, S. and Hyman, A.L. (1974): Influence of corticosteroids on cardiopulmonary responses to catecholamines. In: *Steroids and Shock*, p. 89. Editor: T.M. Glenn. University Park Press, Baltimore, Md.

Kobald, E.E., Lovell, R., Katz, W. and Thal, A.P. (1964): Chemical mediators released by endotoxin. *Surg. Gynec. Obstet., 118*, 807.

Kux, M., Coalson, J., Massion, W.H. and Guenker, C.A. (1972): Pulmonary effects of *E. coli* endotoxin. Role of leukocytes and platelets. *Ann. Surg., 175*, 26.

Lefer, A.M. (1974): Myocardial action of steroids. In: *Steroids and Shock*, p. 53. Editor: T.M. Glenn. University Park Press, Baltimore, Md.

Lefer, A.M., Cowgell, R., Marshall, F., Hall, L.M. and Brand, E.D. (1967): Characteristics of a myocardial depressant factor in hemorrhagic shock. *Amer. J. Physiol., 213*, 492.

Lefer, A.M. and Glenn, T.M. (1972a): Role of the pancreas in the pathogenesis of circulatory shock. In: *The Fundamental Mechanisms of Shock*, p. 367. Editors: L.H. Hinshaw and B.G. Cox. Plenum Publishing Co., New York.

Lefer, A.M. and Glenn, T.M. (1972b): Lysosomal hydrolases and MDF in shock. In: *Shock in Low and High Flow States*. Editors: K.B. Forscher, R.C. Lillehei and S.S. Stubb. Excerpta Medica, Amsterdam.

Lefer, A.M. and Glenn, T.M. (1973): The lysosomal protease-myocardial depressant factor system in circulatory shock. In: *Neurohumoral and Metabolic Aspects of Injury*, p. 367. Editors: A.G.B. Kovach, H.B. Stoner and J.J. Spitzer. Plenum Publ. Co., New York.

Lefer, A.M. and Glenn, T.M. (1974): Corticosteroids and the lysosomal protease-myocardial depressant factor system in shock. In: *Steroids and Shock*, p. 233. Editor: T.M. Glenn. University Park Press, Baltimore, Md.

Lefer, A.L., Glenn, T.M., O'Neill, T.J., Lovett, W.T., Geissinger, W.T. and Wangensteen, S.C. (1971): Inotropic influence of endogenous peptides in experimental pancreatitis. *Surgery, 69*, 220.

Lefer, A.M. and Martin, J. (1970): Relationship of plasma peptides to the myocardial depressant factor in hemorrhagic shock. *Circulat. Res., 26*, 59.

Lefer, A.M. and Rovetto, M.M. (1970): Influence of a myocardial depressant factor on physiologic properties of cardiac muscle. *Proc. Soc. exp. Biol. (N.Y.), 134*, 269.

Levein, J. and Bang, F.B. (1968): Clottable protein in Limulus. Its localization and kinetics of coagulation by endotoxin. *Thrombos. Diathes. haemorrh. (Stuttg.), 19*, 186.

Levein, J., Poore, T., Zanber, N. and Oser, R. (1970): Detection of endotoxin in the blood of patients with sepsis due to gram-negative bacteria. *New Engl. J. Med., 283*, 1313.

Lillehei, R.C., Longerbeam, J.K., Block, J.H. and Manax, W.G. (1964a): The nature of irreversible shock: experimental and clinical observations. *Ann. Surg., 160*, 682.

Lillehei, R.C., Longerbeam, J.K., Block, J.H. and Manax, W.G. (1964b): The nature of experimental irreversible shock with its clinical application. In: *Shock*, p. 139. Editor: S.G. Hershey. Little, Brown and Co., Boston.

Lillehei, R.C. and MacLean, J.D. (1958): The intestinal factor in irreversible endotoxin shock. *Ann. Surg., 168*, 513.

McConn, R. and Nagler, A.L. (1974): Lysosomal enzymes and cardiovascular toxic factor in stored blood. *First World Congress on Intensive Care, London, 1974.*

McNeill, J.R. (1972): Role of vasopressin and angiotensin in response of splanchnic resistance vessels to hemorrhage. *Advanc. exp. Med. Biol., 23*, 127.

Motsay, G., Alho, A.V., Dietzman, R.H., Schultz, L.S., Romero, L.H. and Lillehei, R.C. (1974): Forelimb, small intestine and pulmonary vascular beds in canine endotoxin shock. In: *Steroids and Shock*, p. 151. Editor: T.M. Glenn. University Park Press, Baltimore, Md.

Motsay, G.J., Alho, A., Jaeger, T., Dietzman, R.H. and Lillehei, R.C. (1970): Effects of corticosteroids on the circulation in shock: experimental and clinical results. *Fed. Proc., 29*, 1861.

Movat, H.Z., Steinberg, S.G., Habal, F.M. and Ranadive, N.S. (1973): Demonstration of a kinin generating enzyme in the lysosomes of human polymorphonuclear leukocytes. *Lab. Invest., 29*, 669.

Nagler, A.L. and Levenson, S.M. (1972): Presence of a passively transferable lethal factor in the blood of rats in severe hemorrhagic shock. *J. Trauma, 12*, 10.

Nagler, A.L. and Levenson, S.M. (1974): The nature of the toxic material in the blood of rats subjected to irreversible hemorrhagic shock. *Circulat. Shock, 1*, 251.

Nagler, A.L. and Levenson, S.M. (1975): Cardiovascular toxic factor in patients and its correlation with severe shock. *Circulat. Shock*, in preparation.

Nakano, J. and Schryver, C.D. (1963): Effect of changes in carotid sinus pulse pressure on catecholamine blood levels. *Amer. J. Physiol., 204*, 467.

Nemir, P., Hamilton, W.M., Habboushe, F. and Brody, J.T. (1973): The effect of circulating denatured proteins and vasoactive substances on pulmonary hemodynamics and morphology. In: *New Aspects of Trasylol Therapy. The Lung in Shock*, p. 149. Editors: L. Haberland and D.H. Lewis, F.K. Schattauer Verlag, Stuttgart, New York.

Nemir, P., Hoferichter, J. and Drabkin, D.L. (1963): The protective effect of proteinase inhibitor in acute necrotizing pancreatitis – an experimental and clinical study. *Ann. Surg., 158*, 655.

Nies, A.S., Forsyth, R.P., Williams, H.E. and Melmon, K.L. (1968): Contribution of kinins to endotoxin shock. *Circulat. Res., 22*, 155.

Nykeil, F. and Glaviano, V.V. (1961): Adrenal catecholamines in *E. coli* endotoxin shock. *J. appl. physiol., 16*, 348.

Pierce, C.H., Briggs, B.T. and Gurelius, S. (1972): Methyl prednisolone and phenoxybenzamine in experimental shock: cardiovascular dynamics and platelet function. In: *Shock in Low and High Flow States*, p. 183. Editors: K.B. Forscher, R.C. Lillehei and S.S. Stubbs. Excerpta Medica, Amsterdam.

Ravin, H.R., Schweinburg, F.B. and Fine, J. (1958): Host resistance in hemorrhagic shock. XV. Isolation of toxic factor from hemorrhagic shock plasma. *Proc. Soc. exp. Biol. (N.Y.), 99*, 426.

Reichgott, J.J., Forsyth, R.P. and Melmon, K.L. (1971): Effects of bradykinin and autonomic nervous system inhibition of systemic and regional hemodynamics in unanesthetized Rhesus monkeys. *Circulat. Res., 29*, 367.

Rosenberg, J.C., Lillehei, R.C., Longerbeam, J. and Zimmerman, B. (1961): Studies on hemorrhagic and endotoxin shock in relation to vasopressin. *Ann. Surg. (Chicago), 154*, 611.

Rosenberg, J.C., Lillehei, R.C., Moran, W.H. and Zimmerman, B. (1959): The effect of endotoxin on plasma catecholamines and serum serotonin. *Proc. Soc. exp. Biol. (N.Y.), 102*, 335.

Schayer, R.W. (1960): Relationship of stress-induced histidine decarboxylase activity in histamine synthesis to circulatory homeostasis and shock. *Science, 131*, 226.

Schayer, R.W. (1962): Evidence that induced histamine is an intrinsic regulator of the microcirculatory system. *Amer. J. Physiol., 202*, 66.

Schumer, W., Kapica, S.K. and Teng, T.L. (1969): Validity of the lysosomal theory in oligemic shock. *Arch. Surg. (Chicago), 99*, 325.

Schutz, L., Alho, A.V., Dietzman, R.H., Ersek, R.A., Motsay, G.J., Romero, L.H., Ruiz, J.O. and Lillehei, R.C. (1972): Pharmacological assistance in the low-output syndrome. In: *Shock in Low and High Flow States*, p. 131. Editors: B.K. Forscher, R.C. Lillehei and S.S. Stubbs. Excerpta Medica, Amsterdam.

Shah, J.P., Shah, U.S., Alpert, H.E. and Howard, J.M. (1970): Studies on the release of bradykinin by the splanchnic circulation during endotoxic shock. *J. Trauma, 10*, 255.

Share, L. and Levy, M.N. (1962): Cardiovascular receptors and blood titer of antidiuretic hormone. *Amer. J. Physiol., 203*, 425.

Siegel, J.H., Sonnenblick, E.H., Judge, R.D. and Wilson, W.S. (1965): Occult myocardial failure and vasopressors in shock. *Cardiologia (Basel), 47*, 353.

Slater, T.F. (1969): Lysosomes and experimentally induced tissue injury. In: *Lysosomes in Biology and Pathology*, p. 469. Editors: J.T. Dingle and H.B. Fell. Elsevier, New York.

Spink, W.W. (1960): Adrenocortical steroids in the management of selected patients with infectious diseases. *Ann. intern. Med., 53*, 1.

Spink, W.W. and Anderson, D. (1954): Experimental studies on the significance of endotoxin in the pathogenesis of Brucellosis. *J. clin. Invest., 33*, 540.

Stock, W. and Eigler, F.W. (1969): Wirkung eines Proteinaseninhibitors auf Tourniquet-Syndrom der Ratte. *Z. ges. exp. Med., 151*, 64.

Swingle, W.W., Parkins, W.M., Taylor, A.R. and Hays, H.W. (1938): A study of the circulatory failure and shock following trauma to the healthy vigorous adrenalectomized dog. *Amer. J. Physiol., 124*, 22.

Thomas, L. and Smith, R.T. (1954): Effect of cortisone and antibiotics in lethal action of endotoxins in mice. *Proc. Soc. exp. Biol. (N.Y.), 86*, 716.

Urschel, C.W., Serur, J.R., Forrester, J.A., Amsterdam, E.A., Parmley, W.W., Dembitsky, W. and Sonnenblock, E.H. (1972): Myocardial contractility during hemorrhagic shock, endotoxemia and ischemia. In: *Shock in Low and High Flow States*, p. 77. Editors: B.K. Forscher, R.C. Lillehei and S.S. Stubbs. Excerpta Medica, Amsterdam.

Verrity, M.A., Andiman, R., Munsat, T.L., Smith, R.E. and Szego, C.M. (1973): The lysosome: a role in disease. *Ann. inter. Med., 78*, 725.

Vick, J.A. (1964): Trigger mechanisms of endotoxin shock. *Amer. J. Physiol., 206*, 944.

Vyder, J.K., Nagasawa, K., Corday, E., Parmley, W.W. and Swan, H.J.C. (1974): Hemodynamic aspects of corticosteroid administration in the treatment of acute myocardial infarction. In: *Steroids and Shock*, p. 212. Editor: T.M. Glenn. University Park Press, Baltimore, Md.

Wangensteen, S.L., Geissinger, W.T., Lovett, W.L., Glenn, T.M. and Lefer, A.M. (1971): Relationship between splanchnic blood flow and a myocardial depressant factor in endotoxin shock. *Surgery, 69*, 410.

Wangensteen, S.L., Ramey, W.G., Ferguson, W.W. and Starling, J.S. (1973): Plasma myocardial depressant activity (shock factor) identified as salt in the cat papillary muscle bioassay system. *J. Trauma, 13*, 181.

Webster, M.E. and Clark, W.R. (1959): Significance of the Callicrein–Callidinogen–Callidin system in shock. *Amer. J. Physiol., 197*, 406.

Weil, M.H., MacLean, L.D., Spink, W.W. and Visscher, M.B. (1956): Studies on the mechanism of shock by gram-negative bacteria. *Trans. Ass. med. Physiol., 69*, 131.

Weiner, R. and Zweifach, B.W. (1966): Influence of *E. coli* endotoxin on serotonin contractions of the rabbit aortic strip. *Proc. Soc. exp. Biol. (N.Y.), 123*, 937.

Weissman, G., Zurier, R.B. and Hoffstein, S. (1972): Leucocyte proteases and the immunologic release of lysosomal enzymes. *Amer. J. Path., 68*, 539.

Went, I. and Varga, E. (1952): Experimentelle Untersuchungen über die chemische Gegenregulation des Blutdruckes. *Acta physiol. Acad. Sci. hung., 3*, 377.

White, F.N., Gold, E.M. and Vaughn, D.L. (1966): Renin-aldosterone system in endotoxin shock in the dog. *Amer. J. Physiol., 212*, 1195.

Wilson, J.W. (1974): Cellular localization of ^{3}H-labeled corticosteroids by electron microscopic autoradiography after hemorrhagic shock. In: *Steroids and Shock*, p. 275. Editor: T.M. Glenn. University Park Press, Baltimore, Md.

Wilson, J.M. and Ebert, P.A. (1972): Hemodynamic effects of superior mesenteric artery occlusion: a comparison in anesthetized and unanesthetized dogs. *Ann. Surg. (Chicago), 175*, 214.

Wlodzimierz, F. (1972): Kinin levels in experimental endotoxic shock. *Arch. Immun. exp. Ther., 57*, 135.

Zweifach, B.W. (1962): Tissue mediators in the genesis of experimental shock. *J. Amer. med. Ass., 181*, 160.

Zweifach, B.W., Nagler, A.L. and Thomas, L. (1956): The role of epinephrine in the reactions produced by endotoxin of gram negative bacteria. II. The changes produced by endotoxin in the vascular reactivity to epinephrine in the rat mesoappendix and the isolated perfused rabbit ear. *J. exp. Med., 104*, 881.

Ledingham (ed.). Shock

Monitoring of the patient in shock

M. HILBERMAN and J.J. OSBORN

Introduction

Our concept of monitoring has changed significantly since our school days when we perceived of a monitor as a surrogate teacher frequently more concerned with his own self importance than with our safety or welfare. We now perceive of monitoring as a complex activity which may be used to determine the purity of a city's water supply, the rhythmicity of a patient's heart beat, the financial shenanigans of an election campaign, and somewhere still, we presume, the conduct of children in a classroom. These activities all require the repetitive performance of observations or measurements designed to detect recurrent abberations in the function of the system observed. In addition, when the event monitored for is detected, it will be used to initiate an action or determine the response to some prior action.

Patient monitoring is particularly complex, for the system to be monitored includes the human body, the interface between the body and a variety of support systems, the support systems themselves, and the interaction between the body and a variety of therapies. Monitoring of the various life support systems (e.g. respirators) and of the interface between the life support systems and the patient, is frequently as important as monitoring the patient for intrinsic physiological changes (see Fig. 1). Measurements may be divided

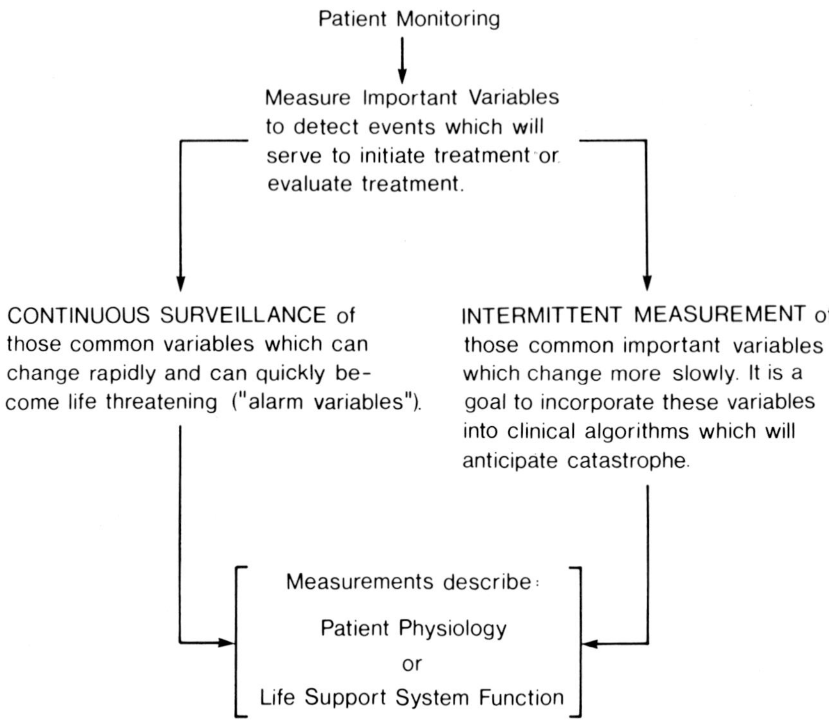

Fig. 1. Patient monitoring consists of the performance of repeated observations of patient physiology or life support system function. These observations may be in the class of continuous surveillance or intermittent measurements.

into two major categories: continuous surveillance and intermittent measurement. Continuous surveillance is considered to occur when measurements are made more often than every 30 minutes; in general, such measurement should be truly continuous if possible. The distinction between continuous surveillance and intermittent measurement should not be dictated by current measurement technology, although it may be. The problem of information overflow at the bedside is acute; estimates should be made of the rates of change of different functions so that the minimum amount of information necessary to detect the event or process is obtained, and not more. A patient monitor is not simply a device for displaying an electrocardiogram on a screen to a patient's bedside. A monitor is a component of a monitoring system, which performs repetitive measurement or observation intended to evaluate, or initiate, some medical action (Table I). A nurse, an oscilloscope, a blood gas machine, or a stethoscope may all function at the same time as monitors; only a small subset

Table I
What is a monitor? An element in a monitoring system: a person or a device which performs a repetitive measurement or observation intended to evaluate or, when appropriate, initiate a medical action.

Mode	Patient status	Life support systems status
Continuous surveillance	Nurse Oscilloscope, with shift register storage for non-fade display of ECG, arterial pressure Pressure and flow sensors Gas analyzers Computer systems	Nurse Pressure and flow sensors Gas analyzers Computer systems
Intermittent	Nurse, physician, therapist Stethoscope, thermometer, sphygmomanometer Clinical laboratory test equipment Radiology equipment Gas analyzers Computer systems	Equipment technicians and their testing devices

of monitors can be considered suitable components of a continuous surveillance system.

The components of the system and the variables monitored may change over time. A patient in shock may be routinely monitored for cardiovascular and respiratory function until bleeding develops. If the cause for this bleeding is disseminated intravascular coagulation (DIC), the patient may require a heparin infusion for control of the bleeding. At this point, another functional subsystem must be monitored and half a dozen more variables added to the list of those already mentioned.

The repetitive nature of the monitoring function suggests that it should be fully automated, with objective measurements substituting for hunches and clinical judgment whenever possible (Sheppard et al., 1974; Osborn et al., 1971). This philosophy does not deny the importance of human observation and skill in providing compassionate patient care or detecting unusual events (Maloney, 1968); it merely takes as a goal quantification of clinical events and automation of the well defined and repetitive tasks of patient monitoring and care so that human skills may be used optimally for integration of the clinical situation, direct patient care, and the management of unusual events.

How Frequently Should Measurement be Made?

Anyone familiar with sampling theory can quickly calculate the number of samples necessary to precisely define a given sinusoidal waveform. We have had difficulties perceiving of a critical illness as a sinusoidal waveform, and have tended to more empiric approaches. If *it* happens fairly often and *it* is serious, then monitor for *it*. If *it* tends to kill quickly, say in less than 10 minutes, then use a continuous surveillance approach, otherwise intermittent measurement is satisfactory. If *it* doesn't happen very often, then don't clutter your bedside with another instrument and your chart with another data element; stay on your toes, and hope you are alert and awake enough to think of *it* at the appropriate time.

The Relationship Between Monitoring and Therapy

Patient monitoring emerged as a concept with the refinement of techniques for cardiac and pulmonary resuscitation. When Zoll presented his techniques for cardiac defibrillation using alternating current in 1956, he also discussed the need for continuous monitoring of the electrical activities of the heart (Zoll et al., 1956). The intrinsic electrical activity of the heart provided a suitable signal around which continuous surveillance systems for cardiac monitoring could be easily built. As the techniques of cardiac monitoring and resuscitation developed together, it became increasingly clear that seconds were precious. The monitors and the techniques were not sufficient; special units with trained personnel and equipment were essential to use the information provided (Hilberman, 1975; Kouwenhoven et al., 1960; Lown et al., 1962). Continuous surveillance of the electrocardiogram began and remains linked to the therapeutic modalities of cardiac resuscitation and the subsequent prophylactic treatment of a variety of cardiac arrhythmias.

The ability to monitor respiratory function was critical to the development of our understanding of respiratory malfunction, and to the utilization of respirators in clinical medicine. The development of devices for respiratory support can be traced back several centuries; by the early twentieth century, several functional mechanical ventilators had been constructed (Mushin and Rendall-Baker, 1953). The absence of instruments for conveniently measuring respiratory volumes and for monitoring gas concentrations in the blood and the inspired air were significantly responsible for the delay in utilization of ventilators. The development of such measuring instruments was critical to the successful application of mechanical ventilators to respiratory care, as characterized in the pioneering developments in Los Angeles (Bower et al., 1950) and in Copenhagen (Astrup et al., 1954). While changes in ventilator support can result in death nearly as rapidly as cardiac arrhythmias, the primary continuous monitor of respirator function has remained the nurse. The development in our hospital of a computer based system for respiratory measurement has made continuous monitoring of respiratory physiology and respirator function available since 1966 (Osborn et al., 1969; Gerbode, 1973). More recently, effective continuous monitors of respirator function have been incorporated in respirator design, noteworthy among these being the monitoring systems of the Elema–Schonander Servo Vent 900 (Nordstrom, 1972), the Ohio 560, and the Searle (Techna) respirator.

The other variables monitored continuously are also related to immediate application of life-saving techniques; the measurement of arterial pressure and the cardiac filling pressure is used to guide intravenous fluid therapy and the administration of cardiac drugs; sudden spikes in temperature are used to initiate vigorous cooling efforts. In a similar fashion, intermittent serial measurement of hematocrit, arterial blood gas tensions, blood lactate levels, the bacterial flora in tracheal aspirates, and regular chest X-rays are closely related to therapeutic manipulations. Furthermore, the events detected (inadequate oxygen carrying capacity, inadequate peripheral perfusion, pneumothorax, atelectasis, respirator maladjustment, etc.) are all serious and occur with sufficient frequency to make monitoring for them worthwhile. It remains true that a number of important changes occur which are of low probability; these are detected by human observation, patient distress, and occasionally cardiac arrest.

What Should Be Monitored?

We have outlined some of the variables which are important to a monitoring scheme in Table II. We think that it is useful to consider variables as existing in modules which tend to be implemented as a group when certain functional abnormalities occur. To discuss each module and each variable in any reasonable depth would require an entire book; here we will discuss a few of the important variables and how they may be used, with considerable emphasis upon our experience in cardiovascular and respiratory monitoring.

Table II
The major modules needed in a monitoring system divided according to the frequency of measurement and the object monitored (patient or equipment). The modules in several are additive. Although there is some redundancy in the shock patient multisystem, failure is frequent, and other modules will be in use from time to time. Thus, hepatic failure or sepsis would introduce the need for a number of other intermittent measures of patient physiology and bacterial flora. The use of extracorporeal membrane oxygenator (ECMO) for temporary support of patients with severe acute respiratory insufficiency introduces continuous measurement of a number of measures of oxygenator function, heparin infusion, and coagulation status. Efforts to monitor the overall environment as provided by a hospital infection central committee are important, but omitted.

Module name	Patient		Life support system	
	Continuous	Intermittent	Continuous	Intermittent
Vital signs	Electrocardiogram Heart rate	Temperature, pulse Respiration, BP		Safety and function of monitors
Mild hemodynamic instability		Arterial pressure (indirect) Pulse rate Pulmonary artery pressure (PAP) Balloon occluded PAP Central venous pressure (CVP) Hematocrit Blood loss		
Serious hemodynamic instability	Arterial pressure (direct) Pulse rate PAP or LAP Blood loss, balance	Hematocrit (blood loss) Balloon occluded PAP Blood lactate Hourly urine output Oncotic pressure	Infusion rate of cardiac drugs	
Potential acute respiratory insuffiency (ARI) (Shock, trauma etc.)	Respiration rate Depth of respiration Color	Respiratory rate (RR) Tidal volume (TV) Yital capacity Arterial blood gases (pH, PO_2, PCO_2) FIO_2 A-a grad Shunt fraction (Q_s/Q_t) Dead space to tidal volume rate (V_D/V_t)		Fraction inspired oxygen (FIO_2)

Table II (continued)

Module name	Patient		Life support system	
	Continuous	Intermittent	Continuous	Intermittent
On ventilator, (being weaned from ventilator)	(RR) (TV) End tidal CO_2	Continue potential ARI measures to establish trends Compliance Tracheal flora	RR TV (expired) Peak pressure End expired pressure FIO_2 or airway O_2	Check parts, tubes, fittings
Metabolic		Weight Fluid balance Serum Na^+, K^+, Cl^- Arterial pH Base excess if disturbance severe, or on hyperalimentation Mg^{2+}, Ca^{2+}	Infusion rate	Pump drip counter or integrity
Renal – if at risk of developing renal failure or in renal failure		Hourly urine volume Free water clearance Serum creatinine, K^+		
Disseminated intravascular coagulation (DIC)		Activated clotting time Platelet count Fibrinogen titer Fibrin split products Clot formation retraction and lysis	Heparin infusion rate	Pump function and integrity

Cardiac Function

The electrocardiogram

Continuous visual monitoring of the electrocardiogram is at the heart of most contemporary monitoring systems, and is useful for the visual detection of arrhythmias and the counting of the heart rate. The new non-fade display systems have considerably improved the usefulness and legibility of the displays. However, computer programs are now available which detect significant arrhythmias more reliably than do clinical personnel; it seems likely that within five years the ECG will be processed automatically and only displayed when it has changes or is distinctly abnormal. For most shock patients, electrocardiographic abnormalities are a late manifestation of respiratory malfunction, acid-base disturbances, or electrolyte abnormalities which should be detected directly.

Arterial pressure

Direct measurement of arterial pressure with an indwelling silastic or teflon catheter, inserted percutaneously, continuously flushed (Gardner et al., 1971), and connected to a pressure transducer, is optimal for the unstable hypotensive patient. The indwelling catheter system improves the accuracy of the measurement, allows for easy withdrawal of blood for pH and gas measurements, permits performance of dye dilution cardiac outputs, and can save an enormous amount of staff time spent finding a faint pulse and making an inaccurate determination of a barely audible pressure. The arterial pressure remains an important index of peripheral perfusion and provides an estimate of cardiac output which is nearly as accurate as many measures of cardiac output derived from analysis of the pulse contour (Jurado et al., 1973). The complication rate from arterial catheterization can be extremely low, particularly if careful percutaneous catheter placement techniques are used. The avoidance of multiple attempts at arterial catheterization at a single entry site, and the removal or reinsertion of an arterial line used for more than five days, have been found to further reduce this low complication rate (Gardner et al., 1974).

Cardiac filling pressure

Central venous pressure (CVP) measurement has guided volume replacement in shock therapy for over a decade. While CVP has been used loosely as a measure of intravascular volume, the measurement and manipulation of the CVP represent a direct clinical application of the Frank–Starling Law of the Heart, and is best understood this way. In 1954 Sarnoff and Berglund published the results of an important series of experiments on the Frank–Starling Law which established a firm basis for much subsequent work on cardiac function. From a clinical point of view, they made several essential observations. They established that right atrial filling pressures did not correlate well with left ventricular function, that there was no descending limb to the curve, and that different myocardial performance levels were best described by a family

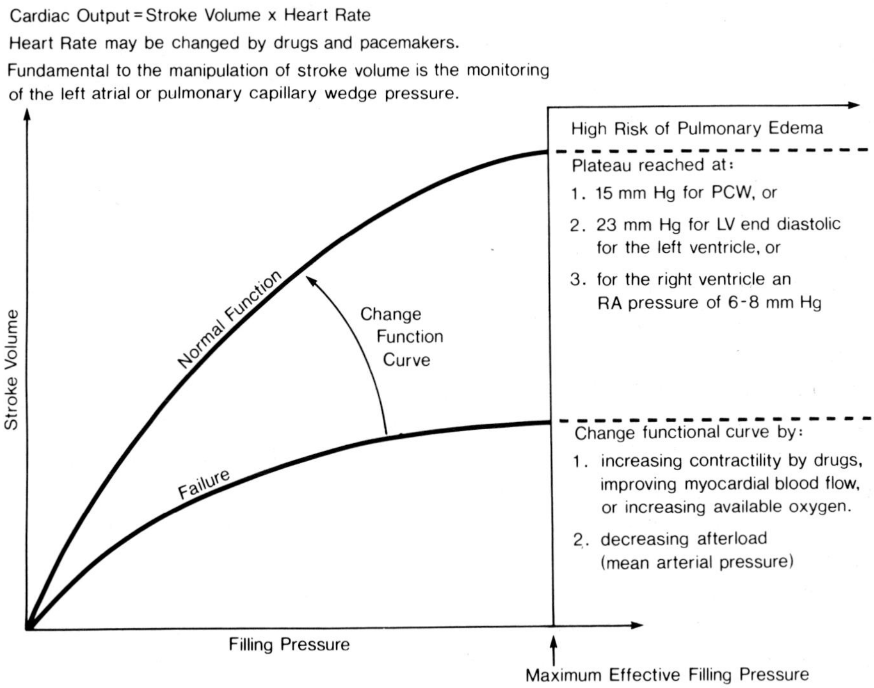

Fig. 2. Relation between filling pressure and stroke volume. An excessive filling pressure does not increase the stroke volume and will usually cause pulmonary edema. The pulmonary capillary wedge pressure (PCW) is a good guide to both left ventricle function and the onset of pulmonary edema. The numbers for the optimum pressure are for patients following myocardial infarction, but seem to be good guidelines for other patients as well.

of curves. The clinical implications of this information and its subsequent augmentation are summarized in Figure 2. While right and left ventricular function are sometimes equally affected in the unstable patient, it is increasingly clear that one cannot assume this to be true in those patients whose cardiac output and LV function are most critical. A low cardiac output associated with a low filling pressure may be increased by increasing the stroke volume; this is achieved by volume infusion to increase the filling pressure of the left ventricle to its optimum. There is a plateau to the stroke volume response beyond which further elevations of filling pressure markedly increase the risk of pulmonary edema, without increasing the stroke volume (Crexells et al., 1973). An actual decrease in stroke volume with increased filling pressure is rarely seen, and then appears primarily related to an increase afterload (mean arterial pressure) (Braunwald, 1965). Stroke volume may be further enhanced after the optimum filling pressure is reached by using drugs to increase the myocardial contractility or decrease the afterload. Subsequent to these manipulations the filling pressure usually declines, and stroke volume may be increased further by once again increasing the filling pressure. The other determinant of cardiac output is heart rate, which may be increased by drugs or cardiac pacing. Development of the Swan–Ganz balloon floatation catheter has made it possible to obtain direct information about the left ventricle in most patients (Swan et al., 1970). Forrester, working in conjunction with Swan, demonstrated that following myocardial infarction, the CVP was not useful in predicting pulmonary edema, while the pulmonary capillary wedge pressure (PCW) determined with a Swan–Ganz catheter was an excellent predictor (see Fig. 3). The greater reliability afforded by the PCW as a guide to fluid administration in shock and trauma patients has recently been documented by De Laurentis et al. (1973). The reliability of the PCW in the face of severe pulmonary pathology is uncertain. Lozman et al. (1974) have found that in cardiac surgical patients supported by mechanical ventilation, levels of positive end expiratory pressure (PEEP) of 10 cm H_2O or greater render the PCW unreliable, at a time when they found evidence for the onset of left ventricular failure. Serial measurements of CVP still appear useful for the early detection of a decrease in venous return secondary to fluid loss or the peripheral redistribution of blood. The available data suggest that it is an inaccurate measure to use in the difficult patient or as a guide to stopping transfusion and avoiding pulmonary edema.

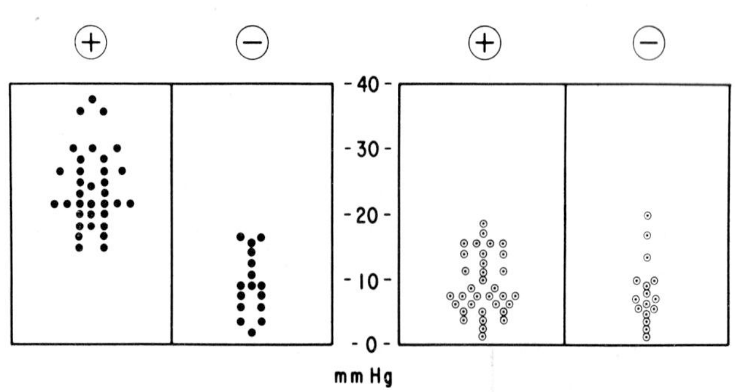

Fig. 3. Correlation between ventricular filling pressures and the presence (+) or absence (−) of radiologic pulmonary congestion, at the time of admission to the coronary-care facility. A level of PCW pressure (●) of 18 mm produced an excellent separation of the two X-ray groups. CVP (⊙) failed to distinguish the same patient groups. (From Forrester et al., 1971, reprinted with permission.)

Perfusion measurements

Blood flow may be measured intermittently using the indicator dilution technique with indocyanine green as the indicator. The use of an automated system for data acquisition, filtering and computation significantly reduces the human error in this technique, and permits the determination of sequential cardiac outputs which differ by only 2% (Hilberman and Hogan, unpublished observations). It seems likely that the thermal dilution technique will replace the older indocyanine green technique.

The measurement of core temperature is useful for a number of reasons; one of the more interesting is as a reference for measurement of skin temperature. The reaction of the autonomic nervous system to blood flow and temperature serves to make serial measurement of the difference between skin and core temperature a useful guide to the adequacy of perfusion (Eberhart and Trezak, 1974; Ibsen, 1967; Joly and Weil, 1969).

The hourly measure of urine output is a simple and extremely valuable measure of peripheral blood flow. In some patients the insidious development of high output renal failure obscures the value of this measure, and the monitoring of free water clearance has been suggested as a measure of early renal failure to be used in conjunction with the output measurement (Baek et al., 1973).

Measurement of the hematocrit, and the maintenance of the hematocrit in the range of 35–45, is important in the assessment and management of perfusion problems. Lower values will excessively reduce the supply of available oxygen (Nunn and Freeman, 1964) and higher values will excessively increase blood viscosity, and may thereby reduce perfusion significantly (MacLean et al., 1971). More recent information on the relationship between haematocrit and oxygen transport is described elsewhere in this monograph (chapter 12).

The extent of peripheral hypoxia is reflected in the arterial pH and the blood lactate. The latter is particularly useful because it is not affected by the administration of bicarbonate, or by hyperventilation. Both initial levels and directional changes in blood lactate levels are important prognostic indicators (MacLean et al., 1971; Peretz et al., 1964; Weil and Affifi, 1970). Measurement of the arteriovenous oxygen difference also provides an index of the adequacy of the circulation to the tissue needs, and the ability of the peripheral tissues to utilize oxygen. A wide difference reflects a lowered cardiac output, while an unusually narrow A-V difference is sometimes seen in sepsis, and reflects peripheral A-V shunting, or an inability of the peripheral tissues to utilize oxygen. Obtaining a true mixed venous sample is important;

this may best be obtained from a catheter in the main pulmonary artery, or by slow withdrawal through a Swan–Ganz catheter with the balloon deflated.

Respiratory Function

Advances in our knowledge of resuscitation, volume replacement, and the treatment of acute renal failure, have resulted in the survival of many patients through the critical early stages of shock. This has led to the emergence of respiratory failure as a leading cause of morbidity and mortality in these patients (Peters and Hilberman, 1971; Powers et al., 1972; Proctor et al., 1970). In Figure 4 we have diagrammed our basic conception of the respiratory monitoring and treatment process. If we begin at the top, we note that the routine care of the shock patient includes basic pulmonary care; physiotherapy and intermittent positive pressure breathing as indicated for the particular patient. At this level there are few good transducers which can be usefully connected to the patient for continuous respiratory monitoring; continuous surveillance consists primarily of direct human observation of the depth of respiration, respiratory rate, respiratory effort and color. Intermittent assessment of respiratory status is indicated in all shock patients at an interval of one to 24 hours, depending upon the patient's condition and stability, until it is clearly established that there is no risk of acute respiratory insufficiency. Measurement of the following variables is desirable: arterial blood gases, tidal volume, vital capacity, maximum inspiratory force, and if possible, venous blood gases and mean expired CO_2 with subsequent calculation of shunt fractions and dead space to tidal volume ratio. It is necessary to perform these measurements on a recurrent basis so that trends and directional changes in pulmonary status may be observed. The most important question to be answered by obtaining these data is whether the patient needs a respirator. Objective criteria for answering this question have been suggested; however, additional data are necessary to provide reliable guidelines (Hilberman et al., 1974; Peters and Hilberman, 1971). If the patient is not in need of a ventilator, one reassesses the adequacy of the conservative treatment given, and may decide to increase or decrease the frequency of physiotherapy and inhalation therapy, as shown in the loop returning to the top in the left.

For the patient in profound shock, prophylactic ventilation support may be preferable to careful monitoring of pulmonary status. Thus, in an animal model of the shock-lung developed by Drs. Blaisdell and Murray and their associates, it was found that all animals expired of pulmonary insufficiency

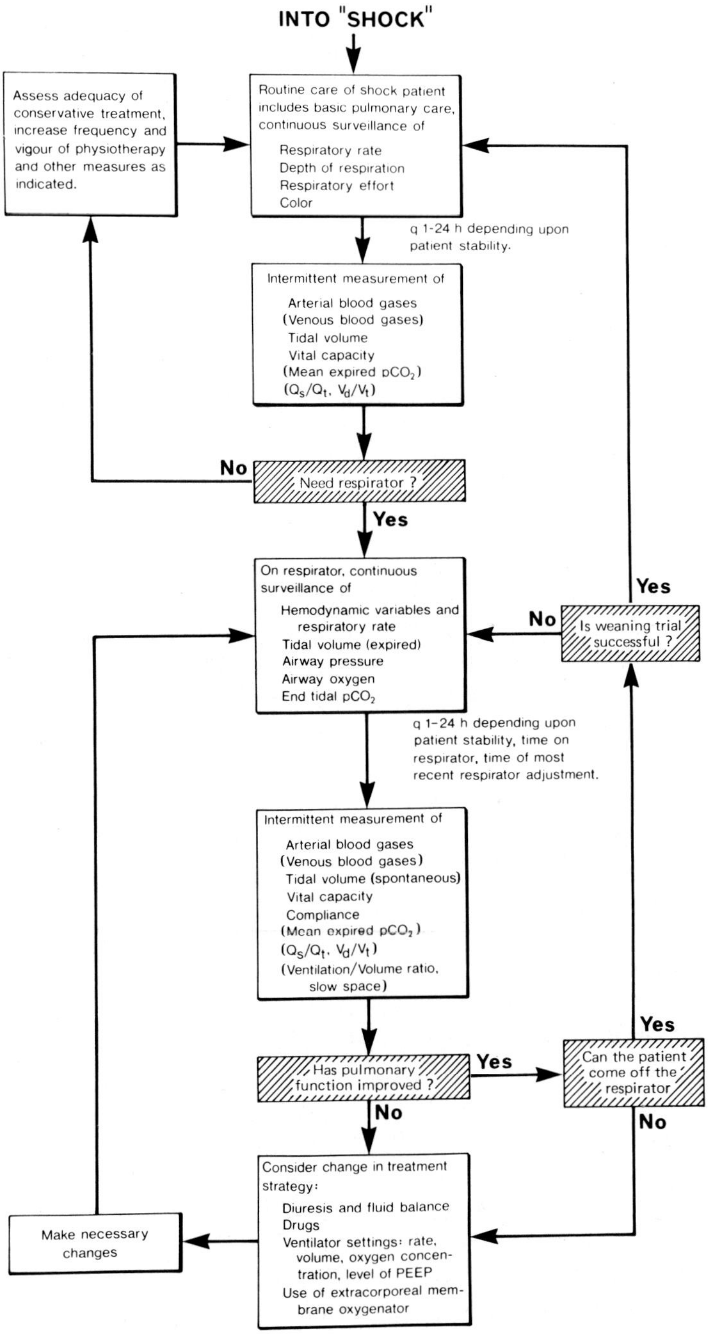

Fig. 4. Flow diagram indicating the major components and decision points in a respiratory monitoring system. For clarity, the decision logic related to the use of antibiotics, diuretics and extracorporeal oxygenation has not been included.

within 24 hours of the release of an aortic clamp which had been in place for four hours. In a second series of experiments, the animals were mechanically ventilated, in order to study the changes in pulmonary mechanics which accompanied the development of the shock-lung syndrome: no animal expired (Stallone et al., 1968; Murray, J.F., personal communication). It is difficult to extrapolate these dramatic observations directly to the care of critically ill humans, but they seem worth careful consideration.

When the patient is mechanically ventilated, the process of monitoring changes abruptly, as illustrated in the lower portion of Figure 4. Continuous hemodynamic monitoring must continue, because mechanical ventilation may decrease cardiac output, particularly in the volume-depleted patient. There is additionally a great need for continuous surveillance of airway pressure, air flow, and gas composition, and it is easy to introduce the equipment needed to make these measurements into the mechanical airway. In our experience, monitoring these basic variables is extremely useful, and has frequently led us to detect changes in ventilator performance before these were detectable by the more traditional methods (Gerbode, 1973; Osborn et al., 1969, 1971). The full test of respiratory variables available using a computer based monitoring system is shown in Table III. It is important to note that we have found the simplest of these variables the most useful: respiratory rate, expired tidal volume, airway pressure, airway oxygen, and end tidal PCO_2.

Periodically (the interval is very much dependent upon patient stability, the length of time the patient has been on the respirator, and the time of the most recent respirator adjustment), it is necessary to assess more completely the physiological status of the pulmonary system, in order to determine the patient's pulmonary status, and his ability to be weaned from mechanical ventilation (see Fig. 4, bottom). Intermittent measurement of spontaneous tidal volume, vital capacity, maximum inspiratory force and compliance, and arterial and venous blood gases are important. The mean expired PCO_2 is useful to calculate the dead space/tidal volume ratio, and arterial and venous blood gas data allow calculation of extremely valuable information about the extent of blood shunting within the lungs. Recently, Lozman and Powers and their colleagues developed a two-compartment model of the lung which considers ventilation as occurring in a fast (high turnover) space and in a slow (low turnover) space. In the hands of these workers, measurement of the ventilation to volume ratio in the slow space is extremely useful in following the patient course, and in determining ventilator settings (Lozman et al., 1974). If there has been no improvement in pulmonary function, it is necessary to reassess the adequacy of ventilation and oxygenation, and to consider changes in therapeutic strategies. After this assessment is completed, the necessary

Table III
Variables routinely monitored by the computer based measurement system in use in the Cardiopulmonary Unit of Pacific Medical Center, San Francisco, California. The last four primary signals (Pulmonary artery pressure on down) are analyzed only on demand; the other measurements are made continuously.

Primary signal	Derived variable
Airway pressure	Respiratory
Air flow	Tidal volume Minute volume Work of inspiration Compliance Resistance Maximum inspiratory pressure Static pressure End-expiratory pressure
Airway oxygen	End-tidal oxygen, FIO_2
Airway carbon dioxide	End-tidal carbon dioxide
Oxygen, carbon dioxide and flow	Oxygen uptake Carbon dioxide production Respiratory quotient
ECG	Heart rate VPC's
Aortic pressure waveform	Systolic pressure Diastolic pressure Mean pressure dp/dt Pulse rate
Pulmonary artery pressure	Mean pressure Diastolic pressure
Cardiogreen densitometer	Cardiac output
Thermal dilution catheter	Cardiac output
Appropriate blood gases	Fick cardiac output Q_s/Q_t V_D/V_t A–a gradient A-V difference

adjustments are made and the patient continues on continuous surveillance. Again, depending upon the extent of the adjustments, it will be necessary to repeat the 'in-depth' physiological observations at an appropriate time. If pulmonary function has improved, one can ask the question: Is the patient ready to come off the respirator? If the patient is not ready to come off the respirator, one again assesses the respirator settings, makes any necessary adjustments, and continues with continuous surveillance. The question of how one assesses the ability of the patient to come off the ventilator is a complex one. The standard techniques for assessment are based primarily upon the accumulation of clinical experience, and have been recently reviewed (Hodgkins et al., 1974). Recently Lozman has suggested that the ventilation to volume ratio of the slow space is the best criterion available in his unit to assess improvement or deterioration in pulmonary status and the ability of the patient to sustain spontaneous ventilation. We have no experience with this variable, but have recently completed a study of ventilator weaning following cardiac surgery (Hilberman et al., 1974). Of the 91 variables studied, the vital capacity and the maximum inspiratory force proved the most predictive of the measurements which can be made at the bedside. When combined, these variables offer a useful means for predicting the ability of the patient to come off the ventilator. It is noteworthy that the arterial blood gases were not good predictors. If the weaning trial is not successful, continuous surveillance of the basic measurements is indicated as respiratory therapy is continued. If the weaning trial is successful, the patient becomes a member of the basic shock population, and should have recurrent estimates of the pulmonary states made until such time as he can be considered well.

In our experience with respirator monitoring, it is clear that such monitoring should be an integral part of any ventilator. We have successfully used a computer based measurement system for providing these measurements before they were incorporated in many ventilators. While ventilators continue to be manufactured which do not contain such warning systems, there will probably be a diminishing role for these unmonitored devices in the modern therapy of the critically ill. Accidents due to ventilator malfunction and tubing disconnection continue to occur. The difference in cost between the least expensive ventilator and the most expensive and best monitored ventilator is small compared to the labor costs in providing respiratory care, and is insignificant when compared to the increased rate of cardiac arrests and patient mortality which can be anticipated with unmonitored machines.

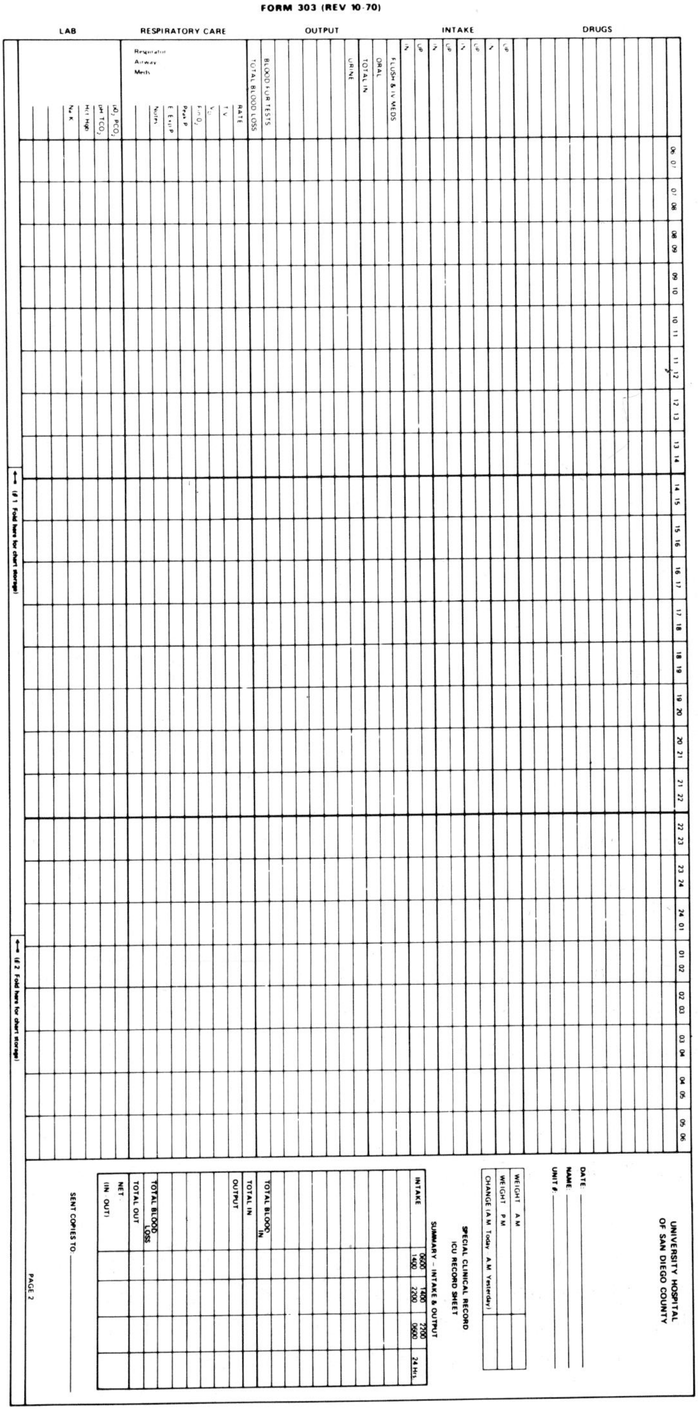

Fig. 5. Intensive Care Unit flow sheets.

Simple Methods for Data Collection Analysis and Display

With the exception of the devices necessary for the continuous measurement of airway gas concentrations, the measurements outlined are accessible to anyone in a modern hospital. There are two problems which need to be addressed to make the measurements generally useful: the data must be recorded in a retrievable fashion, and certain physiological variables must be calculated. In Figure 5 we have reproduced the second page of a flow sheet developed at the University Hospital in San Diego to accomplish this task. The two sheets serve as the basic record keeping system for the nurses, and provide most of the information which the physician will desire about a critically ill patient. A graphic display of vital sign data is combined with the nurses' notes on page one. The sheets may be tailored to the monitoring needs of individual patients by utilizing peel-off labels to relabel the various rows of data (Hilberman and Peters, 1975). These sheets provide an essential organization for the wealth of hourly data; however, they need to be supplemented by a summary sheet which permits following of the progress of a patient over several days or weeks in the intensive care environment.

It is necessary to perform a number of calculations to obtain the maximal amount of physiological information from these primary measurements. We have included in the Appendix calculations useful in assessing cardiac and respiratory physiology in the critically ill. One of the inexpensive, pocket electronic calculators now available should be on every intensive care unit. The calculators allow the performance of all of the necessary physiological calculations in a relatively straightforward fashion, and can be used for the addition of fluid balance data, with a significant increase in the accuracy of these data. Now available for under $1000 is a programmable pocket calculator from Hewlett–Packard (the HP-65). Two basic programming packages are available which contain statistical and medical calculations which can be used frequently in the care of the critically ill.

Computer Based Monitoring

The speed, computational capability, storage capacity, and display capabilities of the general purpose digital computer led investigators to explore the application of these machines to the care of the critically ill, beginning approximately ten years ago. These efforts shared a desire to use the capabilities of the digital computer to provide new physiological information to the clinician at the bedside although they have differed in emphasis. Thus, Weil and Shubin used the computer to calculate physiological variables in critically ill patients in a shock unit. They emphasized the flexibility and display handling abilities of the computer in a system dedicated to the care of two extremely sick patients (Shubin et al., 1971). Homer Warner and his colleagues used an algorithm for the calculation of cardiac output from the aortic pressure pulse wave as the basis for developing an intensive care monitoring system (Warner et al., 1968). Computer systems have been developed to act in a consultative role which may be of value in the teaching of medical students and house officers (Siegel and Stromm, 1974). The ability of digital computers to make measurements and to follow clinical algorithms has been exploited by Kirklin and Sheppard and their collaborators in the development of a system for the automated treatment of patients following cardiac surgery. These investigators have explored the hypothesis that clinical medicine is best practiced following defined rules. When feasible, they have implemented the resultant clinical algorithms in the computer. One result of this approach is that for the past 7 years in Dr. Kirklin's unit, the majority of the blood transfusions following cardiac surgery has been under computer control (Sheppard et al., 1968, 1974). Recently other investigators have established that this approach results in a smoother postoperative course due to a more physiological regulation of the blood transfusion (Morgan et al., 1973). Several approaches to respiratory system assesment have been taken. Peters and Hilberman, using a small computer system, developed a mobile instrumentation set for measuring respiratory mechanics, cardiac outputs, ventilation–perfusion relationships, and gas exchange in the critically ill. These investigators emphasized ease of use of the system and the ability to provide the measurements on a variety of patients in a variety of locations within an intensive care unit, a hospital, or a region (Hilberman et al., 1972; Peters et al., 1972). Powers and his colleagues working in a two bed shock and trauma unit, have emphasized the precise measurement of functional residual capacity and other variables which describe pulmonary function. Their primary purpose has been to obtain measurements for clinical research (Powers et al., 1972, 1973).

We will complete our discussion of shock monitoring by describing in some detail the system in use at Pacific Medical Center in San Francisco, California (Gerbode, 1973; Hilberman et al., 1974; Osborn et al., 1969). The system is built around an IBM 1800 which is a reliable 10-year-old. 16-bit per word, general purpose digital computer. The computer supports nine beds of computer based monitoring at the Pacific Medical Center, two beds of computer based monitoring at Mt. Sinai Hospital in New York, linked by telephone line, and a remote pulmonary laboratory and single bed monitoring system at a local community hospital, which is linked to our system by telephone lines. In addition to these monitoring functions, the system supports the pulmonary function and clinical pathology laboratory in our hospital (the bedside equipment configuration is shown in Figure 6). Input to the computer of ECG and various blood pressures is obtained from standard bedside monitoring equipment. In addition, for all patients on a respirator, a modified Fleisch Pneumotachograph is placed in the airway. This device has been modified to permit gas sampling. The control of electronics and gas analyzers are shared between two beds. Respiratory air flow, airway pressure, instantaneous airway oxygen, and carbon dioxide concentrations are all available as signals to the computer. In addition, special purpose measurements may be obtained from devices such as the Swan–Ganz pulmonary artery catheter used for pulmonary artery pressure monitoring and the performance of thermal dilution cardiac outputs. The complete list of the input signals and the computer variables on the system, as well as the frequency of calculation, is given in Table III.

The system has frequently alerted the staff to deterioration in patient status, or to respirator malfunction. It serves as an important aid to record, review,

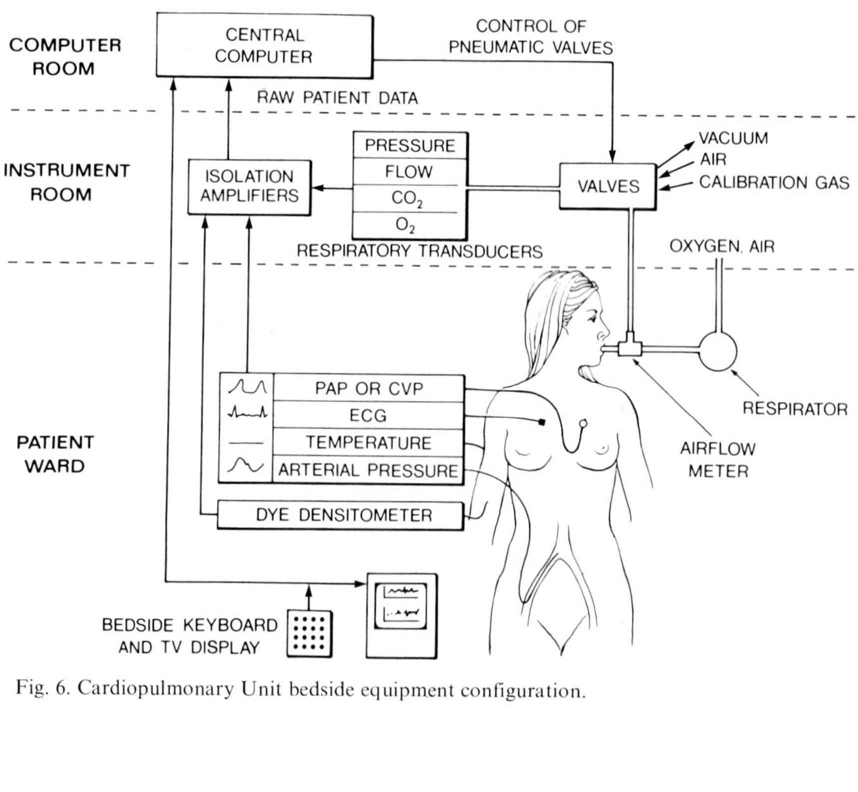

Fig. 6. Cardiopulmonary Unit bedside equipment configuration.

and communicate with the laboratory, and is in heavy use throughout the day with an average of 12 interactions occurring between the clinical staff at the bedside and the computer system each hour for 12 hours following cardiac surgery, and the average then dropping to a sustained level of 6 interactions per hour. The heavy system usage has recently been documented, although a statistical impact on morbidity and mortality has been impossible to establish (Hilberman et al., 1975). The heaviest use of the system at the bedside is to obtain physiological information already calculated by the computer, or to have the computer calculate some additional physiological variables. In Figure 7 a typical output format is shown. This compact 4-hour display with basic trend information is one of the most frequently used displays. The ability to present information in ways designed to aid trend detection is an important aspect of the system. Data display is available in a numeric format, and a larger and more precise graphics display is also available.

The ability of the system to provide data which is current up to the past 30 seconds is particularly useful when nurse and physician are 'trouble-shooting' for the cause of a malfunction. This is illustrated in Figure 8. A malfunctioning valve in a volume-closed respirator caused a reduction in minute volume, and a rise in expired PCO_2, which was detected within 5 minutes by the nurse. For about 15 minutes, she observed the patient and the readings, while she checked the respirator, and looked for difficulties. At

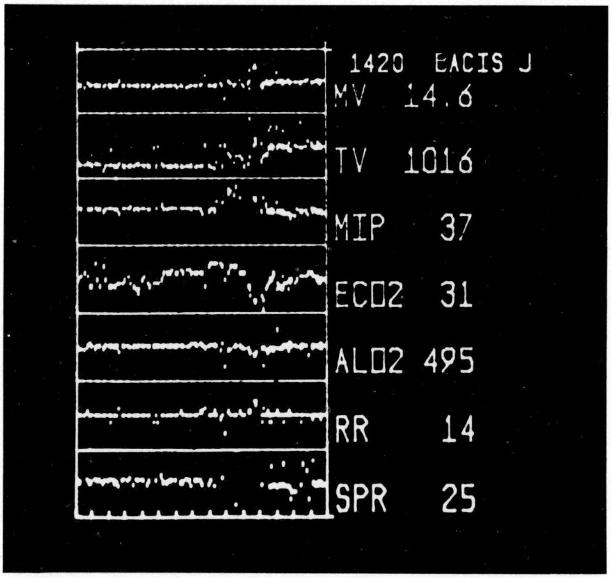

Fig. 7. Four-hour routine respiratory measurement plots.

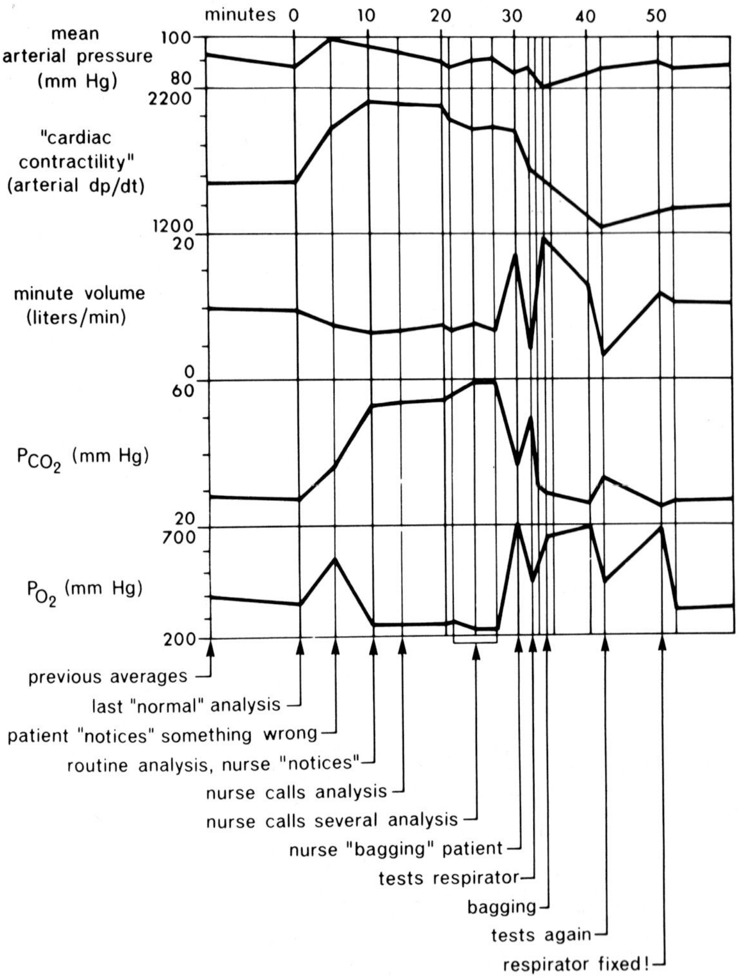

Fig. 8. Redrawn computer based measurement system used in finding patient equipment malfunction. The data are redrawn from the original plots. For details see text.

the 20-minute point, it was obvious that she had not found the cause of trouble, and she called several analyses while she checked various elements of the respirator. At 27 minutes she hand-ventilated the patient with an anesthesia bag, and noted that the minute volume rose promptly, and the patient's PCO_2 fell immediately. This confirmed that the difficulty was mechanical, and not in the patient's own physiology. At the 32nd minute, a short try on the respirator again confirmed that it was the machine which was faulty, and she returned to hand-ventilation while a technician worked over the respirator. At minute 42, the respirator was finally properly fixed, and the patient began to return to his normal steady-state. This kind of 'trouble-shooting' can certainly be carried out using the information available from blood-gas determinations. It usually takes much longer because of the delay between when the sample is drawn and when the results become known, and because of reluctance to draw too many samples.

It is interesting to note that although considerable effort has gone into designing warning and alarm systems, computer-based alarms have not yet, in our experience, been very effective, and bedside alarm systems add more noise than information. It may be that the alarm system is outdated – the new measurements allow us to avoid many old catastrophies. We are investigating another possibility – that the warning problem must be approached not in terms of variables exceeding limits, but as one of complex real time diagnostic decision making. If this hypothesis is true, and the problem solvable, then we should add considerably to the ability of clinical personnel to utilize the complex of data available to aid in caring for the critically ill.

From our experience at Pacific Medical Center, we are not at all certain that we are measuring all the right parameters. Rather detailed automated tests of pulmonary and cardiac function are presently under investigation. These include the measurement of lung spaces and distribution of ventilation–perfusion ratios. Indirect measurement of right and left ventricular function appears possible, but more difficult. The clinical experience does not exist with which to evaluate the use of this kind of specific testing of organ function, but it seems likely that the resulting rather exact physiological information will present a serious challenge to the stethoscope!

Summary

Monitoring the patient in shock is a complicated process in which current medical knowledge interacts with bedside personnel and current technology to form the content and structure of the monitoring system. It is neither possible nor desirable to construct a system which monitors all patients in the same fashion; rather, it is important to recognize that individual patient problems will require monitoring systems with different contents. It would be foolish to monitor a respirator if one is not being used, or to monitor pulmonary artery pressure in a patient without a hemodynamic problem. We hope that this conceptual discussion of monitoring and the partial discussion of the important cardiac and respiratory variables to be monitored in the critically ill shock patient will provide the reader with a useful basis for constructing other modules of a measurement system and tailoring monitoring to the needs of their patients and their hospital environment. The flexibility afforded by microprocessors and the plummeting cost of computational capability are rapidly changing the availability and utilization of computers in the intensive care environment. At present, the costs of using computers are dominated by the costs of front end instrumentation, and it seems likely that this imbalance will continue for the forseeable future. Small portable devices can aid significantly in organizing and analyzing the myriad of data available in the critically ill. The information provided in the Appendix should aid the user in utilizing some of the truly inexpensive approaches to monitoring and physiological assessment which are now available.

Appendix

Equations for calculation of important cardiac and pulmonary physiological variables using simple methods

To calculate the alveolar (A) to arterial (a) oxygen gradient, it is necessary to obtain an arterial blood gas, measure the inspired oxygen level (FIO_2, as a decimal fraction), and calculate the alveolar oxygen partial pressure.

$$P_AO_2 = (P_b - P_{H_2O}) \cdot FIO_2 - P_aCO_2 \cdot \left[FIO_2 + \frac{1 - FIO_2}{R} \right] \text{ in mmHg} \quad (1)$$

$$P_AO_2 = (P_b - P_{H_2O}) - P_aCO_2 \text{ when on } 100\% \text{ } O_2 \text{ in mmHg} \quad (2)$$

$$\text{A–a } DO_2 = P_AO_2 \text{ in mmHg} - P_aO_2 \text{ in mmHg} \quad (3)$$

To calculate the arteriovenous oxygen difference (A-V difference) and the amount of blood shunted through the lung (Q = flow, s = shunt, t = total, Q_t = the cardiac output), it is necessary to calculate the oxygen contents (C) of arterial (a), venous (v), and pulmonary capillary blood (c). The saturations are best measured directly, but may be calculated from the blood gases.

$$C_aO_2 = S_aO_2 \cdot Hgb \cdot 1.39 + P_aO_2 \cdot 0.0031 \text{ in ml/100 cc} \quad (4)$$

$$C_vO_2 = S_vO_2 \cdot Hgb \cdot 1.39 + P_vO_2 \cdot 0.0031 \text{ in ml/100 cc} \quad (5)$$

$$C_cO_2 = S_aO_2 \cdot Hgb \cdot 1.39 + P_AO_2 \cdot 0.0031 \text{ in ml/100 cc} \quad (6)$$

$$\text{A-V diff.} = C_aO_2 - C_vO_2 \text{ in ml/100 cc} \quad (7)$$

$$Q_s/Q_t = \frac{C_cO_2 - C_aO_2}{C_cO_2 - C_vO_2} \text{ as a percent} \quad (8)$$

$$Q_s/Q_t = \frac{(\text{A–a } DO_2) \cdot 0.0031}{(\text{A–a } DO_2) \cdot 0.0031 + \text{A-V } CO_2 \text{ diff.}} \text{ as a percent} \quad (9)$$

The dead space to tidal volume ratio (V_D/V_t) may be calculated from the arterial blood gases and a measure of the mean expired CO_2 level (P_ECO_2) obtained by gas bag collection or the use of an expired gas mixing chamber.

$$V_D/V_t = \frac{P_aCO_2 - P_ECO_2}{P_aCO_2} \text{ as a percent} \quad (10)$$

$$F_ECO_2 = \frac{P_ECO_2}{(P_{barom} - P_{H_2O})} \text{ as a percent} \quad (11)$$

Once the P_ECO_2 is measured the CO_2 production ($\dot{V}_{CO_2}$) may be calculated by measuring the minute ventilation ($\dot{V}$) and then calculating the fractional content of expired CO_2 (F_ECO_2, as a decimal fraction).

$$\dot{V}_{CO_2} = F_ECO_2 \cdot \dot{V} \text{ in cc/min} \quad (12)$$

The cardiac output (Q_t) may be measured by indicator dilution techniques or by calculation of the oxygen consumption ($\dot{V}_{O_2}$) after measurement of mean inspired and expired oxygen contents (FIO_2, FEO_2, as decimal fractions)

$$\dot{V}_{O_2} = (FIO_2 - FEO_2) \cdot \dot{V} \text{ in cc/min} \quad (13)$$

$$Q_t = \frac{\dot{V}_{O_2}}{\text{A-V diff.}} \text{ in L/min } \dot{V}_{O_2} = \frac{\dot{V}_{CO_2}}{0.85} \text{ if one assumes } R = 0.85 \quad (14)$$

$$\text{Cardiac Index} = \frac{Q_t}{BSA} \text{ in L/min/M}^2\text{, where BSA = body surface area} \quad (15)$$

$$\textit{Stroke Volume} = \frac{Q_t}{\text{HR}} \text{ in cc/beat, where HR = heart rate} \tag{16}$$

$$\textit{Stroke Index} = \frac{\text{SV}}{\text{BSA}} \text{ in cc/beat/M}^2 \tag{17}$$

$$\begin{aligned} \textit{Stroke Work Index} &= \text{SI} \cdot \overline{\text{BP}} \cdot 0.0136 \text{ in g M/M}^2\text{/beat,} \\ \text{where } \overline{\text{BP}} &= \text{mean blood pressure} \end{aligned} \tag{18}$$

$$\textit{Systemic Vascular Resistance} = \frac{\overline{\text{BP}} - \text{CVP (in mmHg)}}{Q_t \text{ (in l/min)}} \cdot 80 \text{ in dynes/sec/cm}^{-5} \tag{19}$$

$$\begin{aligned} \textit{Pulmonary Vascular Resistance} &= \frac{\overline{\text{PA}} - \overline{\text{PW}}}{Q_t} \cdot 80 \text{ in dynes/sec/cm}^{-5}, \\ \text{where } \overline{\text{PA}} &= \text{mean pulmonary artery pressure,} \\ \text{and } \overline{\text{PW}} &= \text{the pulmonary capillary wedge pressure.} \end{aligned} \tag{20}$$

References

Astrup, P., Gotzch, H. and Neukirch, S. (1954): Lab investigation during the treatment of patients with poliomyelitis and respiratory paralysis. *Brit. med. J., 1*, 780.

Baek, S.M., Brown, R.S. and Shoemaker, W.C. (1973): Early prediction of renal failure and recovery: sequential measurement of free water clearance. *Ann. Surg., 177*, 253.

Bower, A.G., Bennett, V.R., Dillon, J.B. and Axelrod, B. (1950): Investigation on the care and treatment of poliomyelitis patients. *Ann. western Med. Surg., 4*, 561 and 687.

Braunwald, W. (1965): The control of ventricular function in man. *Brit. Heart J., 27*, 1.

Crexells, C., Chatterjee, K., Forrester, J.S., Dikshit, K. and Swan, H.J.C. (1973): Optimal level of filling pressure in the left side of the heart in acute myocardial infarction. *New Engl. J. Med., 289*, 1263.

De Laurentis, D.A., Hayes, M., Matsumoto, T. and Wolferth, C.C. (1973): Does central venous pressure accurately reflect hemodynamic and fluid volume patterns in the critical surgical patient? *Amer. J. Surg., 126*, 415.

Eberhart, R.C. and Trezek, G.J. (1974): Central and peripheral rewarming patterns in post-operative cardiac patients. *Critical Care Med., 1*, 239.

Forrester, J.S., Diamond, G., McHugh, T.J. and Swan, H.J.C. (1971): Filling pressures in the right and left sides of the heart in acute myocardial infarction, *285*, 190.

Gardner, R.M., Schwartz, R., Wong, H.C. and Burke, J.P. (1974): Percutaneous indwelling radial-artery catheters for monitoring cardiovascular function. *New Engl. J. Med., 290*, 1227.

Gardner, R.M., Warner, H.R., Toronto, A.F. and Gaisford, W.D. (1971): A catheter–flush system for continuous monitoring of central arterial pulse waveform. *J. appl. Physiol., 29*, 911.

Gerbode, F. (1973): Computerized monitoring of seriously ill patients. *J. thorac. cardiovasc. Surg., 66*, 167.

Hilberman, M. (1975): The evolution of intensive care units. *Critical Care Med., 3(4)*.

Hilberman, M., Patitucci, P.J. and Peters, R.M. (1972): On-line assessment of cardiac and pulmonary pathophysiology in the acutely ill. *J. ass. advanc. med. Instruments, 6*, 65.

Hilberman, M., Kamm, B., Lamy, M., Dietrich, H.P., Martz, K. and Osborn, J.J. (1974a): The prediction of respiratory adequacy following cardiac surgery. In: *IEEE Proceedings of the Conference on 'Computers in Cardiology'*, Washington, D.C., October 2–4, 1974, IEEE Cat. No. 74 CHO 879–7c.

Hilberman, M., Kamm, B., Osborn, J.J. and Tarter, M. (1975): An evaluation of computer based monitoring at Pacific Medical Center. *Comput. biomed. Res., 8(3).*

Hilberman, M. and Peters, R.M. (1975): A data collection system for intensive care. *Critical Care Med.*

Hodgkins, J.E., Bowser, M.A. and Burton, G.G. (1974): Respirator weaning (review article). *Critical Care Med., 2,* 96.

Ibsen, B. (1967): Treatment of shock with vasodilators measuring skin temperature on the big toe: ten years experience in 150 cases. *Dis. Chest, 52,* 425.

Joly, H.R. and Weil, M.H. (1969): Temperature of the great toe as an indication of the severity of shock. *Circulation, 39,* 131.

Jurado, R., Matucha, D. and Osborn, J.J. (1973): Cardiac output estimation by pulse contour methods: validity of their use for monitoring the critically ill patient. *Surgery, 74,* 358.

Kouwenhoven, W.B., Jude, J.R. and Knickerbocker, G.G. (1960): Closed-chest cardiac massage. *J. Amer. med. Ass., 173,* 1064.

Lown, B., Newman, J. and Amarasingham, R. (1962): A new method of termination of cardiac arrhythmias. *J. Amer. med. Ass., 182,* 548.

Lozman, J., Powers, S.R. Jr., Older, T., Dutton, R.E., Roy, R.J., English, M., Marco, D. and Eckert, C. (1974): Correlation of pulmonary wedge and left atrial pressures in the patient receiving positive end-expiratory pressure ventilation (PEEP). To be published.

MacLean, L.D., Duff, J.H. and MacLean, A.P.H. (1971): The patient in shock. *Canad. med. Ass. J., 105,* 78.

Maloney, J.V. Jr. (1968): The trouble with patient monitoring. *Ann. Surg., 168,* 605.

Morgan, A., Anderson, W., Bevilacqua, R., Cohn, L., Moore, F.D. and Collins, J.J. Jr. (1973): Effects of computer controlled transfusion on recovery from cardiac surgery. *Ann. Surg., 179,* 391.

Mushin, W.W. and Rendall-Baker, L. (1953): *The Principles of Thoracic Anesthesia, Past and Present.* Blackwell Press, Oxford.

Nordstrom, L. (1972): On automatic ventilation. *Acta anaesth. scand., Suppl. 47.*

Nunn, J.F. and Freeman, J. (1964): Problems of oxygenation and oxygen transport during hemorrhage. *Anaesthesia, 19,* 206.

Osborn, J.J., Beaumont, J.O., Raison, J.C.A. and Abbott, R.P. (1969): Computations for quantitative on-line measurements in an intensive care ward. *Computers biomed. Res., 3,* 207.

Osborn, J.J., Raison, J.C.A., Beaumont, J.O., Hill, J.D., Kerth, W.J., Popper, R.W. and Gerbode, F. (1971): Respiratory causes of 'sudden unexplained arrhythmia' in post-thoracotomy patients. *Surgery, 69,* 24.

Peretz, D.I., McGregory, M. and Dosseter, J.B. (1964): Lacticacidosis: a clinically significant aspect of shock. *Canad. med. Ass. J., 90,* 673.

Peters, R.M. and Hilberman, M. (1971): Respiratory insufficiency: diagnosis and control of therapy. *Surgery, 70,* 280.

Peters, R.M., Hilberman, M., Hogan, J.S. and Crawford, D.A. (1972): Objective indications for respiratory therapy in post-trauma and postoperative patients. *Amer. J. Surg., 124,* 262.

Powers, S.R., Burdge, R., Leather, R., Monaco, V., Newell, J., Sardar, S. and Smith, E.J. (1972): Studies of pulmonary insufficiency in non-thoracic trauma. *J. Trauma, 12,* 1.

Powers, S.R., Mannal, R., Neclerio, M., English, M., Marr, C., Leather, R., Ueda, H., Williams, G., Custead, W. and Dutton, R. (1973): Physiologic consequences of positive end-expiratory pressure (PEEP) ventilation. *Ann. Surg., 178,* 265.

Proctor, H.J., Ballantine, T.V.N. and Broussaro, N.D. (1970): An analysis of pulmonary function following non-thoracic trauma. *Ann. Surg., 172,* 180.

Sarnoff, S.J. and Berglund, E. (1954): Ventricular function. I. Starling's Law of the Heart studied by means of simultaneous right and left ventricular function curves. *Circulation, 9*, 706.

Sheppard, L.C., Kirklin, J.W. and Kouchoukos, N.T. (1974): Computer-controlled interventions for the acutely ill patient. *Computers biomed. Res., 4*, 135.

Sheppard, L.C., Kouchoukos, N.T., Kurtts, M.A. and Kirklin, J.W. (1968): Automated treatment of critically ill patients following operation. *Ann. Surg., 168*, 596.

Shubin, H., Weil, M.H., Palley, N. and Affifi, A.A. (1971): Monitoring the critically ill patient with the aid of a digital computer. *Computers biomed. Res., 4*, 460.

Siegel, J.H. and Stromm, B.L. (1974): An automated consultation system to aid the physician in the care of the desperately sick patient. *Computers biomed. Res., 4*, 115.

Stallone, R.J., Herbst, J.J., Cafferata, H.T., Blaisdell, W.F. and Murray, J.F. (1968): Pulmonary changes following regional ischemia: response to treatment. *Amer. Rev. resp. Dis., 98*, 144.

Swan, H.J.C., Ganz, W., Forrester, J., Marcus, H., Diamond, G. and Chonette, D. (1970): Catheterization of the heart in man with use of a flow-directed balloon-tipped catheter. *New Engl. J. Med., 283*, 447.

Warner, H.R., Gardner, R.M. and Toronto, A.F. (1968): Computer-based monitoring of cardiovascular functions in post-operative patients. *Circulation, 17/2*, 68.

Weil, M.H. and Affifi, A.A. (1970): Experimental and clinical studies on lactate and pyruvate as indicators of the severity of acute circulatory failure (shock). *Circulation, 41*, 989.

Zoll, P.M., Liventhal, A.J., Norman, L.R., Pam, M.H., Gibson, W. (1956): Treatment of unexpected cardiac arrest by external electric stimulation of the heart. *New Engl. J. Med., 254*, 541.

Ledingham (ed.). Shock

Advances in bedside measurements with patients in shock

D.W. HILL

Much has been written about the various conditions embraced by the general term 'shock'. Since this can be an unstable state, not only must the therapy be as effective as possible, but an incipient deterioration in the patient's condition must be detected as soon as possible in order that the appropriate actions can be instituted.

Circulatory shock is defined by Guyton and Crowell (1964) as 'a state of the circulation in which the cardiac output is too low to supply the normal nutritional needs of the body's tissues even when the subject is at rest'. These authors delineate six separate effects of shock which act as a feedback producing yet further severity of shock. These are:

1. a decreased coronary artery flow;
2. a decreased brain blood flow;
3. a decreased nutrition of the vascular system;
4. an increased capillary permeability;
5. ischaemia of many different tissues; and
6. an increased clotting ability.

Clearly, in this condition one will be concerned with a reduced cardiac output, blood pressure, myocardial contractility, regional blood flows, blood volume, venous return and oxygen uptake.

On the other hand, in the case of 'shock with sepsis' (Border, 1971), the picture may be quite different. A useful review of the position is that of

Table I
The cardiac output in gram-positive and gram-negative infection patients (From Weil and Shubin, 1971.)

Variable No. of patients	Gram + ve patients (6)	Gram − ve patients (8)	Normals (11)
Systolic BP	67 ± 4.4	60 ± 3.4	120 ± 2.2 mmHg
Diastolic BP	48 ± 4.1	36 ± 3.7	67 ± 2.7 mmHg
CVP	7.1 ± 1.2	7.0 ± 2.0	7.1 ± 0.2 mmHg
Heart rate	103 ± 8	109 ± 6	76 ± 1 beats per minute
Cardiac index	2.81 ± 0.24	1.85 ± 0.21	3.2 ± 0.07 $\lambda/min/m^2$
Mean circulation time	19.9 ± 2.2	21.2 ± 2.6	12.8 ± 0.03 seconds
Total peripheral resistance	1058 ± 52	1649 ± 172	1270 ± 24 $dyne/sec/cm^{-5}$
Excess lactate	2.5 ± 1.1	10.3 ± 2.4	0.2 ± 0.1 mM

Weil and Shubin (1971). They report that in patients with shock associated with gram-negative bacilli, the cardiac output is usually inadequate, whilst it is likely to be normal in patients with hypotension associated with gram-positive infections (Table I). The cardiac output may also not be reduced in patients with peritonitis. Weil and Shubin make the point that during septic shock states, the monitoring of cardiac output may be not more rational than a simple reliance on monitoring the arterial blood pressure. They instance the case of patients with peritonitis, where the cardiac output is not reduced, but the fact that they are in shock presumably represents a defect in the distribution of the available blood flow, presumably due to arteriovenous shunting. The fact that tissue perfusion is not normal can be observed from the high excess lactate value.

Shoemaker (1967) has discussed the clinical evaluation of the shock state and emphasises that the traditional vital signs: blood pressure, heart rate, respiratory rate and body temperature should be monitored at frequent intervals. He makes the point that the central venous pressure is the simplest test of an overtransfusion. He also feels that the blood volume is the best index of the circulatory state as far as the evaluation of blood loss is concerned, and that renal function as manifested by the hourly urine output is a reflection both of the adequacy of blood volume and renal blood flow.

Siegal et al. (1971) consider that the concept of 'net vascular tone' is the most useful index for separating the group of patients whose state of shock arises from sepsis from those in whom the aetiological factor in the shock process is uncomplicated hypovolaemia. Net vascular tone is taken as the summation of the vascular tone in all the perfused vascular beds. This definition includes anatomical or functional precapillary arteriovenous anastamoses which act to shunt blood away from the metabolising capillary circulation. Siegal et al. (1971) make the point that for any given systemic flow, the patient in septic shock has a reduced peripheral resistance, whereas patients in hypovolaemic shock have an increased peripheral resistance. They have found a log–log plot of cardiac index versus total peripheral resistance to be of value in distinguishing between patients in septic and non-septic shock.

In addition to circulatory parameters, it is also necessary to consider blood-gas and ventilatory parameters. Siegal et al. (1967) also found that patients suffering from septic shock who were in a hyperdynamic state had a decreased effective oxygen transport ratio (ml per litre of blood flow) which was associated with an increase in blood pH. This is primarily due to a metabolic alkalosis since in general, in spite of a mild degree of hyperventilation, the arterial blood, CO_2 tension values were normal. The arterial oxygen saturation was normal but the venous saturation was markedly increased giving rise to a low oxygen consumption. Siegal et al. (1967) found that a log–log plot of the effective oxygen transport ratio versus total peripheral resistance separated patients with non-septic shock from those with a hyperdynamic state due to septic shock. A sophisticated system for the computer monitoring of respiratory variables in acutely ill patients has been described by Raison (1971). This was able to perform breath-by-breath calculations of oxygen uptake, carbon dioxide output and the respiratory quotient. Raison makes the point that for patients on ventilators, the chest wall impedance (compliance and resistance) remains remarkably constant for periods of several hours. Major changes observed in the total compliance and resistance (lungs and chest-diaphragm cage) almost always reflect changes which have occurred in the lung values.

Shoemaker et al. (1973) have discussed the patterns of physiological variables observed in surviving and non-surviving shock patients following major surgery. They found that usually the differences in the patterns of haemodynamic variables between the two groups were more pronounced in the early and later period than in the middle period. The average arterial pressures at the lowest point were similar, so that arterial pressure was not a good predictor of survival. In regard to the monitoring of variables on an early warning basis, Shoemaker et al. (1973) suggest that attention be paid to a lower cardiac output, and other measures of cardiac performance, a higher pulmonary vascular resistance, a reduced oxygen transport, acidosis, a higher arterial carbon dioxide tension, and greater reductions in the haematocrit and blood volume. From the viewpoint of predicting survival, Shoemaker et al. (1973) divide their measured variables into groups: Cardiac-related variables – cardiac index, mean transit time, systolic ejection rate, tension time index and right ventricular stroke work; Volume-related variables – blood volume deficit, red cell mass, central blood volume, central venous pressure and stroke index; Neurohumoral-related variables – systemic vascular resistance, and mean pulmonary vascular resistance; Oxygen transport-related variables – arterial PO_2, oxygen extraction ratio, haemoglobin concentration, arteriovenous oxygen content difference, oxygen availability and oxygen consumption; Acid-base-related variables – arterial pH and PCO_2.

From the previous discussion, it can be seen that the primary bedside instrumentation will consist of a reliable patient monitoring system preferably connected to a multi-channel recorder or data logger so that trends can be observed and followed. The system should be of a modular construction and should be able to handle the electrocardiogram, arterial blood pressure (with the facility of giving the mean pressure), central venous pressure, and heart rate from either the ECG or arterial pressure channels. High and low alarm settings should be available on both the ECG and pressure channels. A body temperature monitor using thermistor probes should be available and this should have at least two probes fitted so that core and peripheral temperatures can be monitored simultaneously. A system for the measurement of cardiac output is desirable. This could be based on the indicator dilution technique using thermal dilution or indocyanine green dye dilution or it might be the non-invasive electrical impedance method. Convenient access should be available to a reliable single cuvette type of electrode system for the measurement of blood pH, PO_2 and PCO_2. Since shock patients may have oxygen transport problems, a dual wavelength oximeter for the measurement of blood oxygen saturation will be useful. For those patients who require automatic ventilation of the lungs, an electrically powered ventilator with facilities for measuring the ventilatory volume and various options for the expiratory phase will be needed.

The Measurement of Blood Pressure

In patients with marked hypotension consequent upon shock, the most reliable method of measuring systemic arterial, left atrial or pulmonary artery blood pressures is directly by means of a pressure transducer. A considerable development has occurred in this field and has resulted in small size models such as the Statham Instruments Model P37 (weight 4 g) and the Kent Cambridge Medical Model PT8 (weight 2 g) which can be connected to a catheter or cannula and taped directly to the patient's skin. They can remain in place for extended periods without causing discomfort or prohibiting movement.

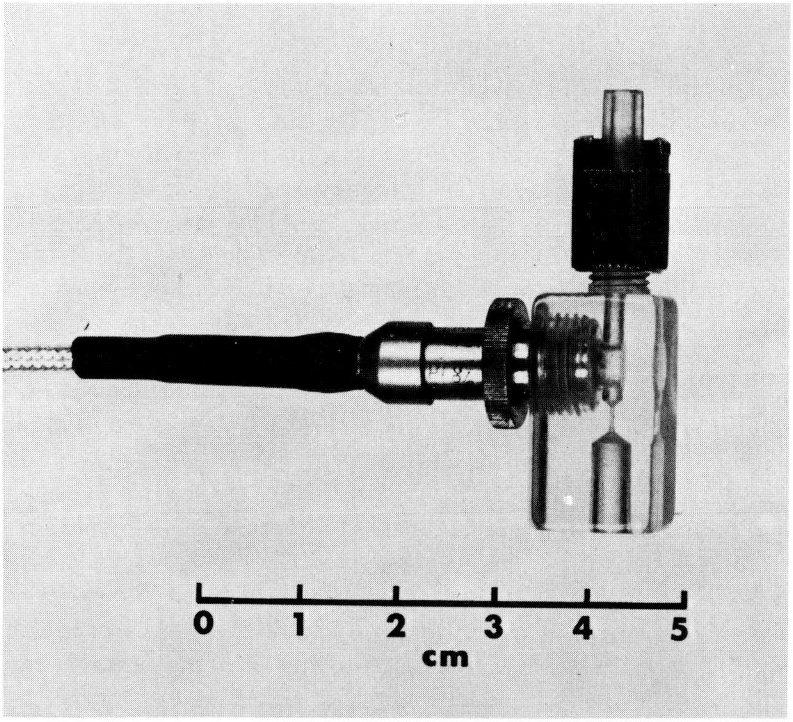

Fig. 1. Model PT8 lightweight silicon–alloy diaphragm blood pressure transducer. (By courtesy of Kent Cambridge Medical Ltd.)

The PT8, shown in Figure 1, uses four semiconductor strain gauges diffused into the rear of a silicon–alloy diaphragm. Temperature compensation resistors are mounted into the transducer's connector. The output is 7 mV per 100 mmHg pressure for a 5 V d.c. excitation, with a thermal drift of not more than 0.2 mmHg per °C over the range 15 to 45°C. The pressure range is −30 to +300 mmHg. When blood pressure transducers are to be used for extended periods it is necessary to flush the catheter or cannula at regular intervals in order to prevent clot formation and a consequent damping of the pressure waveform. A common arrangement is to have a pressurised reservoir of sterile saline connected via a flow restrictor to the transducer cuvette. With a reservoir pressure of 300 mmHg and a flow of 4 to 5 ml per hour it is possible to monitor arterial and venous pressures for several days. Descriptions of flushing systems for long-term pressure recording are given by Grandjean and Perret (1970) and Gardner et al. (1970). For accurate recordings over extended periods, it is necessary regularly to check the baseline and calibration of the pressure channels. If an on-line digital computer system is available, this can be used to monitor the accuracy of the pressure channels (Weil et al., 1972) and also to look for any distortion occurring in the arterial pressure waveform (Klee et al., 1974). An increase in the damping of the trace could arise from clotting of the arterial line or a deterioration in the patient's haemodynamics. The paper by Weil et al. (1972) is a good description of a computer monitoring system applied to shock patients. The blood pressure waveform is displayed on an oscilloscope or recorder to allow the systemic, systolic, diastolic and mean pressures to be determined together with the pulmonary artery diastolic pressure, pulmonary capillary wedge pressure and left atrial pressure in patients with heart failure.

Whilst saline-filled manometers are frequently employed for the measurement of central venous pressure, the use of an electrical pressure transducer enables the CVP to be fed into a data logging system. Unbonded strain gauge transducers are available having sensitivities five or six times that used for arterial pressure recording and are designed for venous pressure measurements.

Blood pressures should be quoted as referred to a particular reference plane, this is normally taken as heart level. The pressure transducers can conveniently be mounted on a vertical metal column adjacent to the patient, so that they can be slid up and down it and locked in the appropriate position. The column also carries bags or bottles of fluids for perfusing the catheters. The choice of reference level becomes important in the case of low pressures, such as the central venous pressure. It may become altered if the patient changes his position. A useful approach is to connect the rear side of the transducer's diaphragm to a plastic tube leading to an otherwise sealed container taped to the patient at heart level. If the patient moves, the reference pressure will alter accordingly and the central venous pressure will still be recorded correctly. The central venous pressure waveform will be modulated by the respiration and with suitable low-pass filtering this can be extracted and used for monitoring the respiratory rate (Meagher et al., 1966). A useful discussion of the role of central venous pressure measurements is that of Guyton and Jones (1973).

Over recent years, much more attention has been paid to the possibility of patients having pacing electrodes or cardiac catheters receiving a microshock which could result in ventricular fibrillation. The philosophy adopted by the Department of Health and Social Security in the United Kingdom is to have all the circuits connected to the patient isolated from earth. Under single fault conditions, the maximum leakage current at the mains supply frequency which is permitted to flow through the patient's heart is not to exceed 50 μA.

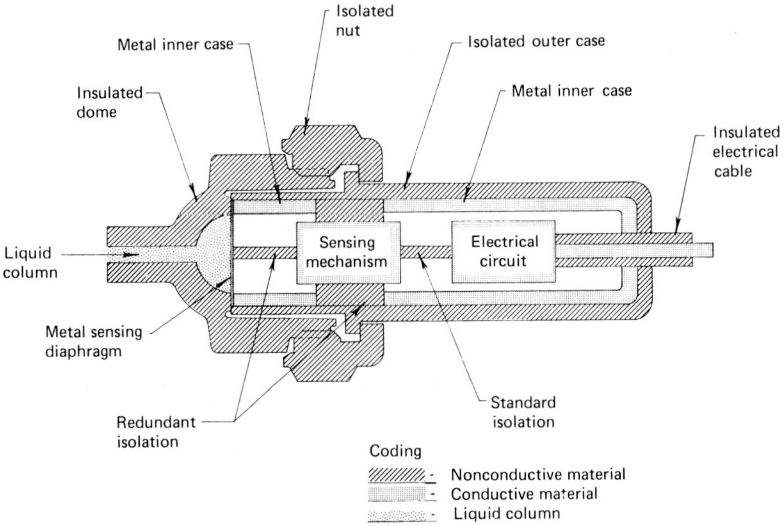

Fig. 2. Model P23 Ia redundant insulation unbonded strain gauge blood pressure transducer. (By courtesy of Statham Instruments Inc., Oxnard, Calif.)

Pressure transducers are now available in which a high degree of insulation is maintained between the catheter fluid and the transducer's mechanism. The Statham Model P23 Ia transducer employs the principle of redundant insulation (Fig. 2). The quoted electrical leakage current is 2 μA maximum at 115 V r.m.s. 60 Hz (5 μA in the case of an internal electrical failure) and a d.c. insulation resistance of 100 mOhm minimum at 50 V.

Patients suffering from shock with sepsis must present a cross-infection hazard. Blood pressure transducers should not be autoclaved but cold-sterilised. Models are now available which have a disposable plastic cuvette which completely separates the catheter fluid from contact with the diaphragm. This reduces cross-infection problems and electrically isolates the patient.

A faithful reproduction of cardiac pressure waveforms is essential if rates of change of pressure and maximum blood ejection velocities are to be used as estimates of cardiac performance. Falsetti et al. (1974) state that the natural frequency of any catheter system used for this purpose must exceed 40 Hz to produce results accurate to 10%.

In severely ill patients with shock, it is usual for the blood pressures to be measured directly with transducers. However, when an indirect measurement of low arterial blood pressures is required, the present method of choice is based on an inflation cuff used with a transcutaneous ultrasonic doppler shift probe to sense the arterial wall motion (Tahir and Adriani, 1973). Buggs et al. (1973) have investigated the method in hypotensive patients and state that "the doppler technique yielded systolic blood pressure values when the blood pressure could not be obtained by auscultation or palpation, especially in noisy environments". A smaller version of the cuff is available for use with children.

The Monitoring of Heart and Pulse Rate

The heart rate is usually obtained from the R-waves of the ECG and the heart rate meter is normally fitted with bradycardia and tachycardia alarm limits. A time delay of about 5 seconds should be provided before the upper limit alarm operates. This is desirable because artefacts arising from the patient's movements in bed may give rise to transient peaks on the ratemeter. It is also desirable that the nurses be able to deliberately mute the alarms for a pre-set time interval whilst they are turning the patient, giving him a bed bath or physiotherapy is in progress. Since the ECG only indicates the presence of electrical and not mechanical activity from the heart, a finger photo-plethysmograph is commonly used to record the peripheral pulse waveform. A photo-plethysmograph can also be mounted on the ear lobe. Stern (1974) used a reflected light transducer on a finger and both reflected and transmitted light transducers on the ear lobe. He found that in response to a series of stimuli presented to his subjects, the ear lobe showed little change in pulse volume whereas the finger showed marked degrees of vasoconstriction. Conventional pick-ups based on an incandescent bulb can suffer from the effects of ambient lighting and finger burns can result when the circulation is badly impaired. The situation has been improved with the modern use of light emitting diodes and gallium arsenide photo-detectors. Modulation of the diode output eliminates the effect of room lighting. Detection of the peripheral pulse can also be performed by means of passing a radiofrequency current through a finger and detecting the diminution in impedance which occurs with each systole. The incidence of false alarms can be greatly reduced by making the sounding of an alarm require the presence of two simultaneous alarm conditions, e.g. an elevated heart and pulse rate (Raison et al., 1968).

In the past, the presence of a heart rate alarm or of extrasystoles has been used to dump the previous 5 seconds of ECG from an endless loop of magnetic tape on to an ECG recorder for inspection. The continuous running of the tape led to the formation on it of bald patches. A much greater degree of reliability is now obtainable by the use of a solid-state shift register which is continuously up-dated with digitised ECG data points. When a fault condition is detected on the ECG, the input to the shift register is stopped and its contents can be dumped on to a recorder or shown on an oscilloscope as a 'frozen' ECG tracing.

The Measurement of Cardiac Output and Related Variables

The most commonly used techniques for the measurement of cardiac output are based upon the dilution by the cardiac output of an 'indicator' substance injected into the venous circulation, or preferably the right side of the heart for the best accuracy, the arrival of the bolus of indicator is detected in the systemic circulation. One approach uses an injection of about 4 ml of cool (0.5°C) saline (coolth) via a special thin-walled catheter into the right ventricle. The tip of the catheter is closed, but there are six side openings at the end which gives an almost complete mixing of the saline with the blood. Detection of the bolus of cool saline is made by a thermistor bead located at the top of another catheter placed in the pulmonary artery. The cardiac output can be found from a knowledge of the volume of coolth injected and its temperature at the tip of the injection catheter, the temperature of the cooled blood in the pulmonary artery, the densities of the saline and the blood, the specific heats of the saline and blood, and the area under the dilution curve traced out by the recorder fed from the output of the thermistor bridge circuit. After the coolth has been injected, the period of the so-called 'appearance time' has to elapse before the recorder deflects to a peak (corresponding with the lowest blood temperature), the deflection then following an exponential curve to its pre-injection value if there is complete mixing of the blood and indicator within the heart and no regurgitation. By the time the cooled blood has completed its first traverse of the circulation it will have warmed to body temperature, so that no subsidiary peak corresponding with re-circulation is seen on the recorder with this method. This renders the measurement of the area under the curve easy to perform with an electronic integrator and has led to the development of compact analogue computers which can be used at the bedside to give a direct reading of the cardiac output (Roberts, 1969; Cowell and Bray, 1970). A critical account of the factors which can affect the accuracy of the thermal dilution technique, particularly in the case of serial determinations of cardiac output over prolonged periods is that of Wilson et al. (1972). The technique is also discussed by Ellis et al. (1972).

The other indicator substance which is widely used for cardiac output determinations is indocyanine green dye (Fox and Wood, 1957). It offers the advantage over earlier dyes that it is rapidly cleared from the circulation – approximately 3% of the dose remaining in the circulation 20 minutes after injection (Cherrick et al., 1960) – and that it absorbs light in the 800 nm region of the spectrum which is where both oxygenated and reduced haemoglobin have the same optical absorption. Hence the absorption of light at 800 nm is unaffected by the degree of oxygenation of the patient's blood. By means of a venous catheter placed into the right atrium, a bolus injection is made of typically 5 mg of dye in 1 ml of solvent for an adult. Meanwhile an electrically powered constant withdrawal syringe is used to draw about 0.4 ml per second of arterial blood through the cuvette of a two-wavelength densitometer (Sutterer and Wood, 1962). When blood containing dye arrives in the cuvette, the recorder driven from the densitometer describes a dilution curve similar to that obtained for thermal dilution. However, for dye dilution, there will be a second re-circulation peak. For the calculation of cardiac output, the area ('area A') lying under the primary curve without re-circulation is required. Assuming that the downslope of the dye dilution curve is a simple exponential, this can be re-plotted on semi-logarithmic graph paper to yield a straight line which can be extrapolated downwards to provide the ordinates required to complete the downslope to one percent of the peak concentration value. The area under the curve 'A' expressed in mg/l × seconds can then be measured with a planimeter and the cardiac output in litres calculated from the expression $Q = 60 \times \text{mg}/\text{A}$, where mg is the number of milligrams of dye injected. This method of calculating the cardiac output is too tedious for repeated determinations. On the assumption that the downslope is a simple exponential a number of algorithms exist for the calculation of 'A' without the need for re-plotting the downslope (Shubin et al., 1967). Siegal et al. (1968) used this approach in conjunction with an electronic calculator for the bedside measurement of cardiac output and haemodynamic variables in patients in shock. A number of commercially available analogue cardiac output computers operate on this type of algorithm. Sullivan et al. (1973) describe an electronic calibration of the integrator used to measure the area under the curve. It is based on the use of a known voltage–dye concentration factor. However, the algorithm may be impracticable with patients who have a low output with a non-exponential downslope or who have a re-circulation peak which occurs early. Under these circumstances it is possible to use the 'forward triangle method' of Hetzel et al. (1958) and Thorburn (1961). Hill et al. (1973)

found the forward triangle method slightly overestimated (0.3% ± 1.2%) compared with the classical extrapolation method.

If a digital computer fitted with an analogue-to-digital converter can be connected by suitable cables at the bedside to the densitometer and the curve sampled at 5 per second, then a program can easily be arranged to calculate the cardiac output, cardiac index, appearance time, and mean circulation time. If the mean arterial blood pressure and central venous pressure are known, the left ventricular stroke work and total systemic resistance can also be calculated (Gil-Rodriguez et al., 1970; Shubin et al., 1967). The right ventricular stroke work can be calculated from the stroke volume, mean pulmonary artery pressure and central venous pressure.

Considerable interest has been shown in possible indices which could be derived from the central aortic pulse waveform and which would be proportional to the stroke volume on a beat-by-beat basis. Such an approach has been reported in computer-based patient monitoring systems (Warner, 1972). However, Starmer et al. (1973) found that while the method worked over a range of stroke volumes when the variation was produced by a single perturbing factor, none of the indices proposed performed adequately when multiple perturbations were involved. Hence the clinical application was markedly limited.

Electrocardiography

ECG electrodes

The regular monitoring of the electrocardiogram over periods of several days is important with many patients, particularly those suffering from shock. In spite of the fact that patients may be delirious, restless and perspiring, it is necessary to be able to obtain good quality ECG signals, particularly if a computer-based arrhythmia analysis system is to be operated. Most electrodes now in use are based upon a lightweight plastic cup filled with a non-irritant electrode cream or jelly and containing a silver–silver chloride or silver disk. This arrangement minimises motion artefacts arising at the electrode–electrolyte interface. The electrodes are usually disposable. A good skin preparation, by abrading the outer horny layer and removing surface grease with an ether–meth mixture, should always be followed if time permits. The electrode cup is attached to the patient's skin by means of a double-side adhesive paper ring or a micro-pore plastic. Albisser et al. (1971) have described an atraumatic disposable electrode for cardiac monitoring, with particular reference to neonates. A new development has occurred with dry, insulated, ECG electrodes which rely upon a capacitive coupling to the patient's body. They do not require a conducting jelly or paste and they block any d.c. potential which may be present at the skin–electrode interface. A high input impedance amplifier is used and with integrated circuit techniques this may be fabricated on the rear of the electrode. David and Portnoy (1972) used an amplifier with a 100 mOhm input impedance and obtained a lower cut-off frequency between 0.01 and 1 Hz depending upon the nature and thickness of the electrode's dielectric layer. Other forms of insulated electrode have been described by Lagow et al. (1971).

ECG arrhythmia monitoring

Commercial arrhythmia monitors have been designed to give warning of runs of premature and widened beats, but these do not seem to have found favour in most intensive care units. A more reliable approach appears to be that based on an on-line minicomputer patient monitoring system (Cox et al., 1972; Feldman et al., 1971). This may well allow a better administration of anti-arrhythmic drugs. Unfortunately the monitoring of arrhythmias does not appear to always provide a reliable warning of an imminent cardiac arrest.

The Measurement of Respiratory Variables

Most modular patient monitoring systems (Fig. 3) provide some means of monitoring the respiratory rate. This is often accomplished by means of a thermistor bead placed under a nostril so as to respond to changes of temperature between the inspired and expired tidal gases. The method usually works well except in the case of restless patients who will not tolerate anything placed on their face. Other approaches are to use the respiratory movements of the thorax to open and close a switch connected to a belt fastened around the chest. An approach currently in favour is to pass a small high frequency current across the chest at approximately 100 kHz and to detect the changes in thoracic impedance which occur with respiration (Baker and Hill, 1969). This technique of rheography only measures chest wall motion directly and does not monitor tidal air flow. Hence, it will not respond directly to a respiratory obstruction but only indirectly to the consequent abnormal chest wall

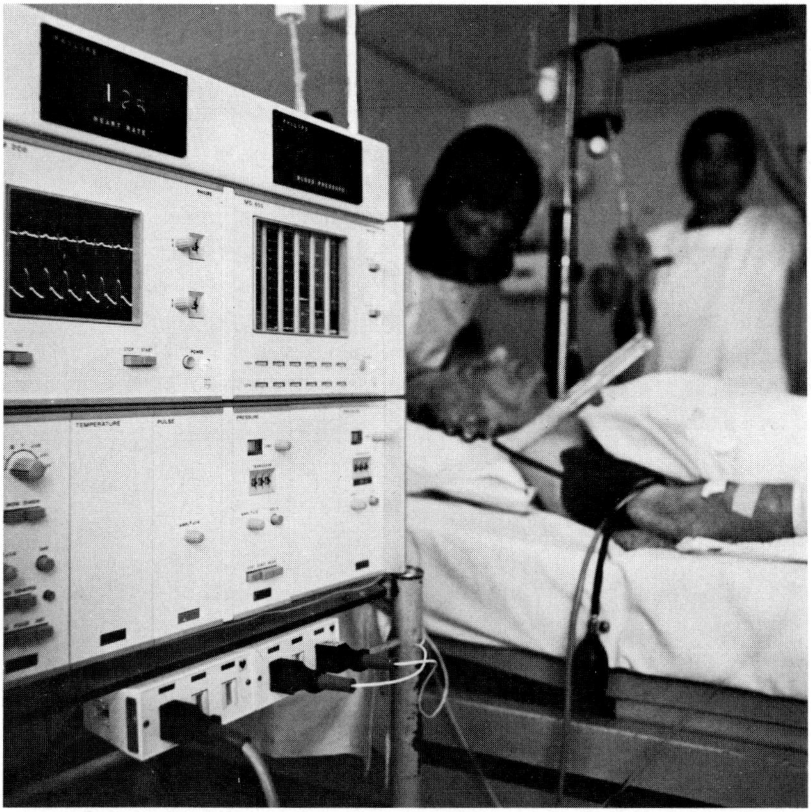

Fig. 3. Modular bedside patient monitoring system. All connections to the patient are made via isolation amplifiers to remove the risk of an accidental micro-shock to the heart. (By courtesy of Philips Medical Systems Ltd.)

motion. Respiratory minute volume is usually measured by means of a device such as the Wright respirometer (Wright, 1955). This is a turbine system with the vane motion coupled to a watch-type display via a gear train. It is convenient to use, but prone to damage (Lunn and Hillard, 1970). A later version now provides an electrical output signal by means of a lamp and photocell to generate pulses as the vane rotates. A similar arrangement may be used to provide an electrical output from a gas meter to record minute volumes (Boocock et al., 1971).

Raison (1971) describes the use of an integrating pneumatachograph for the measurement of tidal volume, together with a rapidly responding oxygen electrode and a digital computer system to measure the breath-by-breath oxygen uptake. By means of an infra-red CO_2 analyser, the carbon dioxide output could also be determined and thus the respiratory quotient calculated. The system was routinely used with acutely ill patients. The breath-by-breath methods contrast for speed with the conventional Fick method for oxygen consumption which requires a knowledge of the cardiac output obtained by dye dilution and of the arteriovenous oxygen content difference found from the value of the haemoglobin and oxygen saturations.

Meade and Owen-Thomas (1973) have developed an ingenious technique for the measurement of carbon dioxide concentrations in respiratory gas mixtures which can contain nitrous oxide. The method is based on the use of a paramagnetic oxygen analyser. With both oxygen and carbon dioxide concentrations known it is possible to calculate oxygen consumption; carbon dioxide output and the respiratory quotient. Meade and Owen-Thomas have used this bedside method with neonates.

pH and blood-gas measurements

These are of particular importance in the treatment of seriously ill patients and most intensive care units have their own combined pH/blood-gas analyser, so that the results can be readily available on a 24-hour basis. Modern automatic analysers, such as the Model 313 pH/blood-gas system by Instrumentation Laboratories, can handle 25 samples of less than 0.4 ml each for pH, PCO_2 and PO_2 analyses per hour. The blood sample is drawn through the common cuvette by means of a peristaltic pump and three digital displays indicate the final data 68 seconds after the sample introduction. Automatic monitoring circuits indicate a membrane failure of the PCO_2 or PO_2 electrodes or a deviation of more than 0.15°C in the controlled temperature. After each blood sample has been analysed, the instrument automatically washes the sample from the cuvette and returns to the calibration mode.

The flushing cycle removes the blood from the cuvette using a cleaning solution to prevent the build-up of protein deposits. It is arranged that the flushing solution is equilibrated with the (5% CO_2, 12% O_2, 83% N_2) calibration gas. This ensures that during flushing the electrodes remain as close to their sample equilibration values as possible, thus ensuring that the instrument has a short response time. It is very suitable for busy intensive care units. Hill and Tilsley (1973) have evaluated the comparative performance of five commercial blood-gas and pH electrode systems.

Considerable progress is now being made in the development of in-dwelling catheter tip oxygen electrodes (Parker et al., 1971). Meldrum et al. (1973) describe a version based on a No. $3\frac{1}{2}$ French catheter. The electrode catheter is sterilised by gamma radiation and is designed to be disposable. Parallel developments are in hand to produce a similar sized CO_2 electrode. Bedside mass spectrometers are now available for the continuous monitoring of respiratory gas tensions and blood-gas tensions (Wald et al., 1970).

In intensive care situations, a knowledge of a patient's pH, PCO_2 and PO_2 may be required at short notice, to ensure a high degree of reliability, the electrode systems should be always left in the standby position with the water baths at body temperature and calibration gases and buffers available. Only a limited number of experienced staff should use the equipment. They can report to the technician-in-charge if there appears to be any change in its performance.

The availability in intensive care units of on-line terminals connected to hospital computer systems is stimulating the development of interactive computer programs aimed at providing management guidelines in the care of patients suffering from acute respiratory failure (Menn et al., 1973). As an example, for a given type of ventilator, the program will recommend a suitable inspired oxygen concentration and suggest the settings which should enable this to be achieved. The program will also look at the tidal volume, respiratory rate and mechanical deadspace and suggest the tidal volume and rate required for an optimal carbon dioxide elimination. Advice can also be given as to whether the patient's condition is such that it is likely to be capable of being weaned from the ventilator. Maas et al. (1972) describe a program for the calculation of the acid base parameters of blood samples which can be run on a minicomputer in the intensive care unit.

Fibre optic oximeters

Reflection type oximeters are now available based on a No. 5 or No. 7 French fibre optic cardiac catheter, containing three separate bundles of fibres (Johnson et al., 1971). One bundle transmits light at 685 nm from a gallium–arsenide–phosphide light emitting diode and the other light at 920 nm from a gallium–arsenide diode. The diodes are pulsed alternately at 200 Hz. The third bundle returns light reflected from the blood to a silicon photodiode and ratio circuit which continuously displays on a recorder the ratio of the reflected intensities at 920 nm and 685 nm. The oxygen saturation is given by the equation:

$$\%\ \text{SAT} = A - B(I_{685}/I_{920})$$

where A, B are constants. The oximeter calibration was linear to within $\pm 2.7\%$

and was independent of temperature variations between 20.5 and 37°C and haematocrit variations for haematocrits greater than 40%.

Disposable fibre optics mounted in a Swan–Ganz balloon catheter are now available for this type of oximeter. The catheter can be floated into the main pulmonary artery in order to continuously monitor the mixed venous oxygen saturation. This reflects the efficiency of the cardiac circulation, provided that the arterial oxygen saturation remains sensibly constant (Martin et al., 1973). Normal mixed venous oxygen saturations would be about 70% indicating an adequate cardiac output and tissue perfusion.

Osmometry

An osmometer is useful for the assessment of oliguric states and the state of renal function in shocked patients. It can be employed to measure the urine/plasma osmolality ratio which provides a guide to the instantaneous clearance of sodium ions. Thus an osmometer can assist in the differentiation between oliguria, secondary to dehydration, poor perfusion states and acute renal failure. Modern osmometers require a sample volume of only 0.15 ml and a measurement time of approximately 2 minutes. Measuring ranges of 0–400, 0–800 and 0–1600 mOsm/kg are available.

Body Temperature Measurements

Electronic thermistor thermometers having several probes for the measurement of core and peripheral temperatures are of considerable value in the monitoring of patients in shock. Weil et al. (1972) with patients in shock monitor the rectal, right toe and left toe skin temperatures and the ambient temperature. Some commercial patient monitoring systems now include a temperature difference module. Typically an output signal corresponding to a temperature difference of ± 3°C is available over the range 20–42°C. Temperature probes are now used in conjunction with isolation amplifiers to ensure that leakage currents of any significance in respect of ventricular fibrillation cannot flow via the probe. Jolly and Weil (1969) have shown the temperature of the great toe can provide a useful indication of the severity of shock in patients.

The Measurement of Urine Volume

The monitoring of an adequate urine volume becomes important with patients in shock and a number of devices have been developed for this purpose. In one arrangement, increments of 5 ml of urine are collected in a measuring cell fitted with an air vent and a capacitive detector. When 5 ml has been collected, a signal from the detector causes the cell contents to be pumped to a reservoir and cell filling to recommence. The total volume collected is displayed on a counter in 10 ml steps, and alarms can be given if the urine flow falls below 5 ml in either 10 or 20 minutes. Weil et al. (1972) displayed the urine output over the last 5 minutes and the last hour together with the cumulative urine volume. Meagher et al. (1966) have described a suitable urinometer for monitoring by a digital computer. Sheppard et al. (1968) have employed a digital computer in a closed loop mode in selected patients to automatically infuse a suitable diuretic agent when the urine output fell below a pre-set limit.

The Monitoring of Cerebral Function

Particularly in patients with hypovolaemic shock, the possibility exists of an inadequate cerebral perfusion and consequent loss of cerebral function. Prior et al. (1971) have reported on a simple cerebral function monitor which gives a continuous recording of the mean amplitude and variation of the cerebral activity in the range 2–15 Hz, the EEG activity being picked up from two silver–silver chloride electrodes attached to the parietal regions on both sides of the head. Schwartz et al. (1973) discuss the application of the cerebral function monitor.

The Detection of Trends in a Patient's Condition

Patients in marked shock are likely to be in an unstable state and some means are required for reliably indicating trends in their individually monitored physiological variables and the combination of these trends into some form of patient condition index. The subject is well discussed by Taylor (1971). Using bedside analogue circuitry, he produced an indication of both short and long-term trends in a particular variable based on an exponentially smoothed version of the signal for comparison purposes. Hope et al. (1973) using an on-line computer system calculated a so-called patient condition factor using exponential smoothing and Trigg's (1964) tracking signal. The patient condition factor takes into account the mean value for the variable concerned and the upper and lower limits set for it by the physician. Digital computers are also being applied to provide a discriminant analysis of the measured variables of patients in shock, e.g. age, diastolic pressure, mean venous pressure, cardiac index, plasma volume and lactate levels, with the aim of calculating the patient's probability of survival. Warner (1970) has described a computer generated data-trend and bargraph display for patient monitoring.

References

Albisser, A.M., Jackman, W.S., Pask, B.A. and Lutz, C.G. (1971): Atraumatic electrodes for cardiac monitoring. *J. Ass. Advanc. med. Instrum., 5*, 73.

Baker, L.E. and Hill, D.W. (1969): The use of electrical impedance techniques for the monitoring of respiratory pattern during anaesthesia. *Brit. J. Anaesth., 41*, 2.

Boocock, G., Swindler, M.R.M. and Tidswell, B.M. (1971): An automated gas meter. *J. sci. Instrum., 4*, 611.

Border, J.R. (1971): Changes in cardiopulmonary function in the severely stressed patient. In: *Septic Shock in Man*, p. 239. Editors: S.L. Hershey, L.R.M. Del Guercio and Rita McConn. Little, Brown, Boston.

Buggs, H., Johnson, Jr. P.E., Gordon, L.S., Balguma, F.B. and Wettach, G.E. (1973): Comparison of systolic arterial blood pressure by transcutaneous doppler probe and conventional methods in hypotensive patients. *Anaesth. Analg. Curr. Res., 52*, 776.

Cherrick, G.R., Stein, S.W., Leevy, C.M. and Davidson, C.S. (1960): Indocyanine green: observations on its physical properties, plasma decay and hepatic extraction. *J. clin. Invest., 39*, 592.

Cowell, T.K. and Bray, D.G. (1970): Measuring the heart's output. *Electron. Power, 14*, 150.

Cox, J.R., Jr., Nolle, F.M. and Arthur, R.M. (1972): Digital analysis of the electroencephalogram, the blood pressure wave and the electrocardiogram. *Proc. I.E.E.E. (New York), 60*, 1137.

David, R.M. and Portnoy, W.M. (1972): Insulated electrocardiography electrodes. *Med. biol. Engng, 10*, 742.

Ellis, R.J., Gold, J., Rees, J.R. and Lillehet, C.W. (1972): Computerised monitoring of cardiac output by thermal dilution. *J. Amer. med. Ass., 220*, 507.

Falsetti, H.L., Mates, R.E., Carroli, R.J., Gupta, R.L. and Bell, A.C. (1974): Analysis and correction of pressure wave distortion in fluid-filled catheter systems. *Circulation, 69*, 165.

Feldman, C.L., Amazeen, P.G., Klein, M.D. and Lown, B. (1971): Computer detection of ventricular ectopic beats. *Computers biomed. Res., 3*, 666.

Fox, I.J. and Wood, E.H. (1957): Application of dilution curves recorded from the right side of the heart or venous circulation with the aid of a new indicator dye. *Proc. Mayo Clin., 32*, 541.

Gardner, R.M., Warner, H.R., Toronto, A.F. and Gaisford, W.C. (1970): Catheter-flush system for continuous monitoring of central arterial pulse waveform. *J. appl. Physiol., 29*, 911.

Gil-Rodriguez, J.A., Hill, D.W., Horny, J.R., Lundberg, S. and Wilcock, A.H. (1970): A comparison of some methods for estimating the area under a dye dilution curve. *Brit. J. Anaesth.*, *42*, 981.

Grandjean, T. and Perret, C. (1970): Long-term monitoring of the arterial blood pressure. In: *Patient Monitoring*, pp. 90–95. Editors: F.J. Crul and J.P. Payne. Excerpta Medica, Amsterdam.

Guyton, A.C. and Crowell, J.W. (1964): Cardiac deterioration in shock: its progressive nature. In: *Shock*, pp. 1–11. Editor: S.G. Hershey. Little Brown, Boston.

Guyton, A.C. and Jones, C.E. (1973): Central venous pressure: physiological significance and clinical implications. *Amer. Heart J.*, *86*, 431.

Hetzel, P.S., Swan, H.J.C., De Arellano, A.A.R. and Wood, E.M. (1958): Estimation of cardiac output from first part of arterial dye-dilution curves. *J. appl. Physiol.*, *13*, 92.

Hill, D.W. and Tilsley, C. (1973): A comparative study of the performance of five commercial blood-gas and pH electrode systems. *Brit. J. Anaesth.*, *45*, 647.

Hill, D.W., Valentinuzzi, M.E., Pate, T. and Thompson, F.D. (1973): The use of a compartmental hypothesis for the evaluation of cardiac output from dye-dilution curves and the analysis of radiocardiograms. *Med. biol. Engng*, *11*, 43.

Hope, C.E., Lewis, C.D., Perry, I.R. and Gamble, A. (1973): Computed trend analysis in automated patient monitoring systems. *Brit. J. Anaesth.*, *44*, 440.

Johnson, C.C., Palm, R.D. and Stewart, D.C. (1971): A solid state fibre optics oximeter. *J. Ass. Advanc. med. Instrum.*, *5*, 77.

Jolly, H.R. and Weil, M.H. (1969): Temperature of the great toe as an indication of the severity of shock. *Circulation*, *39*, 131.

Klee, G., Ackerman, E. and Leonard, A. (1974): Computer detection of distortion in arterial pressure signals. *I.E.E.E. Trans biomed. Eng.*, *BME-21*, 73.

Lagow, C.H., Sladek, H.J. and Richardson, P.C. (1971): Anodic insulated tantalum oxide electrocardiogram electrodes. *I.E.E.E. Trans. biomed. Eng.*, *MBE-15*, 162.

Lunn, J.N. and Hillard, E.K. (1970): The effect of repairs on the performance of the Wright respirometer. *Brit. J. Anaesth.*, *42*, 1127.

Maas, A.H.J., Kreuger, J.A., Hoelen, A.J. and Visser, B.F. (1972): A computer program for calculating the acid base parameters in samples of blood using a minicomputer. *Pfung. Arch. Europ. J. Physiol.*, *334*, 264.

Martin, W.E., Cheung, P.W., Johnson, C.C. and Wong, K.C. (1973): Continuous monitoring of mixed venous oxygen saturation in man. *Anaesth. Analg. Curr. Res.*, *52*, 784.

Meade, F. and Owen-Thomas, J.B. (1973): A paramagnetic method for measurement of the carbon dioxide content of a gas mixture. *Proc. physiol. Soc. (Lond).*, *234*, 12.

Meagher, P.F., Jensen, R.E., Pearcy, M.G., Weil, M.H. and Shubin, H. (1966): Automated urinometer for on-line monitoring of patients with circulatory shock. *Med. Res. Eng.*, *5*, 38.

Meldrum, S.J., Watson, B.W. and Becker, G.A. (1973): A catheter tip transducer for continuous measurement of blood oxygen tension in neonates. *Bio-med. Engng*, *8*, 470.

Menn, S.J., Barnett, G.O., Schmechel, D., Owens, W.D. and Pontoppidan, H. (1973): A computer program to assist in the care of acute respiratory failure. *J. Amer. med. Ass.*, *223*, 308.

Parker, D., Key, A., Scopes, J.W. and Marcovitch, H. (1971): A disposable catheter-tip transducer for continuous measurement of blood oxygen tension in vivo. *Bio-med. Engng*, *6*, 313.

Prior, Pamela, F., Maynard, D.E., Sheaff, P.C., Simpson, B.R., Strunin, L., Weaver, E.J.M. and Scott, D.F. (1971): Monitoring cerebral function: clinical experience with new devices for continuous recording of electrical activity of the brain. *Brit. med. J.*, *2*, 736.

Raison, J.C.A., Beaumont, J.O., Russell, J.A.G., Osborn, J.J. and Gerbode, F. (1968): Alarms in an intensive care unit: an interim compromise. *Computers biomed. Res.*, *1*, 556.

Raison, J.C.A. (1971): Respiratory measurements in acutely ill patients: a new system for study. In: *Septic Shock in Man*, pp. 59–68. Editors: S.L. Hershey, L.R.M. Del Cuercio and Rita McConn. Little Brown, Boston.

Roberts, V.C. (1969): An analogue computer for thermal dilution flow measurement. *Med. biol. Engng*, *7*, 373.

Schwartz, M.S., Collin, M.P., Prior, Pamela, F., Strunin, L., Simpson, B.R., Weaver, E.J.M. and Scott, D.F. (1973): The cerebral function monitor: its use for predicting the neurological outcome in patients undergoing cardio-pulmonary by-pass. *Anaesthesia, 28*, 611.

Sheppard, L.C., Kouchoukos, N.T., Kurtts, M.A. and Kirklin, J.W. (1968): Automated treatment of critically ill patients following operation. *Ann. Surg., 168*, 596.

Shoemaker, W.C. (1967): *Shock – Chemistry, Physiology and Therapy*. Thomas, Springfield, Ill.

Shoemaker, W.C., Prirten, K.J., Amato, J.J., Monson, D.O. and Carey, J.S. (1967): Hemodynamic patterns after acute anaesthetized and unanaesthetized trauma. *Arch. Surg.(Chicago), 95*, 492.

Shoemaker, W.C., Montgomery, E.S., Kaplan, E. and Elwyn, D.H. (1973): Physiolgical patterns in surviving and non-surviving shock patients. *Arch. Surg. (Chicago), 106*, 630.

Shubin, H., Weil, M.H. and Rockwell, M.A. Jr. (1967): Automated measurement of cardiac output in patients by the use of a digital computer. *Med. electron. biol. Eng., 5*, 353.

Siegal, J.H., Greenspan, M. and Del Guercio, L.R.M. (1967): Abnormal vascular tone, defective oxygen transport and myocardial failure in human septic shock. *Ann. Surg., 165*, 504.

Siegal, J.H., Greenspan, M., Cohn, J.D. and Del Guercio, L.R.M. (1968): A bedside computer and physiological nomograms: guides to the management of the patients in shock. *Arch. Surg. (Chicago), 97*, 480.

Siegal, J.H., Goldwyn, R.M. and Del Guercio, L.R.M. (1971): Patterns of cardiovascular response in septic shock. In: *Septic Shock in Man*, pp. 239–251. Editors: S.L. Hershey, L.R.M. Del Guercio and Rita McConn. Little Brown, Boston.

Starmer, C.F., McHale, P.A., Cobb, F.R. and Greenfield, Jr., J.C. (1973): Evaluation of several methods for computing stroke volume from central aortic pressure. *Circulat. Res., 33*, 139.

Stern, R.M. (1974): Ear lobe photo plethysmography. *Psychophysiology, 11*, 73.

Sullivan, F.J., Mroz, E.A. and Miller, R.E. (1973): Electronic calibration of indocyanine green dye-dilution curves. *Amer. Heart J., 85*, 506.

Sutterer, W.F. and Wood, E.H. (1962): A compensated dichromatic densitometer for indocyanine green. *I.E.E.E. Trans., BME-13*, 200.

Tahir, A. and Adriani, J. (1973): Usefulness of the ultrasonic technique of blood-pressure determination. *Anaesth. Analg., 52*, 699.

Taylor, D.E.M. (1971): Computer assisted patient monitoring systems. *Biomed. Engng, 6*, 560.

Thorburn, G.D. (1961): Estimation of cardiac output from forward part of indicator dilution curves. *J. appl. Physiol., 16*, 891.

Trigg, D.W. (1964): Monitoring a forecasting system. *Operational Res. Quarterly, 15*, 271.

Wald, A., Hass, W.K., Siew, F.P. and Wood, D.H. (1970): Continuous measurement of blood gases in vivo by mass spectrography. *Med. biol. Engng, 8*, 111.

Warner, H.R. (1970): A data-trend log and bargraph display for physiological monitoring. *Comput. biomed. Res., 3*, 285.

Warner, H.R. (1972): A computer based information system for patient care. In: *Hospital Information Systems*, pp. 293–332. Editors: G.A. Bekey and M.D. Schwartz. Marcel Dekker, New York.

Weil, M.H. and Shubin, H. (1971): Hemodynamic mechanisms of septic shock. In: *Septic Shock in Man*, pp. 219–230. Editors: S.G. Hershey, L.R.M. Del Guercio and Rita McConn. Little Brown, Boston.

Weil, M.H., Shubin, H., Cady, Jr., L.D., Carrington, H., Palley, N. and Martin, R. (1972): Use of automated techniques in the management of the critically ill. In: *Hospital Information Systems*, pp. 333–381. Editors: G.A. Bekey and M.D. Schwartz. Marcel Dekker, New York.

Wilson, E.M., Ranieri, Jr. A.J., Updike, O.L. and Dammann, J.F. (1972): An evaluation of thermal dilution for obtaining serial measurements of cardiac output. *Med. biol. Engng, 10*, 179.

Wright, B.M. (1955): A respiratory anemometer. *J. Physiol. (Lond.), 127*, 25P.

Ledingham (ed.). Shock

Disseminated intravascular coagulation

P. OLSSON

The numerous and complex problems associated with disseminated intravascular coagulation (DIC) are frequently encountered by the clinician treating severely ill patients. The significance of DIC and the difficulties involved in understanding its pathogenesis and treatment may be judged by the vast literature on the subject. Each specialist views the syndrome in the light of his own particular interest. The haematologist, for example, describes the trigger mechanisms of plasma coagulation and consequent activation of fibrinolysis, while the pathologist mainly interests himself in the occurrence of fibrin formation and emboli in the microvasculature. The following text is intended primarily for the clinician, who wishes to recognise DIC at an early stage and, if possible, to find ways and means of treating the disease before it becomes the fatal complication of a critical illness.

Pathogenesis and Pathophysiological Findings

According to the classical theory, DIC is a pathological process produced by extensive thrombin generation in the systemic blood. Platelets and coagulation factors are consumed by the circulating thrombin. The result is that bleeding occurs and small vessels are obstructed by platelet aggregates and fibrin, in turn leading to multiple necrosis and organ dysfunction (Hardaway, 1966; McKay, 1965; Robb, 1963). Thus, it is obvious that diagnosis of the disease is often confirmed at autopsy. The formation of fibrin is, however, the final phase in the coagulation process and is preceded by a number of reactions which may induce specific pathophysiological changes detectable at an early stage in the disease.

According to current opinion, haemostasis at the site of a vascular lesion takes place in the following manner. The exposed collagen initiates adhesion and aggregation of platelets. The platelets react with the release of adenosine diphosphate and platelet factor 3. The former accelerates the aggregation and release-reaction of the platelets. Platelet factor 3 – a lipid factor – triggers plasma coagulation and thrombin is finally generated. The thrombin further accelerates platelet aggregation and transforms fibrinogen to fibrin. A firm haemostatic plug of platelets and fibrin is then formed at the site of the vascular lesion. In order to prevent the process from developing into a vicious circle with total intravascular thrombus formation as a result, inhibitory mechanisms must be present. Antithrombin in plasma inactivates circulating thrombin. The fibrinolytic mechanism is activated secondarily or simultaneously with the coagulation mechanism and the fibrin formed in the circulation is digested. It may be assumed for teleological reasons that an inhibitory mechanism exists between the platelet release-reaction and the activation of plasma coagulation.

Activation of the haemostatic process in systemic blood must comprise all these components, irrespective of the nature of the trigger mechanism, although some of them may be suppressed. Aggregation and release of platelets alone, when occurring in excess of normal and accompanied by the release-reaction in circulating blood, represent a broader interpretation of DIC. Platelet aggregation can be achieved by many factors apart from adenosine diphosphate, collagen and thrombin, e.g., antigen–antibody complexes, endotoxin, epinephrine, fatty acids, foreign surfaces, trypsin and decreased pH. The effects of platelet aggregation with the associated release-reaction and plasma coagulation must obviously be considered separately when studying the pathophysiological sequelae of DIC.

In man the first 24–28 hours after a traumatic or shock episode are frequently associated with progressive changes in lung function, i.e. increased respiratory effort, decreased arterial oxygen tension and elevated pulmonary vascular resistance. During a later stage, when the patient manifests severe respiratory insufficiency, X-ray examination reveals scattered lung infiltrates which tend to coalesce. This condition is named ‘shock lung’, ‘fat embolism’, ‘white lung syndrome’, ‘respiratory lung’, etc. Respiratory distress syndrome (RDS) has been suggested as a general term (Ashbaugh et al., 1969; Blaisdale et al., 1970; Blaisdale and Schlobohm, 1973). The presence of micro-emboli on histological examination has suggested a relationship between RDS and DIC and much experimental work has been devoted to investigating the significance of platelet aggregation and intravascular fibrin formation in the pathogenesis of these conditions.

In the dog, infusion of a dose of thrombin large enough to cause a substantial decrease in fibrinogen or even complete defibrinogenation results in increased airway resistance, elevated pulmonary vascular resistance (Olsson et al., 1970; Rådegran, 1972; Rådegran et al., 1972) and transient platelet and fibrin deposition in the lungs (Bergentz et al., 1972; Busch et al., 1973; Busch, 1974). If the animals are treated with inhibitors of fibrinolysis, the changes in respiratory variables, e.g., diminished lung-compliance, decreased arterial oxygen tension, increased base excess, will be more long-lasting and the pulmonary microscopic appearances similar to that seen at autopsy in patients with fatal RDS (Arfors et al., 1972). The functional state of the fibrinolytic mechanism is thus of the utmost importance in preventing permanent deposition of fibrin in the pulmonary vasculature (Saldeen, 1966; Bergentz et al., 1972). It would also seem to be of importance in the clinical situation. Inhibition of fibrinolysis is frequently seen in patients following trauma (Borowiechi and Sharp, 1969; Innes and Sevitt, 1964; Lilienberg et al., 1970). The development of fatal RDS has been associated with insufficient fibrinolytic capacity (Rammer and Saldeen, 1970). At this end-stage of DIC, all the pulmonary changes can be attributed to mechanical obstruction of the pulmonary blood vessels, which in fact act as the filter for all fibrin and cell-aggregates formed on the venous side of the circulation.

A slow thrombin-induced depletion of fibrinogen and platelets in the dog without inhibition of fibrinolysis results mainly in an increased ventilatory pressure. The microscopic picture is then characterized by numerous micro-atelectases, but there is no fibrin in the lungs (Olsson et al., 1974). The findings indicate that alterations in the terminal airways may occur in states of DIC.

Studies on rapidly induced platelet aggregation in animals have revealed the importance of platelets in the development of respiratory dysfunction. A brief intravenous infusion of thrombin in the dog gives rise to increased pulmonary vascular resistance, elevated airway resistance and diminished arterial oxygen tension. Simultaneously, there is a reduction of platelets and fibrinogen in the circulating blood. The result, however, is qualitatively and quantitatively the same when the experiments are performed on reptilase-defibrinogenated animals (Rådegran et al., 1972). Thus, the formation of circulating fibrin is not a major aetiological factor in the pulmonary changes.

Rapidly induced intravascular platelet aggregation by agents other than thrombin, e.g., protamine (Rådegran et al., 1971a, b; Rådegran and McAslan, 1972), adenosine diphosphate (Vaage et al., 1974b), collagen (Bø and Hognestad, 1972; Vaage et al., 1974a, b) or antiplatelet serum (Vaage et al., 1974a), elicit identical changes. The pulmonary response to thrombin and protamine-induced platelet aggregation is completely abolished when the animal is given acetylsalicylic acid before the platelet challenge (Fig. 1). The decrease in platelet count in the circulating blood and accumulation of platelets in the lung, however, remain the same as prior to treatment with acetylsalicylic acid (Rådegran et al., 1971a; Rådegran, 1972; Rådegran and McAslan, 1972; Rådegran et al., 1972). The conclusions to be drawn from such experiments are that platelet aggregates per se do not mechanically obstruct the pulmonary vessels and that platelets in intact functional state are a prerequisite for the production of pulmonary reaction.

The haemodynamic and ventilatory changes during this initial phase of DIC can be explained only on the assumption that smooth muscle stimulating mechanisms are active. The increased pulmonary vascular resistance must therefore be caused by vascular constriction. Micro-angiographic studies following induced platelet aggregation indicate increased tone in precapillary vessels and constriction of small intrapulmonary veins seems to result from endotoxin (Alho et al., 1971; Stein and Thomas, 1967), collagen (Vaage et al., 1974a), protamine and thrombin (Rådegran et al., 1974) induced platelet aggregation. The latter observation explains the reported increase of pulmonary blood volume at the peak of the pulmonary response (Vaage et al., 1974a) and the congestion of the lungs (Rådegran and McAslan, 1972) following induced platelet aggregation. The increased airway resistance depends on reduction in dynamic lung compliance and pulmonary resistance, which indicates that both larger and smaller airways are constricted (Rådegran and McAslan, 1972; Vaage et al., 1974b). There is a slow return to normal of all the variables after the peak pulmonary response. Hyperinsufflation of the lungs during this period, however, will immediately restore the changes to the initial levels, especially lung compliance and pulmonary resistance (Fig. 1). Simultaneously, the decreased arterial oxygen tension, which is due to intrapulmonary arteriovenous shunting through micro-atelectases, returns to normal – an indication of recruitment of terminal airspaces (Rådegran, 1972; Rådegran and McAslan, 1972; Vaage et al., 1974a).

The pharmacologically active compounds released from platelets are believed to include adenosine diphosphate, adenosine triphosphate, histamine, serotonin and possibly a hitherto unidentified substance which stimulates smooth muscle and increases vascular permeability (Packham et al., 1968).

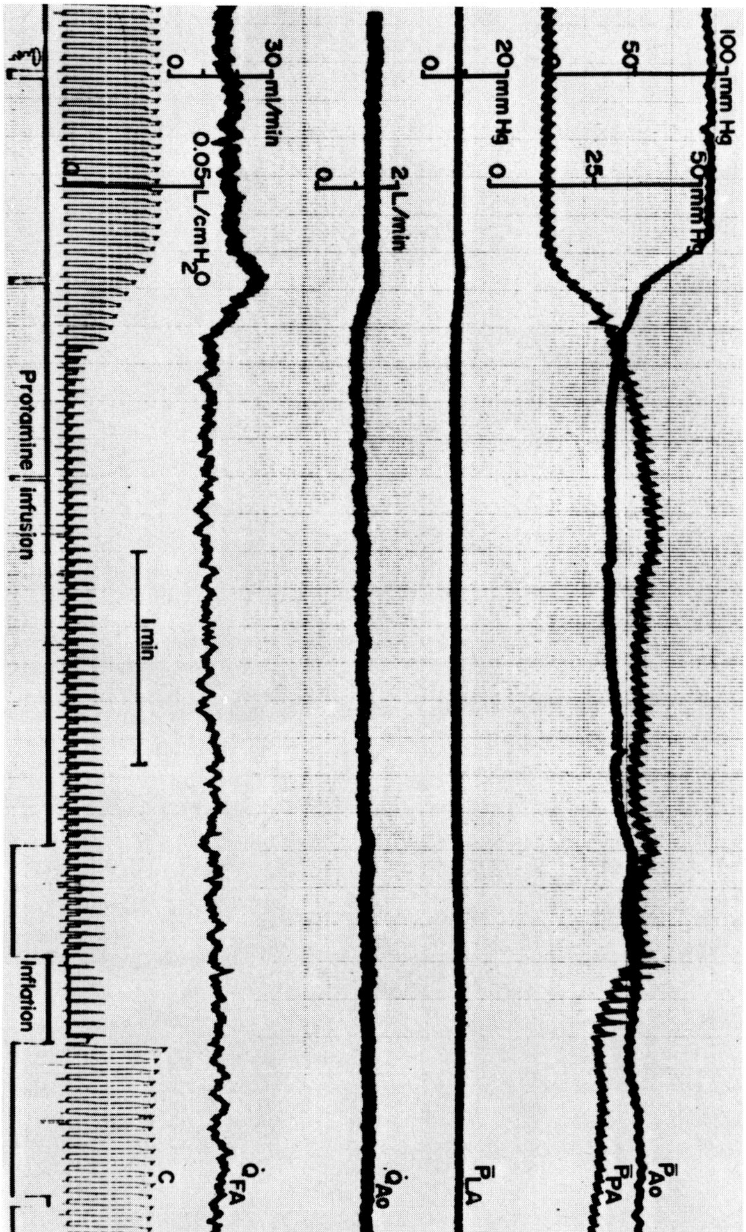
100 mm Hg
50
50 mm Hg
25
20 mm Hg
0
0
2 L/min
0
30 ml/min
0.05 L/cm H2O
0
Protamine infusion
1 min
Inflation
$\bar{P}_{Ao}$
$\bar{P}_{PA}$
$\bar{P}_{LA}$
$\dot{Q}_{Ao}$
$\dot{Q}_{FA}$
C

Fig. 1a.

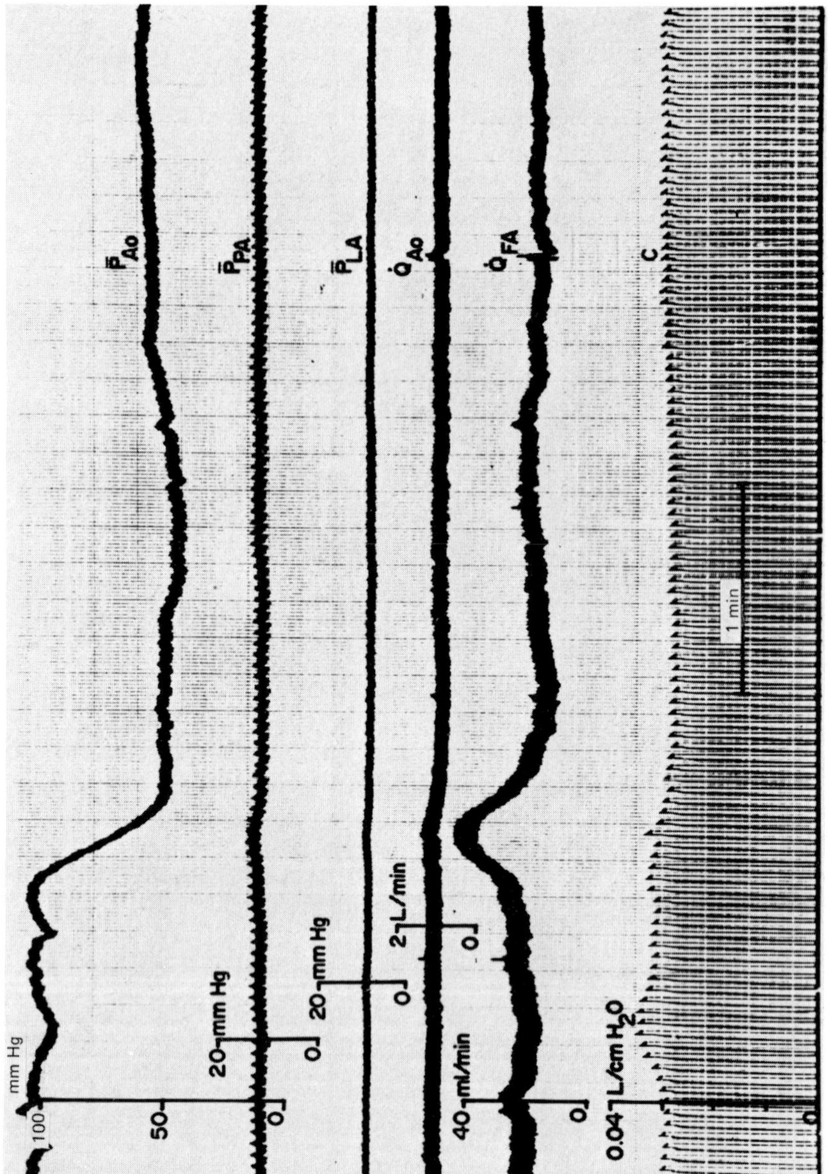

mm Hg
100
50
0
20 mm Hg
0
20 mm Hg
0
2 L/min
0
40 ml/min
0
0.04 L/cm H_2O
0
$\bar{P}_{Ao}$
$\bar{P}_{PA}$
$\bar{P}_{LA}$
$\dot{Q}_{Ao}$
$\dot{Q}_{FA}$
C
1 min

Fig. 1b.

The platelet release reaction is further linked with the synthesis of prostaglandin E_2 and $F_2\alpha$ (Smith and Willis, 1971).

Some authors regard adenosine diphosphate and adenosine triphosphate as pulmonary vasoconstrictors and adenosine diphosphate has been reported to be a bronchodilator in low concentrations and constrictor in high concentrations. Large amounts of adenosine diphosphate are also reported to decrease compliance of the lung and increase resistance to gas flow. In the dog, infusion of adenosine diphosphate and adenosine triphosphate in concentrations that could be expected to be released from platelets, causes a decrease in pulmonary vascular resistance, probably as a passive effect of an increase in cardiac output with recruitment of closed capillary channels (Swedenborg et al., 1971). Histamine is present only in minute amounts in canine and human platelets and may therefore be of negligible importance in these species. Similarly, serotonin does not seem to be an essential mediator of the pulmonary response, although in the dog it causes an increase in pulmonary vascular resistance when infused in physiological concentrations (Rådegran et al., 1971a; Rådegran, 1972), and in the rabbit both serotonin and histamine seem to contribute to the decrease in arterial oxygen tension following thrombin infusion (Groth, 1966). Prostaglandin E_2 dilates bronchi (Said, 1967) and thus exerts an effect quite different from that of a sudden platelet release reaction. $F_2\alpha$, however, causes an increase in both airway resistance and pulmonary vascular resistance which is at least partly due to constriction of intrapulmonary veins (Said, 1967). It is, therefore, possible that prostaglandin $F_2\alpha$ is the mediator of the pulmonary reaction to platelet aggregation. Recent experiments in this laboratory have demonstrated an increased plasma level of prostaglandin metabolites concomitant with the pulmonary response to protamine and thrombin-induced platelet aggregation. After administration of acetylsalicylic acid, the levels of both prostaglandin metabolites and pulmonary function remain unchanged in the dog. It is known that the synthesis of prostaglandin is inhibited by acetylsalicylic acid (Smith and Willis, 1971; Vane, 1971). The prostaglandin appearing in plasma after platelet challenge may originate from lung tissue as a consequence of the effect of platelet aggregates on the pulmonary blood vessels. It has been demonstrated that micro-embolization of the lungs with artificial material releases prostaglandin (Piper and Vane, 1971). On the other hand, similar experiments on platelet-free animals give rise to a very weak pulmonary reaction (Bø et al., 1974; Thomas et al., 1965), suggesting that the prostaglandin synthetised by the platelets themselves is of importance.

A number of laboratory models have been designed to reproduce the clinical situations in which DIC might be involved. These experimental studies have shown that accumulation of platelets and fibrin in the lungs occurs after trauma (Berman et al., 1971; Ljungquist et al., 1971; Saldeen, 1966a, b), endotoxin shock (Alho et al., 1971; Kuida et al., 1958) and haemorrhagic shock (Allardyce et al., 1969). Concomitantly there is a rise in pulmonary vascular resistance, apparently due to both pre- and postcapillary vascular constriction, and the lungs become congested and red (Alho et al., 1971; Buckberg et al., 1970; Cook and Webb, 1968; Kuida et al., 1958). During haemorrhagic shock there is increased ventilatory work, due to increases in respiratory rate, ventilatory pressure and arteriovenous shunting (Cook and Webb, 1968; Wahrenbrock et al., 1970).

In man, trauma, shock and surgical interventions which cause intravascular coagulation activity also occasion respiratory dysfunction (Webb, 1969). The former is recognised by reduced platelet count, elevated or diminished fibrinogen, consumption of prothrombin and factor V and an increase in degradation products in the circulating blood (Attar et al., 1966; Godal, 1962; Olow, 1963; Pepper and Lindsay, 1960; String et al., 1971). The latter takes the form of decreased functional residual capacity, increased arteriovenous shunting in the lungs and reduced arterial oxygen tension (McLaughlin et al., 1969; Powers et al., 1972; Wilson et al., 1969, 1970). During a standardized orthopaedic surgical procedure, it has been demonstrated that accumulation of platelets and fibrin in the lungs and increased thromboplastic activity in pulmonary arterial blood occur at the same time as arterial oxygen tension diminishes (Modig et al., 1974). Studies in patients with fractures have also shown that the alveolar–arterial oxygen difference increases in proportion to the decrease in platelets (Bradford et al., 1970; McCarthy et al., 1973). The similarity between the respiratory disturbances following rapidly induced platelet aggregation and experimental and clinical trauma and shock thus provides strong evidence that the platelet-release reaction in DIC may be one of the factors initiating RDS.

DIC with intravascular fibrin formation in the kidneys has been considered a cause of posttraumatic renal insufficiency (Hardaway, 1966; McKay, 1965). In cases of acute renal failure, renal biopsies frequently reveal deposits of fibrin with aggregated and disintegrated platelets in the glomerular capillaries (Clarkson et al., 1970). Furthermore, excretion of high molecular fibrin degradation products has been found regularly in such patients (Larsson et al., 1971). Inhibition of the fibrinolytic system in animals delays the elimination of intravascular fibrin after infusion of thrombin (Bergentz et al., 1972; Busch et al., 1973), and in patients with acute renal failure inhibition of the fibrinolytic system is a frequent finding (Larsson et al., 1971; Wardle and Taylor, 1968). It is also reported that treatment with inhibitors of fibrinolysis during DIC may cause renal damage (Naye, 1962). It is not known, however, whether fibrin deposition in the kidney is the primary cause of posttraumatic renal insufficiency. In rats with thermal injuries, impaired renal failure function, as measured by glomerular filtration rate, showed no connection with the plasma coagulation disturbance (Rammer, 1973). It is, however, apparent that primary renal vasoconstriction occurs in DIC. Infusion of thrombin in small amounts into the renal artery of the dog gives rise to increased vascular resistance in the renal circulation and decreased urinary output. These changes will not occur if a vasodilator, such as bradykinin, is simultaneously infused with the thrombin (Rådegran et al., 1970). Defibrinogenated animals with a normal platelet count will respond in the same way. Fibrin deposition in the kidney is perhaps a sequel of vasospasm. It can be demonstrated that renal denervation and α-blocking agents protect against renal cortical necrosis provoked by DIC secondary to the Schwartzman reaction (Fine et al., 1959; Palmerio et al., 1962). The substance responsible for the vascular constriction in the kidney has not hitherto been identified. The incidence of posttraumatic renal insufficiency seems to have decreased during the last decade, presumably due to more adequate fluid therapy. The mechanism by which the maintenance of a good diuresis might protect the kidney against DIC is as yet unknown.

The possible involvement of blood vessels elsewhere in the body in DIC is also illustrated by experimental studies. Infusion of thrombin into the femoral artery causes vasodilatation in the vessels of the leg. The substance mediating this effect seems to be adenosine diphosphate released from the platelets at the site of thrombin-induced platelet aggregation (Olsson et al., 1969; Swedenborg, 1970). Intra-aortic or intravenous thrombin will result in an initial fall and a later rise in total peripheral resistance (Olsson et al., 1970). The initial reaction may be ascribed to the release of adenosine diphosphate and the latter to compensatory mechanisms. Intra-arterial infusion of thrombin also causes vasodilatation in the area supplied by the superior mesenteric artery (Høie and Schenk, 1972) and, following intravenous thrombin infusions, vasodilatation in the coronary circulation has been observed (Høie and Schenk, 1971). The mechanisms underlying these latter reactions have not been clarified and the clinical importance of the findings is unknown. The reactions, however, further demonstrate the complexity of the pathophysiological sequelae of DIC.

Diagnosis

The initial changes in platelet count and coagulation factors after trauma or surgery may be regarded as a natural consequence of injury, irrespective of whether the changes represent a transient phase of DIC or a local consumption of coagulation factors on a large wound surface. The development of the full-blown syndrome of DIC is due either to sustained activation of platelets or plasma coagulation or to the fact that the mechanisms counteracting DIC are inactive. The former may result from the presence in the circulation of endotoxin, fat emboli or fatty acids or from increased thromboplastic activity. The latter may relate to the observation that patients who develop a fulminant RDS or posttraumatic renal insufficiency often have inhibition of fibrinolysis. Otherwise, it would appear that the significance of the inhibitory mechanisms in the progression of DIC have not been studied.

Analysis of the coagulation profile in a posttraumatic, postoperative or septicaemic patient with a bleeding tendency, multiple thromboses and functional organ disturbances, i.e., the classical indications of DIC, will very probably show low platelet count, low concentrations of fibrinogen, prothrombin, factors V and VIII, increased level of fibrin degradation products and the presence of fibrin monomers in the circulating blood. Confirmation of the diagnosis at this stage is belated.

An early diagnosis of DIC, as distinct from the inevitable non-specific initial changes in platelets and coagulation factors after injury, can best be made on the basis of regular frequent examination of the haematological disturbances. The interpretation of the results may be influenced by the fact that the patient in this situation has most probably received blood with varying amounts of platelets and coagulation factors. However, a reduction and perhaps later a prolongation of activated partial thromboplastin time, continued decrease of platelets, fibrinogen, prothrombin, factors V and VIII and increase of fibrin degradation products indicate DIC. The formation of fibrin degradation products may not take place if there is endogenous inhibition of fibrinolysis or if the patient has been treated with fibrinolytic inhibitors. Fibrin formation in the circulating blood can be quickly established by precipitation of fibrin monomers with ethanol (ethanol gelation test) (Godal and Abildgaard, 1966). An even more sensitive method for determination of intravascular fibrin formation is the radio-immune assay of fibrinopeptide A (Nossel et al., 1974). Positive findings in these tests confirm the diagnosis of DIC in respect of plasma coagulation. However, fibrin monomers are apparently eliminated swiftly from the blood through the reticulo-endothelial system (Lee, 1962) and fibrinopeptide A has a biological half-life of only 3–5 minutes.

If activation of DIC takes place intermittently, negative results do not therefore rule out the presence of DIC. Furthermore, the ethanol gelation test is difficult and must be performed carefully under well standardized conditions.

The assay of fibrinopeptide A is time-consuming and cannot be used at present for therapeutic guidance.

Current methods do not allow easy recognition of an isolated pathological platelet release-reaction in systemic blood. A rapid method for measuring a release product from the platelets would perhaps be of real clinical value. Platelet factor 4, which is liberated during the release-reaction has been shown to increase in plasma following induced low-grade intravascular coagulation in animals (Fuster et al., 1974) as well as in humans with various intravascular coagulation syndromes (Fuster et al., 1972).

An adequate indication of activation of circulating platelets, however, may simply be the above-mentioned respiratory changes. The injured, postoperative or critically ill patient, who develops respiratory dysfunction in the form of increased respiratory effort and lowered arterial oxygen tension, should be suspected of being in an early stage of DIC and examined and treated accordingly, provided no other definite reason for pulmonary dysfunction exists. Determination of respiration rate, arterial oxygen tension and even alveolar–arterial oxygen difference, together with frequent platelet counts, are simple measures when compared with repeated, time-consuming determinations of coagulation factors. Furthermore, in the initial phase the latter have not undergone changes distinct from those in the uncomplicated post-traumatic or postoperative case.

Treatment

Naturally, immediate efforts should be made to prevent the development of DIC, i.e., long bone fractures should be immobilized, devitalized tissue removed, hypovolaemia corrected, shock and infection combated etc. (Blaisdale and Schlobohm, 1973). When pathologically increased coagulation activity is detected in the circulating blood, it should be arrested by heparin in sufficient doses to prolong activated partial thromboplastin time. However, the dosage necessary to achieve this result may vary considerably, one reason for which may be the release of heparin-neutralizing platelet factor 4. Another reason may be that patients with DIC have varying levels of plasma antithrombin. Heparin exerts its principal anticoagulant effect by activation of a slow thrombin-inhibiting antithrombin (antithrombin III) (Olsson, 1963). In order to maintain activated partial thromboplastin time at the desired level during prolonged heparin therapy for DIC, it is frequently appropriate to keep the heparin dosage constant and supplement it daily with antithrombin III in the form of plasma.

It is clear that heparin therapy involves an added risk of haemorrhage. However, in many cases, this can be regarded as a less serious complication than progressive DIC. If a consumption coagulopathy with generalised bleeding occurs, heparin may even dramatically reduce the bleeding tendency by eliminating fibrinolysis secondary to increased coagulation activity. This fibrinolysis dissolves newly-formed clots and the resultant fibrin degradation products inhibit the haemostatic function of the platelets (Olsson and Johnsson, 1972). Furthermore, heparin inhibits the platelet consumption effect of thrombin and thrombocytopenia can be improved.

It would seem desirable to produce primary inhibition of the platelet release-reaction, particularly when factors other than pathologically increased plasma coagulation activity affect the platelets. Acetylsalicylic acid, dipyridamole, phenylbutazone, indomethacin, sulfinpyrazone and related anti-inflammatory drugs have received much attention as inhibitors of platelet function and may perhaps be used when DIC threatens. Inhibition of the release-reaction, however, involves abolition of the haemostatic function of the platelets. The use of platelet-inhibiting agents is thus contraindicated where there is the least suspicion of acquired plasma coagulopathy. Nevertheless, low molecular weight dextran, because of its effect on the aggregability of the platelets (Bygdeman and Eliasson, 1967), has been employed as an alternative (Blaisdale and Schlobohm, 1973).

The functional respiratory disturbances, which are clearly both early and serious sequelae of DIC, must be counteracted. As previously mentioned, the mechanism of these disturbances is not fully understood and even less is known about appropriate pharmacological treatment in the clinical situation. However, in cases of inadequate lung function after trauma, major surgery and during septicemia, positive pressure ventilation with end-expiratory pressures of 5–15 cm H_2O results in elevated arterial oxygen tension, increased functional residual capacity and improved compliance, all of which indicate the recruitment of terminal airspaces (Ashbaugh et al., 1969; Falke et al., 1972; Pontoppidan et al., 1972). Ventilation with positive end-expiratory pressure is recommended for patients in whom respiratory problems can be anticipated, i.e., after severe trauma, major operations and in critical illness, in order to prevent the development of RDS (Pontippidan et al., 1972). This treatment should be maintained until respiratory function shows substantial improvement (Boyd, 1972; McLaughlin, 1971; Pontoppidan et al., 1972).

The question arises as to whether prevention of the development of RDS by positive end-expiratory pressure ventilation per se stops the further progression of DIC. The literature provides no answer to this question and further experimental and clinical research is clearly necessary to examine the possible relationship between adequate oxygenation and satisfactory haemostatic function.

References

Alho, A., Motsay, G.J. and Lillihei, R.C. (1971): Comparison of lung changes in haemorrhagic and endotoxin shock. *Ann. Chir. Gynaec. Fenn.*, *60*, 202.

Allardyce, B., Hamit, H.F., Matsumuto, T. and Moseley, R.V. (1969): Pulmonary vascular changes in hypovolemic shock: radiography of the pulmonary microcirculation and the possible role of platelet embolism in increasing vascular resistance. *J. Trauma*, *9*, 403.

Arfors, K.E., Busch, C., Jakobson, S., Lindquist, O., Malmberg, P. and Saldeen, T. (1972): Pulmonary insufficiency following intravenous infusion of thrombin and AMCA (tranexamic acid) in the dog. *Acta chir. scand.*, *138*, 445.

Ashbaugh, D.G., Petty, T.L., Bigelow, D.B. and Harris, T.M. (1969): Continuous positive pressure breathing in adult respiratory distress syndrome. *J. thorac. cardiovasc. Surg.*, *57*, 31.

Attar, S., Mansberger, A.R., Irani, B., Kirby, W., Masaitas, C. and Cowley, R.A. (1966): Coagulation changes in clinical shock. II. Effect of septic shock on clotting times and fibrinogen in humans. *Ann. Surg.*, *164*, 41.

Bergentz, S.-E., Ljungqvist, U. and Lewis, D.H. (1972): The distribution of platelets, fibrin and erythrocytes in various organs following thrombin infusions. An experimental study in dogs with and without antifibrinolytic therapy. *Surgery*, *71*, 190.

Berman, I., Smulson, M.E., Pattengale, P. and Schoenback, S.F. (1971): Pulmonary microembolism after soft tissue injury in primates. *Surgery*, *70*, 246.

Blaisdale, F.W., Lim, R.C. and Stallone, R.J. (1970): The mechanism of pulmonary damage following traumatic shock. *Surg. Gynec. Obstet.*, *130*, 15.

Blaisdale, F.W. and Schlobohm, R.M. (1973): The respiratory distress syndrome. A review. *Surgery*, *74*, 251.

Borowiechi, B. and Sharp, A.A. (1969): Trauma and fibrinolysis. *J. Trauma*, *9*, 522.

Boyd, D.R. (1972): Monitoring patients with posttraumatic insuffiency. *Surg. Clin. N. Amer.*, *52*, 31.

Bradford, D.S., Foster, R.R. and Nossel, H.L. (1970): Coagulation alterations, hypoxemia and fat embolism in fractured patients. *J. Trauma*, *10*, 307.

Buckberg, G.D., Lipman, C.A., Hahn, J.A., Smith, M.J. and Hennessen, J.A. (1970): Pulmonary changes following hemorrhagic shock and resuscitation in baboons. *J. thorac. cardiovasc. Surg.*, *59*, 450.

Busch, C. (1974): Quantitative determination of pulmonary microembolism in the dog. *Upsala J. med. Sci.*, *79*, 72.

Busch, C., Lundqvist, H. and Saldeen, T. (1973): Quantitative determination of intravascular coagulation in vivo in various organs in the dog. *Thrombos. diathes. haemorrh. (Stuttg.)*, *29*, 94.

Bygdeman, S. and Eliasson, R. (1967): Effect of dextrans on platelet adhesiveness and aggregation. *Scand. J. clin. Lab. Invest.*, *20*, 17.

Bø, G. and Hognestad, J. (1972): Effects on the pulmonary circulation of suddenly induced intravascular aggregation of blood platelets. *Acta physiol. scand.*, *85*, 523.

Bø, G., Hognestad, J. and Vaage, J. (1974): The role of blood platelets in pulmonary responses to microembolization with barium sulphate. *Acta physiol. scand.*, *90*, 244.

Clarkson, A.R., MacDonald, M.K., Fuster, V., Cash, J.D. and Robson, J.S. (1970): Glomerular coagulation in acute ischemic renal failure. *Quart. J. Med.*, *39*, 585.

Cook, W.-A. and Webb, W.R. (1968): Pulmonary changes in hemorrhagic shock. *Surgery*, *64*, 85.

Falke, K.J., Pontoppidan, H., Kumar, A., Leith, D.E., Geffin, B. and Laver, M.B. (1972): Ventilation with end-expiratory pressure in acute lung disease. *J. clin. Invest., 51*, 2315.

Fine, J., Rutenberg, S. and Schweinburg, F.B. (1959): The role of the reticuloendothelial system in hemorrhagic shock. *J. exp. Med., 110*, 547.

Fuster, V., Bowie E.W.J., Kazmier, F.J. and Owen, C.A. (1974): Platelet consumption in chronically induced plasma platelet factor-4 like activity reflecting rate of intravascular coagulation in dogs. *Thrombos. Res., 4*, 247.

Fuster, V., Cash, J.D., Owen, C.A. and Kazmier, F.J. (1972): Plasma platelet factor-4 in diagnosis of intravascular coagulation. *Third Congress of International Society on Thrombosis and Hemostasis, Washington D.C.*, p. 41.

Godal, H.C. (1962): Quantitative and qualitative changes in fibrinogen following major surgical operations. *Acta med. scand., 171*, 687.

Godal, H.C. and Abildgaard, U. (1966): Relation of soluble fibrin in plasma by ethanol. *Scand. J. Haemat., 3*, 342.

Groth, C.G. (1966): The effect of infused thrombin on the tissue oxygen tension. II. The possible role of 5-hydroxytryptamine and histamine. An experimental study in the rabbit. *Acta chir. scand., 132*, 15.

Hardaway, R.M. (1966): *Syndromes of Disseminated Intravascular Coagulation.* Thomas, Springfield, Ill.

Høie, J. and Schenk, W.G. (1971): Impact of disseminated intravascular coagulation on central hemodynamics and cardiac performance: An experimental study in dogs. *Surgery, 70*, 685.

Høie, J. and Schenk, W.G. (1972): Hemodynamics of disseminated intravascular coagulation. *Arch. Surg. (Chicago), 104*, 838.

Innes, D. and Sevitt, S. (1964): Coagulation and fibrinolysis in injured patients. *J. clin. Path., 17*, 1.

Kuida, H., Hinshaw, L.B., Gilbert, R.P. and Visscher, M.B. (1958): Effect of gram-negative endotoxin on pulmonary circulation. *Amer. J. Physiol., 192*, 335.

Larsson, S.O., Hedner, U. and Nilsson, I.M. (1971a): On coagulation and fibrinolysis in acute renal insufficiency. *Acta med. scand., 189*, 443.

Larsson, S.O., Hedner, U. and Nilsson, I.M. (1971b): On fibrinolytic split products in serum and urine in uraemia. *Scand. J. Urol. Nephrol., 5*, 234.

Lee, L. (1962): Reticuloendothelial clearance of circulating fibrin in the pathogenesis of the generalized Schwartzman reaction. *J. exp. Med., 115*, 1065.

Lilienberg, G., Rammer, L., Saldeen, T., Thorén, L. and Uddströmmer, L. (1970): Intravascular coagulation and inhibition of fibrinolysis in fat embolism. *Acta chir. scand., 136*, 87.

Ljungquist, U., Bergentz, S.-E. and Lewis, D.H. (1971): The distribution of platelets, fibrin and erythrocytes in various organs following experimental trauma. *Europ. surg. Res., 3*, 293.

McCarthy, B., Mammen, E., Leblanc, L.P. and Wilson, R.F. (1973): Subclinical fat embolism: a prospective study of 50 patients with extremity fractures. *J. Trauma, 13*, 9.

McLaughlin, J.S. (1971): Physiologic considerations in shock and trauma. *Ann. Surg., 173*, 667.

McLaughlin, J.S., Suddhimondala, C., Mech, K., Llacer, R.L., Houston, J., Blide, R., Attar, S. and Cowley, R.A. (1969): Pulmonary gas exchange in shock in humans. *Ann. Surg., 169*, 42.

McKay, D.G. (1965): *Disseminated Intravascular Coagulation.* Hoeber Medical Division, Harper and Row, New York, Evanston and London.

Modig, J., Busch, C. and Olerud, S. (1974): Circulatory and respiratory dysfunction during total hip replacement. *Acta anaest. scand., 18*, in press.

Naye, R.L. (1962): Thrombotic state after haemorrhagic diathesis, a possible complication of therapy with epsilon-aminocaproic acid. *Blood, 19*, 694.

Nossel, H.L., Yndelman, I., Canfield, R.E., Butler, V.P., Spanondis, K., Wilner, G.D. and Quereshi, G.D. (1974): Measurement of fibrinopeptide A in human blood. *J. clin. Invest., 54*, 43.

Olow, B. (1963): Effect of streptokinase on postoperative changes in some coagulation factors and the fibrinolytic system. *Acta chir. scand., 126*, 197.

Olsson, P. (1963): Exogenous heparin and the heparin co-factor. *Acta chir. scand., Suppl. 319.*

Olsson, P. and Johnsson, H. (1972): Interference of acetylsalicylic acid heparin and fibrin degradation products in hemostasis of reptilase defibrinogenated dogs. *Thrombos. Res., 1,* 135.

Olsson, P., Rådegran, K. and Taylor, G.A. (1970): Haemodynamic changes resulting from thrombin induced intravascular coagulation. *Cardiovasc. Res., 4,* 443.

Olsson, P., Swedenborg, J. and Lindquist, O. (1974): Effects of slow defibrinogenation on the canine lung. *J. Trauma, 14,* 325.

Olsson, P., Swedenborg, J. and Teger-Nilsson, A.-C. (1969): The role of adenine nucleotides in the peripheral vasodilating effect of thrombin. *Acta physiol. scand., 76,* 137.

Orell, S.R. (1971): Lung pathology in respiratory distress following shock in the adult. *Acta path. microbiol. scand., 79,* 65.

Packham, M.A., Nishizawa, E.E. and Mustard, J.F. (1968): Response of platelets to tissue injury. *Biochem. Pharmacol., Suppl. 17.*

Palmerio, C., Ming, S.C., Frank, E. and Fine, J. (1962): The role of the sympathetic nervous system in the generalized Schwartzman reaction. *J. exp. Med., 115,* 609.

Pepper, H. and Lindsay, S. (1960): Responses of platelets, eosinophils and total leucocytes during and following surgical procedures. *Surg. Gynec. Obstet., 110,* 319.

Piper, P. and Vane, J. (1971): The release of prostaglandins from lung and other tissues. *Ann. N.Y. Acad. Sci., 180,* 363.

Pontoppidan, H., Gettin, B. and Lowenstein, E. (1972): Acute respiratory failure the adult. *New Engl. J. Med., 287,* 690, 743, 799.

Powers, S.R., Burdge, R., Leather, R., Monaco, V., Newell, J., Sardar, S. and Smith, E.J. (1972): Studies of pulmonary insufficiency in non-thoracic trauma. *J. Trauma, 12,* 1.

Rådegran, K. (1972): The effect of acetylsalicylic acid on the peripheral and pulmonary vascular response to thrombin. *Acta anaesth. scand., 16,* 140.

Rådegran, K., Bergentz, S.-E., Lewis, D.H., Ljungqvist, U. and Olsson, P. (1971a): Pulmonary effects of induced platelet aggregation. Intravascular obstruction or vasoconstriction? *Scand. J. clin. Lab. Invest., 28,* 423.

Rådegran, K., Cronestrand, R. and Olsson, P. (1970): The effect of regional thrombin infusion in the renal vascular resistance. *Europ. surg. Res., 2,* 460.

Rådegran, K., Drugge, U. and Olsson, P. (1974): Pulmonary venoconstriction by induced platelet aggration. *Acta anaesth. scand., 18,* 243.

Rådegran, K. and McAslan, C. (1972): Circulatory and ventilatory effects of induced platelet aggregation and their inhibition by acetylsalicylic acid. *Acta anaesth. scand., 16,* 76.

Rådegran, K., Swedenborg, J. and Olsson, P. (1972): Effect of defibrinogenation and acetylsalicylic acid on the circulatory response to thrombin. *Acta chir. scand., 138,* 441.

Rådegran, K., Taylor, G.A. and Olsson, P. (1971b): Mode of action of protamine in regard to its circulatory and respiratory side effects. *Europ. surg. Res., 3,* 139.

Rammer, L. (1973): Renal function in burned rats with reference to the effect of intravascular coagulation. *Scand. J. Urol. Nephrol., 7,* 74.

Rammer, L. and Saldeen, T. (1970): Inhibition of fibrinolysis in posttraumatic death. *Thrombos. diathes. haemorrh. (Stuttg.), 25,* 68.

Robb, H.J. (1963): The role of micro-embolism in the production of irreversible shock. *Ann. Surg., 158,* 685.

Said, S. (1967): Some respiratory effects of prostaglandins E_2 and $F_{2\alpha}$. *Prostaglandin Symposium of the Worcester Foundation for Experimental Biology,* p. 267. Interscience publisher, New York.

Saldeen, T. (1966a): Experimental investigation of fat embolism and intravascular coagulation. *Acta path. microbiol. scand., 66,* 271.

Saldeen, T. (1966b): Further studies on fat embolism and intravascular coagulation. *Acta path. microbiol. scand., 67,* 591.

Saldeen, T. (1967): The occurrence of fibrin in the lungs in an autopsy material. *Virchov Arch. path. Anat., 343,* 20.

Smith, J.B. and Willis, A.L. (1971): Aspirin selectively inhibits prostaglandin production in human platelets. *Nature New Biol., 231*, 235.

Stein, M. and Thomas, D.P. (1967): Role of platelets in the acute pulmonary responses to endotoxin. *J. appl. Physiol., 23*, 47.

String, T., Robinson, A.J. and Blaisdell, F.W. (1971): Massive trauma. Effect of intravascular coagulation on prognosis. *Arch. Surg. (Chicago), 102*, 406.

Swedenborg, J. (1970): Vasoactivity of adenine nucleotides released in vitro from blood cells by thrombin. *Acta physiol. scand., 79*, 359.

Swedenborg, J. (1971): Thrombin induced vasoconstriction in the pulmonary circulation. *Scand. J. clin. Lab. Invest., 27*, 231.

Swedenborg, J., Taylor, G. and Olsson, P. (1971): Hemodynamic changes of adenosine diphosphate, adenosine triphosphate and thrombin in relation to their platelet aggregating activity. *Scand. J. clin. Lab. Invest., 27*, 213.

Thomas, D.P., Tanabe, G., Khan, M. and Stein, M. (1965): *Humoral Factors Mediated by Platelets in Experimental Pulmonary Embolism*, p. 59, *Pulmonary Embolic Disease*. Grune and Strutton, New York.

Vaage, J., Aarseth, P., Enge, I. and Hognestad, J. (1974a): Changes in pulmonary vascular volumes after induced intravascular aggregation of blood platelets. *Acta physiol. scand., 92*, 84.

Vaage, J., Bø, G. and Hognestad, J. (1974b): Pulmonary responses to intravascular platelet aggregation in the cat. *Acta physiol. scand., 92*, in press.

Vane, J.R. (1971): Inhibition of prostaglandin synthesis as a mechanism of action for aspirin like drugs. *Nature New Biol., 231*, 232.

Wahrenbrock, E.A., Carrico, C.J., Amundsen, D.A., Trummer, M.J. and Severinghaus, J.W. (1970): Increased atelectatic pulmonary shunt during hemorrhagic shock in dogs. *J. appl. Physiol., 29*, 615.

Wardle, E.N. and Taylor, G. (1968): Fibrin breakdown products and fibrinolysis in renal disease. *J. clin. Path., 21*, 140.

Webb, W.R. (1969): Pulmonary complications of non-thoracic trauma: summary of the National Research Conference. *J. Trauma, 9*, 700.

Wilson, R.F., Kafi, A., Ansuncion, Z. and Walt, A.J. (1969): Clinical respiratory failure after shock or trauma. *Arch. Surg. (Chicago), 98*, 539.

Wilson, R.F., Larned, P.A., Corr, J.J., Sarver, E.J. and Barrett, D.M. (1970): Physiological shunting in the lung in the critically ill or injured patient. *J. surg. Res., 10*, 571.

Ledingham (ed.). Shock

The shocked child

A.W. WILKINSON

Although the causes of shock are similar in the human subject at any age there are considerable variations in the way in which some of the manifestations of the shocked state develop according to the age of the patient. The most important factor in the child, as in the adult, is the reduction in the volume of blood in active circulation in the body, whether this is due to bleeding and the loss of whole blood from the vessels, or the loss of plasma after burns or scalds, or of gastro-intestinal secretions in acute diarrhoeal states. Neurogenic shock also occurs in children, in which blood is not lost from the vessels, but as the result of vasovagal dilatation of the vessels in the skeletal muscles is segregated temporarily and the volume in active general circulation is reduced.

Differences between Children and Adults

Perhaps the most important difference between the child and the adult arises from the inverse relationship between surface area and total body mass. The relatively greater surface area of the child in proportion to body weight renders the child much more susceptible to changes in the peripheral circulation in the skin and to the effects of an adverse environment, and particularly to wide fluctuations in ambient temperature. The total body water of a lean adult male is about 60% of his total weight and of a similar woman about 55%. In the so-called 'typical' 3.5 kg newly born baby the water content is about 68% but is 77% at 2.5 kg and 82.5% at 1.5 kg. The distribution of this water in the body is also very different in the newly born baby compared with the adult. Extracellular fluid volume diminishes very rapidly during the first three days after birth and more slowly during the first weeks of life and again at adolescence (Fellers et al., 1949). At birth weights of between 2 and 5 kg the extracellular fluid is about 40% of the body weight and it falls to 32–35% at weights from 5–20 kg and to 23–27% in young adults. The intracellular fluid of the newly born baby is about 30% of body weight compared with more than 40% in the adult. These large differences are associated with equally large differences in sodium and potassium content, sodium being about 50% greater per kg body weight and potassium about 20% less per kg body weight in the neonate than in the adult.

It is often said that the newly born baby has a greater tolerance to injury than an older child or adult, but this may be true only in a limited sense. The larger extracellular fluid and blood volume of the neonate mean perhaps that a large inflammatory exudate may be tolerated with less disturbance of blood volume than in older subjects. It is unfortunate that there is so little objective evidence about the effects of fluid and blood loss in the newly born. Most surgeons and anaesthetists who regularly treat neonates are firmly persuaded of the importance of the maintenance of blood volume within normal limits by the immediate replacement of blood as it is lost during the operation.

Blood Volume

The total blood volume of a normal newborn infant is about 85 ml/kg (Mollison et al., 1950); there is, however, some variation according to the packed cell volume, which is usually much higher than in older children and adults, especially when, by delayed clamping of the cord, more of the placental blood flows into the baby. The haemoglobin concentration or packed cell volume should always be measured before operation on newly born babies and when high (15–20 g haemoglobin per 100 ml) may modify the decision whether or not to replace blood lost at operation. Mollison et al. (1950) found very high plasma volumes in four babies with very low packed cell volumes and these infants were in cardiac failure.

The neonate and young infant do not tolerate excessive blood loss and no operation of any magnitude, such as thoracotomy or laparotomy, on such babies should ever be started until compatible blood is available. The surgeon must also reduce the blood loss to a minimum by the use of the cutting diathermy. If this is done it should be possible to ligate a tracheo-oesophageal fistula and make a primary anastomosis of the atretic oesophagus, or to make a laparotomy for a duodenal or other small intestinal atresia, with the loss of not more than 5 to 10 ml of blood. The size of blood loss which needs replacement varies with the weight of the baby. Losses of more than 10 ml, in a 2 kg baby, or 15 ml in a 3.5 kg baby, are equivalent to 350 and 300 ml respectively in a 70 kg adult, and should be replaced by injecting an equivalent volume of compatible blood into the vein into which a needle was inserted for the injection of anaesthetic agents. Blood should be replaced as it is lost and replacement should always keep pace with the loss, and should be completed in the theatre before the operation is finished. Old or cold blood should not be used for replacement in a baby since the rate of injection is usually faster than in older patients and cardiac arrest may be caused either by the cold blood or its high plasma potassium content, especially when the blood is injected through the umbilical vein.

Measurement of blood loss in the neonate or infant is difficult and inaccurate. The best practical method in older children is probably to weight the blood-stained used swabs against an equal number of similar unused ones. In the neonate however the very small losses increase the inherent inaccuracy of this method. It is better for the anaesthetist and the surgeon to become thoroughly familiar with the appearance of various small volumes of blood on the sort of swabs which are used and to make visual estimates of blood loss on this basis; with practice and honesty this is probably as accurate a method as any other.

In older children the blood volume varies with weight and age and in general the blood volume is about 75–80 ml/kg at one year and 65–70 ml/kg in older children. What is much more important than minute variations with age and weight of the individual patient is the conscious awareness of the anaesthetist and surgeon that blood is being lost, and that the loss should be measured as accurately as possible and be replaced without delay and quantitatively when the loss exceeds 10% of the initial total volume, and that replacement should not fall behind the loss. When a child has to be resuscitated before operation it is essential that restoration of the actively circulating volume of blood is complete before anaesthesia is induced, and that more blood is available for replacement of any loss during operation. The vaso-constriction which is such an important part of the response to reduction in blood volume in the child, does not pass off until replacement is complete.

The induction of general anaesthesia in the presence of vasoconstriction may cause a sudden vasodilatation followed by a sharp and profound fall in blood pressure and rapid deterioration of the peripheral circulation.

Hypertensive Response

In children as in adults there is a wide individual variation in the response to reduction in the blood volume. In general the heart rate rises and the systolic and diastolic blood pressures fall, but some children exhibit the hypertensive response in which the systolic blood pressure may be 160–180 mmHg mercury or more with a diastolic pressure of over 100 mmHg. This is due to intense vasoconstriction as an over-compensation to the reduced volume of blood in the vessels. When eventually even this fails to match the difference between the capacity of the vessels and the blood they contain there is a sudden and very severe fall in blood pressure and collapse of the patient. A hypertensive response should always be regarded with great caution and the patient watched very carefully and closely and it is usually wise to start an intravenous infusion at once. In the hypertensive patient as in others with a reduced blood volume the diastolic pressure may slowly rise with little change in systolic pressure and then suddenly there is a precipitous fall in both pressures. This rise in diastolic pressure is another ominous sign which should not be missed.

Variations in Clinical Features

The clinical picture of the severely shocked child varies very much. One child may lie flaccid and quiet, with waxen, pallid, cold skin, absent peripheral pulses and barely breathing. Another may become maniacally excited with flailing fractured limbs and have to be held down, but it may be noticed that the wounds are not bleeding. In both the most important treatment is rapid expansion of the blood volume. Severely injured children respond very well to adequate transfusion and resuscitation should be specific, adequate and rapid. Drugs should not be used to control restlessness, which subsides when the cerebral circulation is restored. The best treatment of the cold, pale, clammy skin of the severely shocked child is to restore the circulating blood volume by rapid transfusion, while keeping the child covered with a sheet and a blanket.

Heat in any form will cause vasodilatation and is harmful. During an operation the most useful way of assessing the state of the patient, especially in the neonate, is by close and careful observation of the behaviour of the patient, of the colour of the blood in the wound, of the volume of blood which is being lost and the state of the peripheral circulation in the extremities. When the blood in the wound becomes sparse or, worse still, bleeding stops, transfusion is essential and urgent and these signs are more immediate and crucial indicators of its need than any other. So long as rough handling and the use of fixed mechanical retractors are avoided shock is not likely to develop unless there is too much bleeding or the operation and anaesthesia are unduly prolonged. Prevention is better than any cure and the effects of rough handling of tissues last four or five days.

In the newly born and the infant body temperature must be controlled by putting the baby on an electric mattress, combined with the measurement of core temperature with a thermal probe inserted either into the rectum or the oesophagus, or better still in the closed axilla with the arm strapped by the side. Even in older children the repeated measurement of body temperature is worthwhile when operations are very prolonged and there is much exposure of bowel or the thoracic cavity. Direct measurement of blood volume is not feasible in small babies or even in older children, and in general surgical operations we have not found it necessary to measure central venous pressure during operation or at any other time. At the end of a long operation sudden changes in position or rolling the child from side to side may cause deterioration and should be avoided.

Shock due to Burns or Scalds

About 90% of all injuries to children by burning and scalding are small in extent and do not produce severe physical shock. Injuries which involve less than 10% of the body surface area seldom cause much systemic disturbance. Between 10 and 15% there is some reduction in the volume of blood in active circulation, as the result of coagulation in a deep burn, or loss of plasma from the unusually permeable vessels in a more superficial injury. With injuries of more than 15% the patient must be carefully watched for signs of circulatory impairment. Most injuries of more than 20% of the body surface require replenishment of the volume of circulating blood at some stage or another and in all such patients an intravenous infusion should be started as soon as possible after admission of the child to hospital.

In burns or scalds which are superficial the injury involves only the surface layers of the skin and the capillary circulation in the skin is irritated but only very little of it destroyed. This results in intensive inflammatory reaction in the vast cutaneous capillary bed of the skin and the outpouring into the tissues and blisters of a large quantity of fluid which ressembles plasma in its composition. This fluid contains plasma proteins up to a molecular weight of about 125,000. The capillaries are normally slightly permeable to albumin. In superficial burns or scalds, however, the capillaries are as permeable to plasma albumin as they are to sodium and other mineral ions in the extracellular fluid. The rate of outflow of plasma-like fluid from the circulating blood exceeds its rate of return for about 18 to 24 hours after injury, and as a result the amount of exuded fluid increases and causes swelling. From about 30 hours after injury the size of the swelling normally begins to diminish as the rate of return to the circulation of the exuded plasma-like fluid exceeds the rate at which this fluid is being lost from the vessels.

This normal state of affairs can be very much distorted by the kind of treatment which is provided. When attempts are made to increase the circulating blood volume by the infusion of solutions of mineral salts in the manner suggested by Shires (1968) the resulting inflammatory exudate is enormously increased. Even in the normal subject when an isotonic solution of mineral salts is injected intravenously an equilibrium results in which three-quarters of the solution is distributed outside the walls of the capillaries in the extra-vascular space, and only one quarter remains within the vessels. This equilibrium is even more displaced towards the extra-vascular space in patients with an extensive inflammatory exudate due to burning or scalding. Because of the increased capillary permeability to albumin and the other smaller plasma proteins in the injured area the same thing happens when plasma is injected. Very little of the injected plasma remains within the vessels, most of it passes out into the inflammatory exudate and accumulates there at least during the first 24 to 30 hours after injury. It follows that in order to produce an increment in the volume of blood actually circulating within the vessels of the rest of the body, which is necessary to maintain oxygen carriage and gas exchange between the tissues and the lungs and the expired air, very large volumes of solutions of mineral salts or human plasma must be administered. It is in this situation that the use of 6% gum acacia in 0.9% saline was of such value in former times and dextran of an average molecular weight of 150,000 in 0.9% saline is now the fluid of choice. In such a preparation the molecular weight of about 55% of the total dextran is more than 125,000 and about 45% is between 125,000 and 150,000. The majority of dextran of this molecular weight will remain in circulation for at least 48 hours and it is thereafter slowly broken down and excreted in the urine. The use of dextran preparations with weight average molecular weights of 40,000 and 70,000 have little more effect on blood volume than a similar volume of 0.9% saline or plasma though they do have some effect on the movement of red cells in the peripheral capillaries.

It has been claimed that the use of low molecular weight dextran will improve blood flow through the kidneys and therefore the volume of the urine which is produced, but this is not borne out by the observation of the thick syrupy urine which some patients pass after infusions of dextran, indicating that while dextran is well excreted by the kidneys the water which may come out with it is subsequently reabsorbed. Before dextran is administered blood should be taken for compatibility testing, but if this cannot be done accurate cross-matching can still be carried out provided the red cells are first washed with saline to remove dextran.

Many means of judging the circulatory state of the burned or scalded child have been used. The peripheral blood pressure, measured with a cuff of suitable size, gives valuable information but at a later stage than the close study of peripheral circulation. The rate which colour returns to the skin or nail bed of fingers or toes, or of the ear lobe, and the quality of the colour, are important indications of the state of the blood flow through those parts of the peripheral circulation. Normally colour should return within a second or two of release of compression. The colour should be normal red or pink. When the skin is cyanotic or the colour takes more than three seconds to return, the deeper the cyanosis and the slower the return the more serious is the impairment of circulation and the more urgent is the treatment to restore the circulating volume. Such observations of peripheral circulation and of the pulse rate or heart rate are usually all that is needed to maintain a critical watch on the peripheral circulatory state of even the very severely injured child and to form the basis of resuscitation. The addition of measurements of the peripheral blood pressure are an advantage but not essential. Delay in return beyond three seconds is an indication for the immediate administration, at as fast a speed as possible, of a sufficient volume of 150,000 molecular weight dextran in 0.9% saline to restore the colour of the peripheral skin and the rate of return of that colour to less than two seconds after compression. When this is achieved the dextran can be stopped and the infusion continued at a very slow rate, 10 drops per minute of 6% glucose solution, until further deterioration occurs in the peripheral circulation when more dextran should be given as rapidly as possible in sufficient volume to restore the peripheral colour as before. When the burns are extensive and much of the area involved is deep blood may be used in addition to dextran.

Occasionally on admission the peripheral veins are so constricted that in order to get improvement in the rate of flow of blood in the veins, a less viscous fluid such as 0.9% saline or a balanced electrolyte solution should first be used and as soon as flow improves then the more viscid, slower flowing 6% dextran can be substituted. The measurement of packed cell volume is undesirable in children because it requires frequent finger pricks to obtain blood for micro-estimations. Measurement of the volume of urine produced every hour is also undesirable because it requires insertion of a catheter into the urinary bladder. Even if the flow of urine is a good indication of the volume of blood flow through the kidneys it is doubtful whether this is of any value as an indication of the state of the peripheral circulation in the limbs. The infusion of 6% glucose solution at a very slow rate should be continued for as long as there is any risk of further circulatory deterioration, and in very extensive injuries this means for about 48 hours.

When dextran is used as described above, resuscitation and maintenance of a satisfactory circulating volume of blood can be achieved with much smaller volumes of fluid than with any other preparations. It is unnecessary to administer such large volumes that the resulting inflammatory oedema underneath the coagulated skin in limbs, which are circumferentially injured, is so much increased by the loss of the injected fluid from the vessels that the circulation to the distal parts of the limbs is impaired, and incisions have to be made through the coagulated skin to allow blood to flow. In the case of circumferential injuries of the trunk interference with respiration is not uncommon when the very large volumes of fluid recommended by Shires (1968) are administered in the treatment of burn shock. In deeply burned patients the use of dextran combined with the coagulation of up to 30% of the original total red cells in the burned area may cause severe anaemia, and blood should always be transfused when this occurs. In children the primary cleaning of the burned area can be done without general analgesics; the intramuscular injection of a suitable dose of morphine for the age and weight of the child provides complete relief of pain.

When at a later stage split-skin autografts are applied it is important that the surgeon cuts the grafts as expeditiously as possible and immediately applies suitable pressure dressings to the raw surface from which the grafts have been taken. If this is done quickly blood loss will be negligible and does not need to be replaced. The raw surface to be grafted should be damaged as little as possible to prevent blood loss when debris is removed from it and when the grafts are applied to it. No matter how carefully and rapidly the surgeon works compatible blood for replacement should, however, always be available when extensive burns are grafted.

Other Causes of the 'Shocked State' in Children

Intussusception. Until a few years ago the mortality rate for intussusception in infancy was due almost entirely to strangulation and gangrene of the affected segment of bowel, and the failure to replace adequately the consequent loss of blood into the wall and lumen of the affected segment of gut and the mesentery. This may cause nearly as large a loss of blood as strangulation due to volvulus of the intestine. Resection of the affected length of the gut with the blood it contains can be tolerated only if the volume of lost blood is replaced. Some blood, sufficient to restore the peripheral circulation to normal, must be given before operation is undertaken, even though quite a large part of this transfused volume may be lost into the involved segment of bowel. The transfusion must be continued during the operation to maintain an adequate circulating volume while loss continues into the affected gut and replacement of the whole loss into the bowel and its mesentery and during the operation should be completed during the operation. The blood replacement should also be sufficient to allow for any small continuing loss by post-operative ooze after the transfusion has been stopped.

Volvulus of the midgut. Volvulus of the midgut may result in obstruction of the venous return from the superior mesenteric vein draining the whole or most of the midgut. When the arterial inflow is not also closed off this leads to the progressive loss of more and more of the circulating blood into this segment of the circulation, and a serious and continuing reduction in effective blood volume. The only solution to this problem lies in the reduction of the volvulus by laparotomy and untwisting of the midgut, but before this can be done the circulatory state of the child must be improved by the rapid increase in the actively circulating blood volume by the transfusion of a sufficient volume of compatible blood. At times the urgency for replacement means some risk must be accepted in the use of blood which is used before the full range of modern compatibility tests have been carried out. An alternative is to use dextran 150,000 in the first place but blood must be replaced later. In the newly born the blood should be injected before operation into the umbilical vein, exposed and cannulated in the midline of the abdominal wall, about an inch above the umbilicus where the transverse upper abdominal laparotomy incision will be made later. With this method there is less risk of infection than from using the umbilical vein in the stump of the cord and the transfusion can be continued without interruption during the operation. This sort of resuscitation may also be necessary when much blood is being lost into the dilated distal end of an atretic piece of intestine which has twisted on its vascular pedicle and has caused venous but not arterial obstruction.

Diarrhoea. Severe reduction in circulating blood volume may result from diarrhoea in disaccharide intolerance and should be treated by the rapid expansion of extracellular fluid volume with a balanced electrolyte (Fox et al., 1952) solution until the peripheral circulation is restored. In enterocolitis complicating Hirschsprung's disease there is a large loss of fluid into the affected segment of bowel; this may be part or the whole of the colon and sometimes the small intestine and stomach may also be involved. There is also a loss of blood into the mucous membrane of the affected bowel and the mucosa may later slough and there is consequently a loss of whole blood. The first and most important measure is to raise the extracellular fluid volume as rapidly as possible by the intravenous injection of a balanced electrolyte solution to open up the peripheral vessels. Then large molecular weight dextran and blood should be transfused to restore and maintain blood volume. The quantities of these fluids which should be used must and can only be judged in the individual, by the response to treatment as shown by the changes in the colour and rate of return of colour after compression of the peripheral circulation in the nail beds or finger tips, and by the behaviour of the child. It is necessary also to decompress the bowel by the insertion of a rectal tube but this should not be done until the existing loss of extracellular fluid has been at least partly replaced.

Peritonitis. In peritonitis there may be a large reduction in circulating blood volume because of the extensive inflammatory exudate in the peritoneal cavity, in the parietal peritoneum and on the surface and in the wall of the involved bowel and in the mesentery. The use of electrolyte solutions then does little to improve the circulatory state apart from the initial rapid infusion which delates acutely the constricted vessels. To complete and maintain lasting resuscitation an adequate volume of compatible whole blood must then be transfused. When large quantities of solutions of mineral salts such as 0.9% saline or balanced electrolyte are used most of the administered fluid rapidly passes out of the vessels into the inflamed tissues, and increases the volume of the fluid in the peritoneal cavity, in the lumen of the gut and in the inflammatory oedema of the wall of the bowel. This both causes and prolongs the ileus which delays the return of normal activity and motility in the bowel.

Septic Shock

Septic shock may be a complication of peritonitis but also occurs in infections of other kinds. Altemeir et al. (1967) found that 63% of patients with gram-negative septicaemia were in the first, seventh and eighth decades. More than 60% of those in the first decade were newly born infants, but their mortality rate was only 21% compared with 52% overall and 67% over the age of 40 years. In childhood the clinical picture is similar to that in older patients but the causes differ. Septic shock may occur after gangrene of the bowel especially when there is perforation, in undiagnosed leakage from an intestinal anastomosis, when a colon replacement for the oesophagus sloughs, when infected urine leaks into the peritoneal cavity from a uretero-intestinal anastomosis and only rarely in the child when urinary tract obstruction is complicated by infection. The earliest signs are unusual and unexpected restlessness, a rising pulse rate, sometimes cyanosis and an illness which is difficult to explain, going on to progressive peripheral circulatory failure. The early administration of blood and saline or better, a balanced electrolyte solution is essential, but if the infection can be located, it must be adequately treated surgically as soon as possible. Vasoactive substances, such as isoproterenol, and vasodilators, such as phenoxybenzamine, are not of much if any good in children. Corticosteroids also have unpredictable effects. Provided the peripheral circulation can be restored and the general state is improving and urine is being passed a low blood pressure, which is quite common, is not of any serious significance and usually gradually rises to within the normal range.

Methods of Administration of Fluid

In the neonate the usual practice is to insert a needle into a vein in the scalp or the back of the hand through which relaxants and other drugs used by the anaesthetist can be injected. Blood also can be injected through this needle but it is not our practice to maintain a continuous infusion during or after operation unless the oral intake of fluid or milk cannot be started within 24 hours of operation. The use of the umbilical vein has been mentioned and is of great value when rapid preoperative resuscitation is necessary, for example in a strangulated volvulus of the midgut or an atresia. In infants or older children the peripheral veins can usually be entered with a needle except when they are tightly constricted. It is then preferable and usually quicker to expose the vein under local anaesthesia and insert a polythene cannula of the largest possible size. For small children some kind of graduated cylinder should be put in the infusion tubing between the reservoir and the drip chamber so that the volume of each fluid which is given can be accurately measured.

References

Altemeier, W.A., Todd, J.C. and Inge, W.W. (1967): Gram negative Septicaemia: a growing threat. *Ann. Surg., 166,* 530.

Fellers, F.X., Barnett, H.L., Hare, K. and McNamara, H. (1949): Change in thiocyanate and sodium[24] spaces during growth. *Pediatrics, 3,* 622.

Fox, C.L., Winfield, J.M., Slobody, L.B., Swindler, C.M. and Lattimer, J.K. (1952): *J. Amer. med. Ass., 148,* 827.

Mollison, P.L., Veall, N. and Cutbush, M. (1950): Red cell and plasma volume in newborn infants. *Arch. Dis. Childh., 25,* 242.

Shires, G.T. (1968): Fluid and electrolyte needs at operation. *Sth Afr. med. J., 42,* 867.

Ledingham (ed.). Shock

Shock in pregnancy

J. BONNAR

Introduction

Shock still remains the most dangerous and frequent emergency associated with pregnancy and apart from death can result in bilateral renal cortical necrosis, acute tubular necrosis and Sheehan's syndrome. When a pregnant woman suffers shock the reduction in utero-placental blood flow causes hypoxia and shock in the fetus. Modern obstetric practice requires round-the-clock cover for anaesthesia and a senior anaesthetist should be available at all times for obstetric emergencies. Pregnant women require the knowledge and skill of an experienced anaesthetist as they are often gravely at risk and present a more complicated clinical picture on account of the pregnancy. The anaesthetist is a key member of the obstetric team and his advice and assistance are invariably required in the management of a pregnant woman with shock.

The main causes of death directly attributable to pregnancy and childbirth are abortion, pulmonary embolism, haemorrhage and eclampsia or pre-eclampsia. Deaths due to these four major complications have steadily declined over the last twenty years and other causes of maternal death have now assumed increasing importance. These include ectopic pregnancy, infection, amniotic fluid embolism, ruptured uterus and death directly due to anaesthesia. Table I

Table I
Main causes of maternal death in England and Wales (1961–69).

	1961/63	1964/66	1967/69
Abortion	139	133	115
Pulmonary embolism	129	91	75
Haemorrhage	92	68	41
Eclampsia and pre-eclampsia	104	67	51
Ectopic pregnancy	42	42	31
Sepsis, excluding abortion with sepsis	33	57	33
Amniotic fluid embolism	27	30	27
Ruptured uterus	38	30	18
Anaesthetic deaths	24	37	34
Miscellaneous causes	64	24	30
Total	692	579	455

Data compiled for the *Report on Confidential Enquiries into Maternal Deaths in England and Wales* (H.M.S.O. London, 1972).

lists the number of deaths from these various causes in England and Wales in the three-year periods between 1961 and 1969. The major factor leading to death in virtually all these obstetric complications is the state of shock. Many maternal deaths could be prevented if the shock syndrome were recognised early and managed correctly.

Physiological Adaptations in Pregnancy

In hospital practice extensive use is made of laboratory tests for the management of patients. In pregnancy the physiological situation is markedly altered and apparently healthy women may have biochemical measurements which deviate from what is regarded as normal in the non-pregnant state. The accepted range of normality in pregnancy is inevitably wide and indeed adequate knowledge in some areas of the normal range of physiological values in healthy well-nourished pregnant women is still not available.

Cardiovascular function

Cardiac output. In normal pregnant women at rest, but not supine, cardiac output rises during the first ten weeks of pregnancy by about 1.5 l/minute and this rise is maintained for the remainder of the pregnancy. The increase in cardiac output is brought about both by an increased heart-rate and an increased stroke volume (Hytten and Leitch, 1971). The mean cardiac output throughout pregnancy is about 6 l/minute. Previously it had been maintained that the cardiac output showed a fall in late pregnancy but this was shown to be a technical artefact due to measurements being made with the patient supine, in which position the pregnant uterus lies on and occludes the vena cava. When the patient turns on to her side the basal cardiac output is as high at the end of pregnancy as in mid-pregnancy.

Heart rate and blood pressure. The heart rate in pregnancy has been the subject of many studies which have shown that the rate is increased in early pregnancy and does not reach its maximum until the last trimester. An increase of the heart rate of 15 to 20 beats to a maximum of about 85 per minute is usually present by the third trimester of pregnancy (Ihrman, 1960). The position of the patient during pregnancy has an important effect on the level of the arterial blood pressure. The blood pressure is almost always highest when the patient is sitting up and lower when she lies supine. In a small minority of women a massive fall of blood pressure will occur in the supine position – the supine hypotensive syndrome – as a result of the occlusion of the inferior vena cava. The arterial blood pressure is lowest when the patient lies on her side (Trower and Walters, 1968). In the supine position the aorta may be compressed as well as the inferior vena cava. In normal pregnant women both the systolic and diastolic blood pressure fall by 5–10 mmHg or more in the first half of pregnancy. Different workers have reported wide variations in the absolute pressures. In the second half of pregnancy both the systolic and diastolic blood pressures gradually rise towards the non-pregnant level as the women approaches term.

Venous pressure. The venous pressure in the arm remains unchanged in pregnancy, but there is a progressive increase in the femoral venous pressure. This is due to the mounting pressure of the uterus on the vena cava and pelvic veins as well as to the relatively high pressure of the blood discharged from the uterine veins. A considerable quantity of blood can therefore accumulate in the lower limbs in pregnancy. In addition to the greater venous pressure, the veins in pregnancy are considerably more distensible, dilating more for a given internal pressure (Goodrich and Wood, 1964). Pressures in the right side of the heart, right atrium and ventricle, as well as in the pulmonary artery are unaffected by pregnancy (Bader et al., 1955). Central venous pressure is the most effective way of monitoring blood or fluid replacement, particularly in obstetric complications, where a great deal of the blood loss may be concealed or septic shock is suspected. An average pressure of 10 cm H_2O in the third trimester was reported by O'Driscoll and McCarthy (1966). The use of the central venous pressure in the diagnosis of shock will be discussed later.

Peripheral blood flow. In pregnancy the peripheral blood flow is greatly increased, particularly in the hands and feet, the skin being characteristically warm and the hands clammy. The blood flow in the hand shows a substantial increase, the resting blood flow in the skin of the hand increasing from 4 ml/minute/100 ml tissue to as high as 18 ml/minute at term (Ginsburg and Duncan, 1969). Other evidence of increased blood flow in the hand comes from rise of finger skin temperature from an average of 34.2°C in normal non-pregnant subjects to 35.9°C at 36 weeks gestation (Herbert et al., 1958). Palmar erythema and vascular spiders occur commonly in pregnancy and haemangiomas may appear or existing ones increase in size. Raynaud's disease disappears in pregnancy, a phenomenon which was noted by Raynaud himself. Another area of vascular dilatation in pregnancy is the nasal mucus membrane which often provokes blockage or even bleeding from the nose. The normal reaction to stress stimuli is a pressor response, a peripheral vasoconstriction, but in pregnancy there is usually a dilator response (Dolezal and Figar, 1965). What modifies the response is not known but oestrogens, which are at a particularly high level in pregnancy, are known to depress sympathetic activity (Lloyd and Pickford, 1961).

Blood volume

During a healthy pregnancy the plasma volume increases by at least 1250 ml above the average non-pregnant level of 2600 ml. During the first ten weeks little change occurs but after this the volume rises progressively levelling off at about 30–34 weeks gestation. The terminal fall of 200 to 300 ml which was previously described was most likely the result of technical artefact due to measurement of the plasma volume with the patient supine. In general the bigger the fetus the bigger the rise in plasma volume. Pre-eclampsia is associated with a reduced rise in plasma volume and in multiple pregnancy there is a much greater increase than average (Hytten and Leitch, 1971). Red cell volume also increases and the rise begins sometime between 10 and 20 weeks gestation and continues progressively until the end of pregnancy. In healthy pregnant women taking iron supplements the erythrocyte volume rises by about 30%, the average non-pregnant volume of 1400 ml increasing to about 1800 ml.

As with plasma volume the increase is related to the clinical situation and is invariably much larger in multiple pregnancy. The volume of the erythrocytes and the plasma volume bear no fixed relation to one another. In pregnancy the plasma volume presumably rises because increased circulation is needed in the skin to dissipate fetal heat and in the kidneys to increase filtration; erythrocyte volume increases because oxygen transport needs to be enhanced to meet the requirements of the fetus and the additional maternal tissue. The change in the erythrocyte and plasma volume is not in the same proportion and in the last 10 weeks of pregnancy when the increase in plasma volume is greatest the haematocrit falls from the average non-pregnant value of about 40% to a minimum of 33 to 34%.

Serum electrolytes and carbon dioxide output

In normal pregnancy a small but consistent fall occurs in the concentration of serum electrolytes (Newman, 1957). With the exception of the bicarbonate concentration the mean values remain well within the 'normal' clinical range. In early pregnancy the serum sodium falls by 2–3 mEq/l to a relatively constant level and the potassium by 0.2 to 0.3 mEq/l. The bicarbonate concentration falls early in pregnancy by a substantial amount that is consistent with the fall in the PCO_2; a reduction of PCO_2 from 38.8 mmHg to 30.6 mmHg by the end of the second trimester was reported by Lyons and Antonio (1959). This reduction of PCO_2 presumably helps the fetus to dispose of CO_2 by providing a gradient and obviates the fetus having a high PCO_2. For the mother the low PCO_2 has widespread effects: since pH is maintained the plasma bicarbonate must be reduced and this may also account for the lowering of the plasma sodium level. Another consequence of the low PCO_2 for the pregnant women is the sensation of dyspnoea which is a not uncommon complaint (Gilbert and Auchincloss, 1966).

Blood coagulation and fibrinolysis

Two of the vital mechanisms involved in haemostasis are the blood coagulation system which is responsible for staunching blood flow from the vascular tree and the fibrinolytic system which mediates the removal of fibrin. Both these systems undergo extreme changes during pregnancy (Bonnar, 1973). Plasma fibrinogen substantially alters during pregnancy, the total amount of circulating fibrinogen increasing from an average of 10 g in the normal non-pregnant woman to nearly 20 g in late pregnancy; the levels of plasma fibrinogen in late pregnancy and labour are usually 400–600 mg/100 ml. The concentration of coagulation factors VII, VIII and X are also considerably increased in normal pregnancy whereas the levels of prothrombin and factors V, IX, XI and XII appear to be unchanged. In the fibrinolytic system the level of circulating plasminogen activator and the activator content of venous endothelium are both depressed in the latter half of pregnancy. The increased levels of clotting factors during pregnancy probably represent a physiological development to provide for rapid and effective uterine haemostasis during parturition when a blood flow of 600 ml or more per minute to the placental site has to be staunched by a combination of myometrial contraction and explosive fibrin deposition (Bonnar et al., 1970a, b).

The increased levels of coagulation factors and the depressed fibrinolytic activity create a potentially vulnerable situation for intravascular fibrin deposition and a whole spectrum of intravascular clotting may occur in several obstetric complications which provide initiating stimuli (Table II). In conditions such as abruptio placentae, intrauterine death or missed abortion clot-promoting substances enter the circulation and trigger off intravascular clotting. In amniotic fluid embolism massive intravascular clotting may occur with the conversion of all the circulating fibrinogen to fibrin. When plasma concentrations of fibrinogen and coagulation factors fall to very low levels coagulation failure ensues and uncontrollable haemorrhage may occur from any damaged areas of the vascular system. Blood coagulation disorder is now recognised as a major factor in deaths due to haemorrhage arising during pregnancy or childbirth. The presence of a coagulation defect should be considered in those obstetric complications listed in Table II. Screening procedures should therefore be used to give early warning that the haemostatic system is abnormal and to alert the transfusion service to the need for obtaining supplies of fresh compatible blood. In the management of obstetric haemorrhage the most useful tests are those concerned with the level and clottability of the plasma fibrinogen

Table II
Obstetric complications associated with disseminated intravascular coagulation.

1. Abruptio placentae
2. Amniotic fluid embolism
3. Eclampsia and pre-eclampsia
4. Induced (saline) abortion
5. Retained dead fetus or missed abortion
6. Intra-uterine infection – septic abortion
   ante- and postpartum infection.

and with the platelet count. As bedside procedures the *whole blood clotting time* and the *thrombin clotting time* are recommended. The *fibrinogen titre* provides a rapid estimate of the level of plasma fibrinogen. The *platelet count* is of value in indicating the presence of intravascular coagulation and very low levels emphasise the need for obtaining fresh blood. For a rapid assay of the level of fibrin degradation products the latex agglutination method is useful.

Aetiology and Classification of Shock in Obstetrics

Shock in a pregnant woman, or one recently delivered, may be due to a single factor but in many situations more than one may be contributing e.g. in endotoxic shock, hypovolaemic and cardio-pulmonary components may also be present. Table III sets out a classification of shock based on the initiating haemodynamic event and lists the complications which may be responsible.

Table III
Shock in obstetrics.

1. Hypovolaemic	Haemorrhage – ectopic pregnancy, abortion, abruptio placentae, placenta praevia, ruptured uterus, postpartum haemorrhage, amniotic fluid embolism Fluid loss – hyperemesis gravidarum, acute pyelonephritis, excessive diuresis Supine hypotension – compression of vena cava by the gravid uterus Inversion of uterus
2. Endotoxic	Uterine – infected abortion, chorionamnionitis, postpartum sepsis Renal – acute pyelonephritis
3. Cardio-pulmonary and anaesthetic	Cardiac arrest Myocardial infarction Pulmonary embolism – thrombus, amniotic fluid, air Aspiration of gastric contents Hypotension due to regional anaesthesia High or total spinal block Drug reaction

Diagnosis and Evaluation of Shock

A detailed history should be obtained if necessary from a relative – the amount of blood loss, type of abortion or delivery, history of drug allergy, cardiovascular and renal disease. Physical examination will enable an initial assessment of the shock state to be made and may provide information on the source of any infection. The mental state of the patient and the condition of the peripheral circulation are two important signs. Grave signs are cold cyanosed extremities, poor peripheral venous filling and a lethargic or comatose patient.

In evaluating the shocked patient and monitoring response to treatment the observations and measurements listed in Table IV are recommended. In patients with severe endotoxic shock and poor peripheral perfusion blood gas analysis, pH and acid-base status should be determined if possible; a low pH with a metabolic acidosis is characteristic of this condition.

Table IV
Evaluation and monitoring of shock.

Observation	Frequency	Function assessed
Pulse rate	15 min	Cardiac function
Blood pressure	15 min	
Central venous pressure	15 min	Dynamic blood volume
Urine output	60 min	Renal function
Whole blood clotting time Fibrinogen titre Platelet count	60 min	Haemostatic function and intravascular coagulation
Skin colour and temperature	60 min	Peripheral circulation
Blood gas analysis, pH and acid base status	as indicated	Metabolic and respiratory function

Hypovolaemic Shock

Hypovolaemic shock secondary to haemorrhage is by far the most common variety of shock observed in pregnant women. In many situations the deficiency of the circulating blood volume may be due to concealed bleeding such as in ectopic pregnancy, abruptio placentae and uterine rupture. Hypovolaemia due to dehydration and electrolyte imbalance is now uncommon due to the early use of intravenous fluid therapy in patients with severe vomiting in early pregnancy and with acute pyelonephritis.

Haemorrhagic shock

During childbirth a healthy woman can suffer a rapid blood loss of over 1 litre without any evidence of shock. This is most likely due to the increased blood volume during pregnancy and the reduction of blood in the uterine circulation after delivery. Often shock is preceded by repeated haemorrhages or a prolonged steady loss which has a cumulative effect.

In the early phase of shock a pregnant women presents with tachycardia and a relatively normal blood pressure but she appears restless and anxious. If untreated by volume replacement hypotension ensues. In the early decompensated phase the hypotension readily responds to volume replacement. Haemorrhagic shock is characteristically reversible until very late in its evolution and for this reason vigorous therapy should always be employed as soon as the diagnosis is made even in an apparently exsanguinated patient.

Management of haemorrhagic shock. The essentials of management are to arrest the bleeding and restore the circulating blood volume. Control of the bleeding may not be possible without major surgery. When measures to combat shock have been initiated efforts should be directed at achieving haemostasis and the approach will depend on the underlying condition. When evidence of intra-abdominal bleeding is present correction of the hypotension before surgery is often not possible as the increase of the blood pressure provokes further intra-abdominal bleeding. This often creates difficulty for the anaesthetist who is understandably hesitant about anaesthetising a patient with hypotension. When blood volume replacement is under way haemostasis must be achieved and in conditions like ectopic pregnancy or ruptured uterus surgery is essential to control the exsanguinating haemorrhage. In certain desperate situations the systolic blood pressure cannot be raised above 50–60 mmHg despite rapid replacement therapy and in these situations immediate operation is mandatory despite the state of shock. As soon as the bleeding point is secured the blood replacement results in rapid recovery. Rarely an ectopic pregnancy is located in a uterine cornu; in this situation uterine bleeding points may be extremely difficult to control and hysterectomy is required. In severe degrees of haemorrhagic shock the intravascular fluid volume should be replaced with compatible blood. This should be done through a large-bore needle or indwelling polythene catheter (16 gauge), to allow rapid transfusion. When a patient's blood loss is estimated to be as much as 6–8 pints the blood which is given should be as fresh as possible.

In late pregnancy severe haemorrhage is usually associated with bleeding from the placental site e.g. placenta praevia or premature separation of the placenta, or with rupture of the uterus. Profuse bleeding in a patient with placenta praevia is often due to the onset of labour. When it is severe enough to produce a state of shock the patient should be admitted directly to the operating theatre and rapid blood volume replacement commenced using compatible whole blood or, if necessary, screened O negative blood. Vaginal examination of a patient with a suspected placenta praevia can provoke torrential bleeding and must never be performed outside an operating theatre which is fully prepared for immediate Caesarean section. The patient must also have an intravenous infusion running and compatible blood available in theatre. In the presence of life-threatening bleeding due to placenta praevia Caesarean section will be the most effective way of stopping the uterine haemorrhage. Once the uterus is emptied the blood loss from the placental site can be controlled by pressure and if necessary haemostatic sutures can be placed in the lower uterine segment to stop bleeding.

Uterine rupture. Rupture of the uterus can occur during pregnancy, labour or at delivery. Severe haemorrhage which can be rapidly fatal may occur, particularly when the uterine artery or one of its large branches has been lacerated. Often these patients have had previous uterine surgery such as hysterotomy or Caesarean section but in the highly parous patient a previously intact uterus can rupture during labour. Uterine rupture can also occur as a result of such obstetric procedures as internal version or forceps delivery through an incompletely dilated cervix. Where vaginal operative deliveries are performed the uterine cavity and lower uterine segment should be explored and the vagina and cervix carefully inspected. In the patient with uterine rupture the presenting picture will be one of shock and signs of internal haemorrhage. If the rupture occurs in labour the fetus may be palpated outside the uterus. Once the diagnosis has been made blood replacement should be started immediately and preparations made for laparotomy. With uterine rupture delay is unwise as there may be no response to resuscitative measures until the severe haemorrhage from the ruptured uterus is stopped. On entering the blood-filled abdomen manual compression of the aorta against the vertebral column will enable better visualization of the bleeding site after removal of the clots. After locating the rupture the bleeding vessels can be controlled with sutures and where the defect is small a repair may be attempted but usually with a ruptured gravid uterus abdominal hysterectomy is indicated. In certain situations in which hysterectomy is undesirable ligation of the internal iliac arteries may be necessary to control the bleeding. This is best performed by isolating the bifurcation of the iliac arteries where the ureter crosses the pelvic brim. The internal iliac artery is identified and ligated; the ligation can be carried out using chromic catgut and adverse effects from this procedure are rarely encountered. Arteriograms 3–6 months after bilateral internal iliac artery ligation will often show the vessels recanalised or the presence of numerous collaterals around the site of the ligatures.

Amniotic fluid embolism. This rare complication can occur in association with high parity, hypertonic uterine contractions as a result of oxytocin or prostaglandin stimulation of labour, intrauterine death, and traumatic delivery. The clinical picture is that of cyanosis and dyspnoea, convulsions and profuse haemorrhage with incoagulable blood. The condition carries a mortality rate of approximately 80% and at postmortem foetal squames and other elements are found in the pulmonary vessels. Amniotic fluid embolism is the most likely diagnosis if profound shock and a haemorrhagic diathesis develop immediately after delivery in a previously normal patient. Oxygen should be given and treatment guided by the observations listed in Table IV; in particular, central venous pressure monitoring is essential. The right atrial pressure is often increased due to the obstruction in the pulmonary circulation and rapid transfusion can precipitate cardiac failure. The infusion rate should be guided by the response of the central venous pressure. Fresh blood replacement and heparinisation for a short period to stop intra-vascular coagulation is the most logical approach (Bonnar, 1973). If fresh blood is not available stored blood, fresh frozen plasma and platelet concentrates should be used. Digitalization may also be indicated if the central venous pressure is elevated.

Fluid loss – shock

Shock due to severe dehydration and electrolyte loss is now rarely seen in developed countries with modern obstetric services. The situation can arise in association with the excessive vomiting of early pregnancy or vomiting as a result of acute pyelonephritis. In late pregnancy hiatus hernia can be aggravated as a consequence of the pressure of the gravid uterus and this can result in obstruction with incessant vomiting. In gynaecological practice the use of gonadotrophin therapy to induce ovulation may result in hyperstimulation of the ovaries. Over a period of a few days large cystic ovaries and ascites develop with a massive fluid shift from the vascular compartment, hypotension and haemoconcentration. Management consists of adequate fluid and electrolyte replacement and in some patients the administration of intravenous albumen.

Supine hypotensive syndrome

This condition is now recognised as a common complication in late pregnancy and especially where epidural anaesthesia is used in labour. Typically the patient is lying on her back in bed or on a couch and while she is being examined she complains of dizziness, breaks out in a cold sweat and can even lose consciousness. The blood pressure shows a progressive drop and the pulse becomes rapid and barely palpable. In severe cases this syndrome becomes evident within a minute but in some patients the hypotension does not develop for five to ten minutes after the patient has been lying in the supine position. The condition is most frequent in the last trimester, particularly near term. The blood pressure returns quickly to normal when the patient is turned on to her side. Caesarean section is often performed with the patient in the total supine position and apart from the hypotension which this may cause in the mother acute fetal distress may arise from the reduction of utero-placental perfusion. Caesarean section is best performed in the right or left lateral position to avoid aortic and caval compression. This can readily be achieved by tilting the table to the left or placing a folded sheet or pad of foam beneath the patient's buttock. Theatre table attachments are also available which incorporate a padded support to elevate and displace the gravid uterus off the vena cava.

Inversion of the uterus

Acute inversion of the uterus is a rare but important cause of shock and haemorrhage in the third stage of labour. The uterus literally turns inside out and the inverted body and fundus passes through the cervix into the vagina and may prolapse through the vulva. Inversion may take place before, during or after placental separation. The commonest cause is third-stage mismanagement with the attendant pressing on the fundus or pulling on the umbilical cord when the uterus is relaxed. Shock is usually extreme and out of proportion to the blood loss. Death may occur very quickly. Unexplained shock in the third stage of labour should suggest uterine inversion. The diagnosis is made by the body of the uterus being no longer palpable in the hypogastrium and a rounded mass being felt protruding through the cervix. If the placenta has detached severe bleeding may also be present.

Acute inversion has a mortality of about 50%. The uterus must be replaced as fast as possible without waiting for resuscitation. Any delay will increase the mortality and make replacement more difficult as the inverted uterus quickly becomes oedematous. If the mother is in extremis the uterus should be replaced without waiting for anaesthesia but if anaesthesia can be given immediately this is advisable. If the placenta is still attached the uterus can be replaced before detaching the placenta but replacement may be easier if the placenta is stripped off. The uterus is manually pushed back into the proper position; the part which inverted last should be replaced first and the fundus last of all. The inverted uterus can also be replaced by running sterile water into the vagina from a douche-can to create an intravaginal fluid pressure; the entrance to the vagina is closed by the hand. After the uterus is replaced further haemorrhage should be prevented by an injection of ergometrine and a syntocinon infusion. Measures to combat shock as described under 'Management of hypovolaemic shock' should be carried out simultaneously but the first priority is replacement of the inverted uterus.

Endotoxic Shock (Bacteraemic or Septic Shock)

In a young woman endotoxic shock is most often seen in association with pregnancy; the condition is the leading cause of maternal death in the United States (Emmanouel et al., 1973). The syndrome is most commonly seen with infection following illegal or legal abortion, but it can also arise with chorioamnionitis, acute pyelonephritis and postpartum sepsis. Endotoxic shock results from infection with gram-negative bacteria and the most common organisms involved in the obstetric patient are *Escherichia coli, Bacteroides,* especially *fragilis, Proteus, Pseudomonas aeruginosa* and *Clostridium welchii.* Studdiford and Douglas (1956) were the first to draw attention to 'vasomotor collapse' in association with septic abortion. The mortality from septic shock has been variously reported as between 30% and 80% (Murdoch et al., 1968; Neeley et al., 1971); in women suffering from endotoxic shock associated with septic abortion a mortality of 15% has been reported (Morris, 1967). The relatively young woman with septic shock may be expected to respond better to therapy than an older debilitated patient. Recovery is much more likely if the diagnosis is made early and the patient receives intensive care. Pulmonary factors in shock are recognised as being important in determining patient survival as well as lung function afterwards (Wilson, 1972).

Pathophysiology. The two main theories proposed to explain the syndrome of endotoxic shock have been selective vasospasm and disseminated intravascular coagulation. Studies of peripheral resistance in patients with endotoxic shock, however, have yielded conflicting data. Disseminated intravascular coagulation was proposed by McKay (1965) who showed a correlation between autopsy findings in patients dying of endotoxic shock and the changes of the generalised Schwartzman reaction in experimental animals. Cavanagh and colleagues (Cavanagh and Dahm, 1972; Cavanagh et al., 1969; 1970) attempted to clarify the mechanism of endotoxic shock by experimental studies in the baboon. In animals given a single intravenous lethal dose of potent coliform endotoxin, selective vasospasm, disseminated intravascular coagulation and reduced myocardial response to sympathetic stimuli all played an important part in the pathogenesis. In the primate the kidney appears to be a primary target organ in endotoxic shock, and acute tubular necrosis is much more frequently associated with endotoxic shock than with hypovolaemic shock due to haemorrhage (Cavanagh et al., 1970).

Clinical aspects

Prevention. Any patient who has an infected abortion may progress to endotoxic shock and as such warrants effective antibiotic therapy and early removal of the infected products of conception. Evacuation of the uterus within six to twelve hours of the initiation of antibiotic therapy is recommended. When such patients are under general anaesthesia for removal of the retained products, the manipulation involved may provoke bacteraemia. The patient may develop central cyanosis, tachycardia and hypotension. Failure of the patient to regain consciousness following the anaesthetic should also raise the suspicion of endotoxic shock. A coagulation disorder, the result of disseminated intravascular coagulation, may also develop, resulting in persistent uterine bleeding and oozing from venepuncture sites. During pregnancy *premature rupture of the membranes* may occur and a conservative policy is usually adopted if the gestation is less than 37 weeks. *Intrauterine infection* may develop and present a more serious hazard to the baby and mother than that of prematurity. Each patient must be considered individually, but where good facilities are available for the care of premature babies and the fetal maturity is over 34 weeks induction of labour should be considered

24 hours after the membranes have ruptured. *Acute pyelonephritis* in pregnancy may, in rare situations, progress to endotoxic shock. Such a development is extremely unlikely in a patient who receives the appropriate antibiotic therapy and intravenous fluids to correct dehydration and electrolyte imbalance.

Diagnosis of septic shock. A past history of drug allergies, renal disease or cardiovascular disease should be obtained. History and clinical examination will provide vital information regarding the source of the infection and the severity of the shock state. The patient's mental condition and the state of the peripheral perfusion are two valuable signs. Cold cyanosed extremities and coma indicate a grave prognosis.

From a clinical standpoint endotoxic shock may be classified as primary or secondary. Primary shock is subdivided into the early or warm hypotensive phase and the late or cold hypotensive phase. Secondary shock is also known as irreversible shock.

Primary shock – early or warm hypotensive phase. In the early phase the patient is hypotensive, alert and apprehensive. Her face is flushed and her skin is warm. The temperature is usually in the range 38.4°C to 40.6°C. Rigors or 'shaking chills' which coincide with temperature peaks may occur. Moderate tachycardia with a pulse rate of 90 to 110 per minute is usually present but in some patients the pulse rate may be less than 72 per minute. The pulse pressure remains satisfactory and urine output is not reduced.

Primary shock – late or cold hypotensive phase. In this late phase of primary shock, the clinical picture is one of a hypotensive patient who is pale and clammy and often with a subnormal temperature. The patient has tachycardia with a pulse rate usually in excess of 110 beats per minute. The blood pressure drops below 80 mmHg and oliguria is present. On rare occasions dyspnoea due to myocardial failure may be present; this generally arises if the patient is seen late or where hypotension has been assumed to be due to hypovolaemia and the patient is over-transfused.

Secondary irreversible shock. Prolonged cellular hypoxia and anaerobic metabolism which arise with endotoxic shock are manifested by metabolic acidosis and excess blood lactate. Irreversible shock should be suspected in any patient who has elevated arterial blood lactate levels. Anuria, with cardiac or respiratory distress and coma indicate a very serious prognosis.

Management of endotoxic shock

Serial monitoring of the patient in endotoxic shock is essential and such patients are therefore best treated in intensive care units with staff experienced in their management. The observations and measurements of importance in the initial and continuing evaluation of the patient in shock are shown in Table IV. Of these the central venous pressure (CVP) is essential for the proper management. In some patients fluid loss will also have occurred from haemorrhage, sequestration of fluid in the bowel or dilatation of the peripheral vascular bed. An important factor in the restoration of blood pressure is to ensure that the blood volume is normal. The CVP provides a reliable guide and sequential changes are more important than the initial reading. However, a CVP reading of less than 2 cm H_2O at the mid-thoracic level reflects a decreased volume of blood returning to the heart and levels higher than 16 cm imply cardiac failure. The sequential changes of the CVP are also a measure of the ability of the cardiovascular system to handle the increasing intravascular volume. When the CVP begins to rise rapidly with the administration of fluid, the limits of cardiovascular competence have been reached. Hardaway et al. (1967) found that the pulmonary artery pressure increases before the CVP when left heart failure develops. If a patient therefore develops evidence of left heart failure in the absence of a high CVP she should be treated regardless of the CVP. If the systolic blood pressure is 100 mmHg or above, the CVP is better maintained at a low normal level (3 to 4 cm of water) particularly if evidence of disseminated intravascular coagulation is present (Hanson, 1974).

Laboratory studies. The investigations which are indicated in the obstetric or gynaecological patient with endotoxic shock are shown in Table V. Cervical smears should be taken immediately for bacteriological examination and the bacteriology services alerted for their urgent examination and aerobic and anaerobic culture. A specimen of urine should be taken for microscopy, culture and biochemical examination. Blood cultures should be obtained and are best taken at the times of rigors or temperature spikes; Mitchell and Simpson (1973) recommended the storage of empty anaerobic jars for anaerobic culture at 37°C to reduce a long period of growth, and using a warm jar they were able to grow bacteroides overnight. Blood biochemical investigations include serum electrolytes and blood urea; arterial blood lactate, pH, and blood gas analysis are also recommended. A full blood count including platelets and film should be done and a screening test for coagulation defect. The platelet count and the level of plasma fibrinogen as determined by the fibrinogen titre are valuable for assessing progress and other tests such as the whole blood

Table V
Investigations in the obstetric patient with endotoxic shock.

1. Bacteriology	Cervical smear Urine and blood for aerobic and anaerobic culture.
2. Biochemistry	Serum urea and electrolytes Urine/plasma osmolarity ratio Arterial blood lactate pH, blood gas analysis and acid-base status.
3. Haematology	Full blood count and film Platelet count and coagulation tests
4. X-ray	Chest and abdomen
5. ECG	

clotting time, thrombin time and prothrombin time will give a broad indication of the degree of coagulation disturbance. Severe thrombocytopoenia associated with prolonged prothrombin or thrombin time and the low fibrinogen titre indicates a severe coagulation defect due to consumption of the components concerned.

Treatment of endotoxic shock. The aims of treatment are to eradicate the source of infection, to restore an effective blood volume and micro-circulation and to correct any metabolic and haematological abnormalities which have arisen as a consequence of the shock state. The particular treatment for any patient will depend on the predisposing condition. If a removable septic focus is present then its removal will be of primary concern. The aspects of management which are of major importance are as follows:

1) Assess the adequacy of ventilation and the airway. Oxygen should be given and if necessary endotracheal intubation or a tracheostomy should be performed. If the arterial PO_2 does not rise above 70 mmHg with oxygen given via a face mask mechanical ventilation should be considered. Pulmonary changes in endotoxic shock – 'shock lung' – seriously compromise respiratory function and ventilatory support can be life-saving.

2) The electrolyte and acid base status should be assessed and adequate fluid and blood replacement given, using the central venous pressure and the urinary output, as guides to the restoration of circulating blood volume. If a metabolic acidosis is present sodium bicarbonate should be given.

3) Antibiotic therapy should be given immediately and not delayed for the results of bacteriological examination. Large doses given by the intravenous route should be used and the antibiotics selected will depend on the known antibiotic sensitivities in the hospital in which the patient is being treated. In the obstetric patient the infecting organism is frequently *E. coli* or *Bacteroides*

and the most effective antibiotic therapy at present is considered to be combinations of gentamicin sulphate and clindamycin, or tobramycin and clindamycin for short term high dosage therapy (Johnston, personal communication, 1975). Other drugs which may be employed include carbenicillin, chloramphenicol and tetracycline. When oliguria is present nephrotoxicity must be considered. If penicillin is used the sodium salt is preferable as large doses of potassium penicillin could be hazardous in the presence of renal impairment.

4) If the response to fluid and antibiotic therapy is unsatisfactory then pharmacological doses of corticosteroids are advised. Methylprednisolone sodium succinate (solu-medrone) 15–30 mg/kg body weight per day or dexamethasone (Decadron) 3–6 mg/kg body weight per day is recommended given by continuous intravenous infusion after an initial loading dose of 125 mg of methylprednisolone sodium succinate or 20 mg of dexamethasone (125 mg of methylprednisolone sodium succinate is equivalent to 500 mg of hydrocortisone). The precise mode of action of the corticosteroid therapy is not known but these drugs may exert a beneficial effect on endothelium, platelets and the pulmonary circulation. Large doses of corticosteroids improve tissue perfusion by decreasing peripheral vascular resistance. The sudden discontinuation of corticosteroids which have been given for short periods, up to 72 hours, apparently produces no ill-effects and a regimen of gradual withdrawal is not necessary (Cavanagh and Comas, 1975).

Cardiac failure. In the patient with a sustained tachycardia and a central venous pressure above 15 cm of water, digitalisation is indicated. The serum potassium should be normal prior to digitalisation; in the presence of impaired renal function digoxin toxicity may arise. An intitial dose of 0.5 mg digoxin should be given slowly intravenously, preferably under ECG monitoring and a further dose of 0.25 mg may be indicated over the next twelve hours. The digoxin can be discontinued after 48 hours when the patient's condition has improved.

Vasoactive therapy. If shock persists after the use of steroids, the use of isoprenaline has been recommended (Mortsay et al., 1970). Isoprenaline is a pure β-mimetic drug which results in arteriolar dilatation and an increased heart-rate and stroke volume leading to an increased cardiac output. Continuous ECG monitoring is essential to detect cardiac arrhythmia. Isoprenaline should be administered as an infusion in a concentration of 8 μg/ml and the speed of the infusion regulated so that the pulse rate remains below 130 beats per minute. If the tachycardia persists a β-adrenergic blocker such as practolol may be used but in patients with endotoxic shock cardiac arrest can occur.

Renal function. Immediate and continuing assessment of renal function in endotoxic shock is essential. Patients in renal failure are particularly liable to fluid overload, hyperkalaemia and drug toxicity. If oliguria is present and a urine/plasma osmolarity ratio of less than 1 : 1, acute renal failure is likely to develop. Mannitol infusion may save patients with poor renal function from developing acute renal failure. If oliguria persists despite mannitol, large doses of frusemide are recommended in an attempt to induce a diuresis; up to 2000 mg of frusemide may be given intravenously daily at a rate of not more than 250 mg/hour (Hanson, 1974). Renal dialysis may be required and should be started early. Peritoneal dialysis may be successful in patients with septic abortion but if there is any suspicion about intestinal or uterine trauma haemodialysis is preferable. When acute renal failure is diagnosed the dosage of drugs being administered should be reviewed and nephrotoxic antibiotics should, if possible, be avoided.

Haematological aspects. Bacterial endotoxin either directly or indirectly through the effects on the cardiovascular system can trigger disseminated intravascular coagulation. The degree of intravascular clotting will be indicated by the platelet count and the fibrinogen titre. Where haemorrhage is not a problem the use of heparin will arrest the intravascular fibrin deposition and routine heparinisation of patients with septic abortion has been recommended (Margulis et al., 1971). In patients with excessive bleeding the blood loss may be aggravated if heparin is introduced and the replacement of the depleted haemostatic components by fresh blood transfusion is the most appropriate therapy. This will provide coagulation factors and platelets, as well as the coagulation inhibitors, antithrombin III and anti-Xa. When peripheral perfusion has improved as the result of blood volume expansion, coupled with steroid and antibiotic therapy, the consumption of coagulation factors and platelets usually stops. If peripheral perfusion remains poor and evidence of continued consumption of clotting factors is present, then antithrombotic therapy with heparin should be considered. In the presence of intravascular coagulation the low levels of coagulation factors and large amounts of fibrin degradation products will render clotting tests unreliable for assaying heparin. The dosage of heparin is best controlled by monitoring the level in the circulation with a specific test based on its anti-Xa effect (Denson and Bonnar, 1973). A level of heparin in the plasma of 0.2 to 0.5 units/ml as shown by the anti-Xa assay will not compromise local haemostatic function but will inhibit activated factor X; a concept now used in the prophylaxis of thrombosis by low dosage heparin. In a patient with endotoxic shock heparin is best given by intravenous infusion and not by bolus intravenous injection as the latter is followed by dangerously high levels of heparin (Bonnar et al., 1972).

Surgical treatment. At the initial clinical assessment the question of surgical removal of any septic focus should be considered. Medical treatment may improve the patient initially but should there be an extensive nidus of infection medical treatment alone may not save the patient. In cases of septic abortion the uterus should be evacuated as soon as adequate supportive measures are under way and preferably within six hours of diagnosis. The removal of the infected products of conception by digital evacuation of the uterus followed by gentle curettage may be all that is required. Suction curettage is also a rapid and effective way of removing infected products of conception. If, however, the uterus is gangrenous or the infection has advanced to the stage of micro-abscess formation in the myometrium then hysterectomy may be the only effective surgical treatment. Hysterectomy should be considered 1) if the patient continues in shock following curettage and adequate supportive measures, 2) the uterus is over 16 weeks gestational size, 3) the uterus is perforated, 4) an intrauterine *Clostridium welchii* infection is present, or 5) a corrosive toxic douche has been used. An aggressive surgical approach is advocated where signs of extensive pelvic infection are present including X-ray findings of gas in the uterine wall and evidence of intravascular haemolysis (Ledger, 1972). Hysterectomy may be technically difficult due to the presence of inflammation and oedema in the pelvis and the operation should be performed by an experienced gynaecological surgeon. When clostridial infection is present the pedicle size should be kept small to avoid leaving behind any unnecessary devitalised tissue.

In the presence of chorioamnionitis, if vaginal delivery is not achieved within twelve hours, delivery by Caesarean section should be considered. If severe uterine infection or endotoxic shock is present Caesarean hysterectomy may be the best form of treatment. Patients with endotoxic shock are often critically ill and if they are deteriorating rapidly urgent surgery may be mandatory. As soon as the supportive measures are under way and the dynamic blood volume restored operation should be performed under the cover of steroids and antibiotics. These patients are prone to cardiac dysrhythmias and monitoring of the central venous pressure and ECG are essential. A considerable danger of bleeding during the operation is present as a result of intravascular coagulation and compatible fresh blood or fresh frozen plasma should be available to provide a supply of coagulation factors including fibrinogen.

Cardio-Pulmonary Shock and Complications of Anaesthesia

Cardiac arrest may occur due to myocardial infarction, cardiac tamponade or massive pulmonary embolism and in these circumstances treatment will be as in the non-pregnant individual. When cardiac arrest occurs in an obstetric patient it is usually in association with anaesthesia. As other causes of maternal death have declined, anaesthetic deaths have become of major concern in maternal mortality. In obstetric emergency operations the patients are often at considerable risk from the anaesthetic and all too often a junior anaethetist without proper supervision has to take the responsibility. Anaesthetic complications appear to occur more commonly in obese and coloured patients. In the latter hypoxia may not be easily recognised.

Anaesthetic deaths in obstetrics. Of the maternal deaths associated with complications of anaesthesia which were reported in the *Report on Confidential Enquiries into Maternal Deaths in England and Wales* (1972) avoidable factors were present in 34 of the 50 deaths. Over half of the deaths were due to aspiration of regurgitated stomach contents. Difficulties may arise with tracheal intubation and with repeated attempts stomach contents may enter the trachea and result in asphyxia. Aspiration of gastric contents may follow regurgitation or vomiting during recovery from an anaesthetic. Prevention of this serious hazard is a basic principle of all obstetric anaesthetic technique. When a woman is in labour her stomach can never be assumed to be empty – labour, pain, analgesic drugs, all contribute to delayed emptying. Achalasia of the cardia which is common in pregnancy, upward displacement of the stomach due to the gravid uterus and the raised intra-abdominal pressure during labour all favour regurgitation. In his classic studies of the aspiration syndrome, Mendelson (1946) showed that acid contents produced a chemical pneumonitis in the lungs which did not develop if the acidity was neutralised. When emergency general anaesthesia is required in an obstetric patient, 15 ml of a magnesium trisilicate mixture should be given to raise the pH of the gastric contents.

Treatment of aspiration of gastric contents. Immediate action to clear the tracheo-bronchial tree of as much solid or liquid material as quickly as possible, including lavage with a sodium bicarbonate solution, is of vital importance. In the undelivered mother the immediate risk to the child which will result from the delay in the operative procedure must be accepted.

Steroid therapy should be used such as hydrocortisone, 200–400 mg initially and 600 mg daily for maintenance (Kennedy, 1974). Artificial ventilation is required with concentrations of oxygen to correct hypoxia and the patient should be supervised in an intensive care unit. When cardiac arrest is secondary to asphyxia, fatal cerebral damage has usually already occurred.

Hypotension following regional anaesthesia. The principal cause of hypotension in obstetric patients following lumbar or caudal epidural anaesthesia is sympathetic blockade which results in loss of vasomotor tone, peripheral pooling and decreased venous return (Cohen, 1974). An intravenous infusion should always be set up before a regional block is given and the total supine position should be avoided to prevent aortocaval compression. When hypotension occurs the patient must be turned on her side to remove all compression on the vena cava and oxygen administered. The intravenous infusion should be accelerated and the legs elevated to promote venous return. If these measures do not restore the arterial blood pressure intravenous ephedrine or mephenteramine should be given by incremental doses. These drugs do not appear to compromise uterine blood flow.

High or total spinal block. This may occur as a complication of a lumbar or caudal epidural. The onset may be immediate and if not recognised can result in death. Very shortly after the block is given the patient becomes restless, drowsy and dyspnoeic, cannot speak and rapidly loses consciousness. Respiratory arrest, cardiovascular collapse and cardiac arrest can follow within seconds. In a high spinal block with diaphragmatic breathing still present oxygen administration and reassurance of the mother may be sufficient. With a total spinal block, apnoea will develop and loss of consciousness; endotracheal intubation and positive pressure ventilation with 100% oxygen should be instituted immediately.

If the patient is not unconscious light general anaesthesia can be given followed by endotracheal intubation and controlled ventilation. Hypotension should be corrected as described above and with prompt therapy cardiac arrest can be avoided. These life-threatening complications of regional anaesthesia emphasize the necessity of having skilled anaesthetic staff and resuscitation equipment at hand when regional blocks are given.

References

Bader, R.A., Bader, M.E., Rose, D.J. and Braunwald, E. (1955): Hemodynamics at rest and during exercise in normal pregnancy as studied by cardiac catheterization. *J. clin. Invest., 34,* 1524.

Bonnar, J. (1973): Blood coagulation and fibrinolysis in obstetrics. *Clinics in Haematology*, p. 213. Editor: A.S. Douglas. Saunders, London.

Bonnar, J., Denson, K.W.E. and Biggs, R. (1972): Subcutaneous heparin and prevention of thrombosis. *Lancet, 2*, 539.

Bonnar, J., McNicol, G.P. and Douglas, A.S. (1970a): Coagulation and fibrinolytic mechanisms during and after normal childbirth. *Brit. med. J., 2*, 200.

Bonnar, J., Prentice, C.R.M., McNicol, G.P. and Douglas, A.S. (1970b): Haemostatic mechanism in the uterine circulation during placental separation. *Brit. med. J., 2*, 564.

Cavanagh, D. and Comas, M.R. (1975): Shock. *Gynecology and Obstetrics*. Editor: Romney. McGraw Hill (in press).

Cavanagh, D. and Dahm, Jr. C.H. (1972): Endotoxic shock. *Obstet. Gynaec., 1*, 273.

Cavanagh, D., Rao, P.S., Sutton, D.M.C., Bhagat, B.D. and Bachmann, F. (1969): Endotoxic shock in the subhuman primate. I. Hemodynamic and biochemical changes. *Arch. Surg., 99*, 107.

Cavanagh, D., Rao, P.S., Sutton, D.M.C., Bhagat, B.D. and Bachmann, F. (1970): Pathophysiology of endotoxic shock in the primate. *Amer. J. Obstet. Gynec., 108*, 705.

Cohen, H. (1974): Complications of regional anesthesia in obstetrics. *Clin. Obstet. Gynec., 17/2*, 211.

Denson, K.W.E. and Bonnar, J. (1973): The measurement of heparin: a method based on the potentiation of anti-factor Xa. *Thrombos. diathes. haemorrh. (Stuttg.), XXX*, 471.

Dolezal, A. and Figar, S. (1965): The phenomenon of reactive vasodilation in pregnancy. *Amer. J. Obstet. Gynec., 93*, 1137.

Emmanouel, D.S.M., Gonzalez-Loya, J.P. and Katz, A.I. (1973): Renal complications of shock in pregnancy. *J. reprod. Med., II/1*, 6.

Gilbert, R. and Auchincloss, J.H. (1966): Dyspnoea of pregnancy, clinical and physiological observations. *Amer. J. med. Sci., 252*, 270.

Ginsburg, J. and Duncan, S.L.B. (1969): Peripheral blood flow in normal pregnancy. *Cardiovasc. Res., 1*, 132.

Goodrich, S.M. and Wood, J.E. (1964): Peripheral venous distensibility and velocity of venous blood flow during pregnancy or during oral contraceptive therapy. *Amer. J. Obstet. Gynec., 90*, 740.

Hanson, G.C. (1974): Septicaemic shock. *Postgrad. med. J., 50*, 288.

Hardaway, R.M., James, P.M. and Anderson, R.W. (1967): Intensive study and treatment of shock in man. *J. Amer. med. Ass., 199*, 779.

Herbert, C.M., Banner, E.A. and Wakim, K.G. (1958): Variations in the peripheral circulation during pregnancy. *Amer. J. Obstet. Gynec., 76*, 742.

Hytten, F.A. and Leitch, I. (1971): Cardiovascular dynamics. In: *Physiology of Human Pregnancy, 2nd Ed.*, pp. 69–110. Blackwell Scientific Publications, Oxford.

Ihrman, K. (1960): A clinical and physiological study of pregnancy in a material from Northern Sweden. VI. The arterial blood pressure at rest and in orthostatic test during and after pregnancy. *Acta Soc. Med. upsalien., 65*, 315.

Kennedy, R.L. (1974): General analgesia and anesthesia in obstetrics. *Clin. Obstet. Gynec., 17/2*, 227.

Ledger, W.J. (1972): Infections in obstetrics and gynecology. *Surg. Clin. N. Amer., 52*, 1447.

Lloyd, S. and Pickford, M. (1961): The action of posterior pituitary hormones and oestrogens on the vascular system of the rate. *J. Physiol. (Lond.), 155*, 161.

Lyons, H.A. and Antonio, R. (1959): The sensitivity of the respiratory centre in pregnancy and after the administration of progesterone. *Trans. Ass. Amer. Phys., 72*, 173.

McKay, D.G. (1965): *Disseminated Intravascular Coagulation: An Intermediary Mechanism of Disease*. Hoeber-Harper.

Margulis, R.R., Dustin, R.W., Lovell, J.R., Robb, H. and Jabs, C. (1971): Heparin for septic abortion and the prevention of endotoxic shock. *Obstet. Gynec., 37*, 474.

Mendelson, C.L. (1946): Aspiration of the stomach contents into the lungs during obstetric anaesthesia. *Amer. J. Obstet. Gynec., 52*, 191.

Mitchell, A.A.B. and Simpson, R.G. (1973): Bacteroides septicaemia. *Curr. med. Res. Opinion, I*, 385.

Morris, J.A. (1967): Bacteraemic shock in obstetrics. *Advances in Obstetrics and Gynecology, Vol. I.* Editors: S.L. Marcus and C.C. Markus. Wilkins & Wilkins Co., Baltimore.

Mortsay, G.J., Alho, A., Jaeger, T., Rietzman, R.A. and Lillehei, R.C. (1970): Effects of corticosteroids on the circulation in shock. Experimental and clinical results. *Fed. Proc., 29*, 1861.

Murdoch, J.C.McC., Speirs, C.F. and Pullen, H. (1968): The bacteraemic shock syndrome. *Brit. J. Hosp. Med., I/3*, 346.

Neely, W.A., Berry, D.W., Rushton, F.W. and Hardy, J.D. (1971): Septic shock. Clinical physiological and pathological survey of 244 patients. *Ann. Surg., 173/5*, 657.

Newman, R.L. (1957): Serum electrolytes in pregnancy, parturition and puerperium. *Obstet. Gynec., 10*, 51.

O'Driscoll, K. and McCarthy, J.R. (1966): Abruptio placentae and central venous pressures. *J. Obstet. Gynaec. Brit. Cwlth, 73*, 923.

Report on Confidential Enquiries into Maternal Deaths in England and Wales, 1967–69 (1972): Department of Health and Social Security, Her Majesty's Stationery Office, London.

Studdiford, W.E. and Douglas, G.W. (1956): Placental bacteraemia: a significant finding in septic abortion accompanied by vascular collapse. *Amer. J. Obstet. Gynec., 71*, 842.

Trower, R. and Walters, W.A.W. (1968): Brachial arterial blood pressure in the lateral recumbent position during pregnancy. *Aust. N. Z. J. Obstet. Gynaec., 8*, 146.

Wilson, J.W. (1972): Pulmonary factors produced by septic shock cause or consequence of shock lung. *J. reprod. Med., 8/6*, 307.

Ledingham (ed.). Shock

Burn shock

D.M. HEIMBACH

Introduction

In terms of overall care and rehabilitation, there is probably no more challenging patient in all of medicine than the burn victim. On the other hand, his initial care is usually straightforward. Without associated injuries, the etiology of his shock is readily apparent, and the depth and extent of his burns provide predictive value both for the severity of the shock and for resuscitation requirements. The present chapter will deal with the pathophysiology of burn shock, compare the most common resuscitation methods, and, finally, mention some anesthetic problems in the acute post-burn period.

Pathophysiology

The skin is the largest organ of the body and thermal injury destroys all regulatory function. Normal keratin layers and lipid content of the skin prevent the passage of water vapor from the tissues into the environment. Following a full thickness burn, all such function is lost and water evaporates from the tissues at nearly the same rate it would from an open pan. With a partial thickness burn, some vapor barrier is retained, but evaporation still proceeds at an accelerated rate proportional to the depth of burn (Wilson and Moncrief, 1965; Jelenko, 1967; Jelenko et al., 1967, 1968, 1971). With 40% of the skin surface burned, water losses may amount to 100 ml/m^2/hour through the burn itself (Moncrief and Mason, 1964). This evaporative loss increases daily free water requirements by two to three liters over basal requirements of nonburned individuals. It was assumed that the heat production required in evaporation was a major source of the hypermetabolism universally found in the burn patient. More recent work, however, has shown that the hypermetabolic state persists even when evaporative water loss is prevented (Neely et al., 1974; Zawacki et al., 1970).

The shield provided by the skin from assault by environmental bacteria is also destroyed by burning. Sepsis with gram-negative bacteremia and shock is the commonest cause of death after the first ten days following injury. Sepsis as a cause of shock in the early post-burn phase is uncommon except in massively contaminated wounds or burns associated with other systemic injuries. Infection occurring during the first several days post-burn is almost invariably caused by gram-positive cocci (usually streptococcus). Such infections are manifested by spreading erythema beyond the limits of the burn, high fever, and disorientation, but, in contrast to gram-negative sepsis, rarely present as shock. To prevent this serious early complication, some burn centers advocate low dosage prophylactic penicillin given for the first five days following injury.

Full thickness cutaneous injury markedly alters the physiology of the whole organism. In areas of full thickness loss, cells are coagulated and the capillaries are thrombosed. Areas surrounding full thickness burns and areas of partial thickness damage develop marked capillary permeability with intense plasma protein and electrolyte sequestration into the area of injury. Cinephotomicrographs taken by Robb (1967), taken as a burn was produced in the mesentery of rabbits, demonstrate the dynamics of the microcirculation. Arteriolar and venular dilatation are considered first degree changes. Many additional capillaries become visible and carry blood whereas they had been empty before. A second degree state is characterized by precipitation of platelets along the walls of venules. Platelet thrombi and stasis occur in both arterioles and venules in the third degree state. In addition to increased capillary permeability, venous stasis in the presence of continued arteriolar flow enhances edema formation. In small burns edema formation is limited to the burn itself and the immediately adjacent areas. It is well documented, however, both clinically and experimentally, that larger burns are associated with extensive edema formation in unburned areas, regardless of the resuscitation method. The mechanism is not yet understood. Recent studies from Baxter's laboratories (Vaught et al., 1974), using intracellular membrane potentials, demonstrate significant alterations of muscle cell membrane function almost immediately after thermal injury resulting in an intracellular translocation of sodium and, to a lesser extent, water into skeletal muscle cells distant from the burn site. As a result of this additional fluid translocation in areas remote from the burn, the circulating plasma volume is further diminished. Transcapillary refill from 'normal' areas replenishes the plasma volume at the expense of the total body extracellular fluid space. The vicious circle continues as the transiently increased plasma volume is further sequestered as edema fluid. In addition to pure mechanical volume depletion, there are undoubtedly circulating denatured proteins, peptides, kinins, and vasoactive amines, all of which create an unstable vascular space.

The end result of the above factors is a marked depression of cardiac output with consequent decreases in visceral perfusion, leading to classic hypovolemic shock. If untreated, death results from large burns; and in medium sized burns, acute tubular necrosis with anuric renal failure is a common accompaniment. Such tragic consequences are almost entirely preventable if appropriate resuscitation is begun in the early hours post burn. Very large and deep burns may produce free hemoglobin and myoglobin from red cell and muscle destruction. The resultant hemoglobinuria and myoglobinuria only seriously impair renal function in the presence of decreased renal blood flow. The characteristic burgundy urine generally clears after several hours of diuresis. If adequate urine volume is achieved with fluid load, alkalization, and occasionally osmotic diuretics, serious renal sequelae are rare. The same generalized capillary permeability appears to affect the kidney during the early post-burn period, manifested by proteinuria with substances of a molecular weight as high as 150,000 found in the urine by the third post-burn day. As with other capillaries, however, after this period there is a gradual and progressive healing of the lesion. On the other hand tubular integrity as measured by sodium resorption, potassium excretion and ability to handle water, creatinine, and urea remain unimpaired in the presence of adequate resuscitation.

Studies on anesthetized dogs with severe scald burns demonstrate an increased mean arterial blood pressure and pulse rate after the burn but both tended to stabilize with time. Cardiac output showed a precipitous fall immediately after the burn and remained very much decreased throughout the entire post-burn period, while the mean circulation time progressively increased after the burn and the central blood volume progressively decreased (Michie et al., 1963). The maintenance of a relatively stable blood pressure coupled with decreasing cardiac output indicates that peripheral resistance is markedly increased.

This may be due either to peripheral vascular constriction or increases in blood viscosity. 'Sludging' of blood due to a markedly increased viscosity is common (Brooks et al., 1950). The overall pathophysiology thus appears to be increased transudation of fluid through capillary walls with resultant edema formation leading to hemoconcentration and sludging which decreases effective circulatory fluid volume and thereby decreased central blood volume with a decreased cardiac output.

Hematologic Changes

Anemia following severe burns begins during the first week, is progressive, and may be severe. The older literature presumed actual thermal damage to erythrocytes resulting in acute hemolysis and decreased survival of damaged erythrocytes as well as the progressive sequestration of circulating red cells in the wound during the early post-burn phase (Davies and Topley, 1956; Gilmore and Fozzard, 1960; Jones et al., 1956; Moore et al., 1946). Several features of the anemia, however, cast doubt on this mechanistic theory. For example, the disappearance of both autologous and transfused red blood cells occurs at relatively equal rate throughout the first post-burn week (Davies and Topley, 1956). The bizarre shape of red blood cells commonly found in the first post-burn week has been attributed to heat damage, but also reappeared following exchange transfusion in burn patients. An interesting study by Loebl and Baxter (Loebl et al., 1973, 1974) using chromium^{51}-labeled erythrocytes in a crossover study between burn patients and normal controls demonstrated the half life of normal erythrocytes from non-burn donors was very short in burn patients compared to the survival in normal volunteers. The survival time of the patient's own red cells was equally decreased when reinjected into the patient after the chromium^{51} labeling. The survival time of the patient's cells, however, when transfused into unburned individuals was found to be in the normal range. In addition, external counting to measure the distribution of chromium^{51} cells in the burn patient failed to demonstrate progressive accumulation of radioisotope in the burn wound or the spleen implying that these were not selective sites of red cell removal from the circulation. The study implies an ongoing humoral or vascular mechanism resulting in increased erythrocyte destruction as an important feature of the post-burn anemia in addition to the relatively small number of cells actually destroyed and trapped in the burn wound.

A mild form of intravascular coagulation occurs in all full thickness burns, and in large burns, may be of sufficient magnitude to show abnormalities in clotting function. As demonstrated by Gehrke (Gehrke et al., 1971) thrombocytopenia, abnormal platelet function, and plasma clotting factor deficiencies were demonstrated in addition to a circulating anticoagulant with properties similar to those of heparin. In addition, increased fibrin split products have been demonstrated indicating increased fibrinolysis (Baxter et al., 1967). These laboratory changes rarely proceed to clinical bleeding. When they do, some other mechanism of disseminated intravascular coagulation should be sought – usually gram-negative septicemia. It has been recently suggested that heparinization may be useful as routine treatment in the burn patient (Saliba et al., 1973). It would seem, however, that the hazards of such anticoagulation (from GI bleeding, burn debridement, escharotomy, and from tracheostomy if one is required) would far outweigh the benefits in the routine circumstance.

Gastrointestinal Problems

The most common early gastrointestinal problem is a paralytic ileus. Patients behave unpredictably in this regard but many patients with burns over 30% of their total body surface will not tolerate oral intake for the first 48 hours post burn. Gastric distention becomes especially hazardous in patients with facial or oral burns where the resultant edema prevents expulsion of vomitus which may then find its way into the trachea and lead to a severe aspiration pneumonia. For this reason it is the policy of some burn centers routinely to place a nasogastric tube in patients at risk with burns in excess of 35%. Curling's ulcer with massive hemorrhage may occur within 24 hours postburn but usually occurs after the resuscitation period is complete. Massive GI hemorrhage should certainly be considered in any patient who develops shock in spite of apparently adequate fluid resuscitation.

Pulmonary Changes

The term 'respiratory burn' is probably a misnomer. Reflex closure of the glottis, the cooling effect of the upper airway, and the poor heat carrying capacity of air protect the respiratory tree from thermal injury and, experimentally, thermal necrosis of the tracheo-bronchial tree can be produced only by the direct instillation of live steam into the trachea (Moritz et al., 1945) or by direct inhalation of combustible gases. On the other hand, there is no question that the byproducts of combustion, particularly of the newer synthetic fabrics and plastics, can produce intense damage to the lungs. The symptoms of such inhalation injury occur during the resuscitation period and should be differentiated from the pulmonary complications which are among the most common causes of late mortality. The later pulmonary complications share many of the features of 'post-traumatic pulmonary insufficiency' occurring with other forms of trauma and sepsis and are beyond the scope of this chapter (Achauer et al., 1973; Dressler and Skornik, 1972; Foley et al., 1968; Rapaport et al., 1973; Skornik and Dressler, 1970). Inhalation of noxious gases produces a severe tracheo-bronchitis and alveolar damage. The first symptoms of such damage usually occur within 18 to 36 hours post-burn and are manifested by wheezing and bronchospasm. Such symptoms have ominous portent with the reported mortality rates varying from 48% (Stone and Martin, 1969) to 90% (Stone et al., 1967). The injury should be suspected in any patient with a flame facial burn or singed nasal vibrissi. Significant pulmonary damage is uncommon in burns sustained out of doors but should always be suspected in flame burns occurring in a closed space. In a suspect patient, frequent check of arterial blood gases may be the earliest hint of forthcoming problems. While it has been previously demonstrated that a decrease in PO_2 occurs following any significant trauma (Epstein et al., 1963), a significant fall in PO_2 from admission levels occurring after resuscitation has begun may be the earliest manifestation of pulmonary injury. Even with a deteriorating patient, the chest X-ray may remain clear for several days and is of little use. Prompt and vigorous pulmonary therapy is essential to reverse the natural history of the disease which leads to progressive pulmonary edema, infection, and terminal (hyaline) membrane disease. High risk patients may benefit from a 'croup tent' prior to the onset of symptoms. After wheezing begins, the patient may or may not benefit from the usual bronchodilators. Bolus therapy with large doses (20 to 25 mg/kg) of corticosteroid repeated every 6 to 12 hours as necessary may affect the bronchospasm with dramatic results (Stone and Martin, 1969). If the disease progresses in spite of this therapy, control of the airway must be attained either with endotracheal intubation or tracheostomy. At that point a progression of pulmonary therapy should be instituted similar to that commonly used with other forms of post-traumatic pulmonary insufficiency. Fluid therapy is extremely important with patients with inhalation injury and pulmonary edema may be aggravated by whatever resuscitative regimen is used. The use of diuretics and osmotic loads are still controversial, without convincing evidence of either being efficacious.

Initial Patient Evaluation

Whatever resuscitation program is used, there is general agreement about initial patient evaluation and appropriate clinical response to resuscitation. Patients will be seen at varying intervals from the time of injury, but fluids should be started immediately on arrival at the emergency ward. All clothing should be removed and, as with all trauma patients, immediate attention directed to the airway. In the absence of pulmonary injury, it is very rare for a burn patient to need a tracheostomy. Facial burns per se, while not an indication for tracheostomy, should alert the clinician to its possible need during the second 12 to 24 hours. Expectoration of carbonaceous sputum is a warning that inhalation injury may be present, as is history of a flame burn occurring in a closed space. The history is important in searching for associated trauma or underlying diseases that may have caused the burn – myocardial infarction, Stokes–Adams attack, and cerebral vascular accidents are not uncommon causes of burns in the older population. Associated injuries or medical problems may markedly alter the resuscitation plan and, in fact, may take precedence over the burn injury itself. The extent of the burn should then be carefully mapped, using either a standard form (Fig. 1), or, if not available, the 'rule of Nines' provides a satisfactory estimate. The rule of Nines divides the total body surface as follows: each upper extremity, 9%; head and neck, 9%; anterior trunk, 18%; posterior trunk, 18%; each lower extremity, 18%; and genitalia, 1%. When using this rule, note that a child's head is somewhat higher in proportion to his body than an adult's head. For purposes of resuscitation, most authors consider partial and full thickness burns as a unit in calculating fluid requirements. The patient should be weighed on admission and patients with serious burns (those in excess of 25%) should have a Foley catheter placed for monitoring of hourly urine output. Tetanus prophylaxis should be given if the patient has not been immunized within the five year period preceding his burn. All other medications, including narcotics, should be given intravenously since absorption by any other route is uncertain, at best. Patients with underlying heart disease, associated trauma, or large burns (45% and above) should have a central venous catheter placed, either through the subclavian route, or threaded through a large peripheral vein. Less critical burns, however, can be easily managed with urine output alone, and the central venous system should not be violated. The burn wounds should be gently washed, dead skin debrided and blisters broken. Debridement can almost always be accomplished with minimal pain using small doses of intravenous narcotics and should not require general anesthesia. A dilute

DALLAS COUNTY HOSPITAL DISTRICT

DALLAS, TEXAS

BURN RECORD

To be completed upon admission:

Unit # __________

Name __________

Address __________

Birthdate __________

Classification __________

OP ☐ ER ☐ IP ☐ Admit # __________

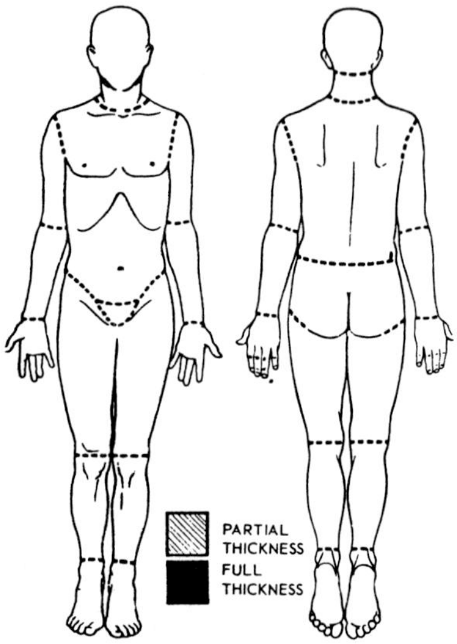

Date: __________

Height: __________ **Weight:** __________

2° ______ + 3° ______ = ______ %

Percent Surface Area Burned
(Berkow Formula)

AREA	1 YR.	1–4 YRS.	5–9 YRS.	10–14 YRS.	15 YRS.	ADULT	2°	3°
Head	19	17	13	11	9	7		
Neck	2	2	2	2	2	2		
Ant. Trunk	13	13	13	13	13	13		
Post Trunk	13	13	13	13	13	13		
R. Buttock	2½	2½	2½	2½	2½	2½		
L. Buttock	2½	2½	2½	2½	2½	2½		
Genitalia	1	1	1	1	1	1		
R.U. Arm	4	4	4	4	4	4		
L.U. Arm	4	4	4	4	4	4		
R.L. Arm	3	3	3	3	3	3		
L.L. Arm	3	3	3	3	3	3		
R. Hand	2½	2½	2½	2½	2½	2½		
L. Hand	2½	2½	2½	2½	2½	2½		
R. Thigh	5½	6½	8	8½	9	9½		
L. Thigh	5½	6½	8	8½	9	9½		
R. Leg	5	5	5½	6	6½	7		
L. Leg	5	5	5½	6	6½	7		
R. Foot	3½	3½	3½	3½	3½	3½		
L. Foot	3½	3½	3½	3½	3½	3½		
TOTAL								

034

FORM NO. 50415

Fig. 1

solution of organic iodine is a useful antiseptic, but hexachlorophene soaps should be avoided in small children because of the danger of systemic absorption and the possibility of convulsions. In patients at risk of ileus and gastric dilatation, a nasogastric tube is placed on low suction. Base line laboratory blood work is drawn and should include hemoglobin, hematocrit, serum electrolytes, clotting studies, arterial blood gases, pH, and type and cross matching for blood. Serial hemoglobin, hematocrit, electrolyte and blood gas determinations are then obtained at intervals of about 6 hours. With resuscitation well under way, the wound is now ready for the preferred local management, including exposure, topical chemotherapy, or 0.5% silver nitrate solution.

Careful notation should be made of any full thickness circumferential burn of the extremities, trunk or neck. If this point is overlooked, disastrous consequences may result. After thermal destruction of elastic fibers, the full thickness burn eschar rapidly becomes an unyielding carapace. Subsequent edema formation expands inward from this closed space and may seriously compromise the circulation distal to its constricting band. Ignorance of this fact has caused loss of unburned distal extremities, and needless tracheostomies on patients whose respiratory difficulty resulted from constriction of the chest wall rather than airway obstruction. The problem is easily relieved by an escharotomy through the burned skin down to subcutaneous tissue in areas of constricting third degree burns. This procedure can be done without anesthesia, since the full thickness burn is anesthetic, and if not performed too deeply, can be done with little blood loss.

Assessment of Resuscitation

The patient with adequate resuscitation should be alert and cooperative. Combativeness usually represents hypoxia, either from diminished blood flow or early inhalation injury. Blood pressure monitoring is frequently difficult with burned extremities, but the heart rate should remain below 110 in adults. Capillary filling should remain prompt in unburned area and the skin should remain warm and pink. Most authors agree that an adult's urine output should be 50 ml per hour and children's output should be no less than 25 ml per hour. In the absence of cardiac disease, urine flow is probably as good a guide as central venous pressure for moderate sized burns (Rubin and Bongiovi, 1970). None of the present methods of resuscitation will prevent the hemoglobin from rising, but the amount of its rise will give some indication as to fluid requirements. These simple clinical parameters are usually satisfactory in guiding resuscitation; the most useful probably being the urinary output. A satisfactory urine output implies a satisfactory renal blood flow and is a reasonable measure of visceral perfusion elsewhere.

Resuscitation

There is no more hotly contested issue in the management of the burn patient than what form the fluid resuscitation should take. Fortunately, all modern programs provide a relatively equal survival rate. We thus are faced with a choice between several satisfactory regimens and must use other parameters for success. The ideal regimen should be easily administered, monitored with minimum laboratory data, use inexpensive fluid, maintain a normal hematocrit and normal level of serum albumin, return all physiological parameters to normal, and produce minimal edema formation. Such a regimen does not presently exist. We unfortunately do not know the best parameters to choose in measuring response to resuscitation. It is certainly comforting to have an alert patient excreting large volumes of good quality urine with a normal cardiac output, but it is difficult to assess the possible harm done by increased edema and the modestly overloaded cardiovascular tree required to achieve these goals. Thus, it may be useful to briefly review the various treatment programs and mention some advantages and disadvantages of each. The composition and rate of administration, rather than the total quantity given provide the basic differences among treatment plans. Composition varies from colloid alone, colloid plus electrolyte solution, isotonic electrolyte solution alone, and hypertonic electrolyte solution.

Resuscitation Programs

Mixtures of colloid and crystalloid

The two most commonly used combination formulas are the Evans (Evans et al., 1952) and the Brooke (Reiss et al., 1953) formulas. Both formulas have been successfully used for twenty years and provide the standard by which newer formulas are judged. Both were derived retrospectively by calculating

Table I
Comparison of Evans and Brooke formulas.

Evans:	Brooke:
First 24 hr	First 24 hr
colloid 1 ml/kg/% burn	colloid 0.5 ml/kg/% burn
crystalloid 1 ml/kg/% burn	crystalloid 1.5 ml/kg/% burn
maintenance water (2000 ml)	maintenance water (2000 ml)
Half given during the first 8 hr	Half given during first 8 hr
Half over the next 16 hr	Half given next 16 hr
Second 24 hr	Second 24 hr
colloid 0.5 ml/kg/% burn	colloid 0.25 ml/kg/% burn
crystalloid 0.5 ml/kg/% burn	crystalloid 0.75 ml/kg/% burn
maintenance water (2000 ml)	maintenance water (2000 ml)
Colloid	Colloid
dextran 70/normal saline solution	plasma or plasma substitute
Crystalloid	Crystalloid
normal saline solution	lactated Ringer's solution
Maximum calculated burn 50%	Maximum calculated burn 50%

actual fluid requirements of burn patients before any standard guidelines were established – hence they became the standard guidelines.

The Brooke formula differs from the Evans formula (Table I) in that the amount of colloid is only one-half as much, the amount of electrolyte solution is one and one-half times as much, and lactated Ringer's solution is used in place of physiologic saline. Both formulas provide the same amount of total fluid during the first 48 hours. Both formulas are based on the fact that albumin rich plasma is lost into the burn wound and that the plasma volume is better restored by replacement with colloid. The adequacy of the Evans formula was rechecked by Hutcher and Haynes in 1972 and not surprisingly in view of the formula's origin was still found to be successful. Advocates of mixture formulas feel that less total fluid is required and consequently less edema is formed and the hazard of pulmonary overload somewhat diminished. On the other hand, when whole blood or plasma is used as the colloid, the risk of hepatitis is increased, the expense is far greater, and keeping track of two or more solutions is more complicated. To obviate the latter difficulty, Stone has devised a composite solution of colloid and crystalloid approximating the Brooke formula (Stone, 1973; Stone et al., 1969). As would be expected, this produced adequate resuscitation and obviated the indecision of what bottle of fluid to hang next. At the present time use of this solution requires a somewhat complicated mixing process prior to administration with the possibility of introducing contamination and carries the same risk of hepatitis and expense. The total volume of fluid given over the first 48 hours averaged 5.4 ml/% burn/kg (see Table II).

In practice, smaller burns can frequently be resuscitated by oral means and thereby require less fluid than these formulas provide, while burns larger than 50% will commonly require larger amounts of fluid than provided by the cut-off at 50% total body surface used.

Colloid alone

Some investigators, primarily in Europe, advocate the use of colloid solution alone (Sørensen, 1973; Sørensen et al., 1967; Sørensen and Thomsen, 1968; Wilkinson, 1973). Wilkinson, at the Burns Unit at the Royal Hospital for Sick Children in London advocates 'bolus' therapy of high molecular weight dextran in quantities just sufficient to maintain a normal blood pressure and capillary refill. Patients are allowed to drink fruit juice with glucose if not vomiting, and he does not measure hourly urine. With the use of this method, he found that a smaller total volume of fluid could be given in smaller injuries. Burns less than 20% received only 40% of the volume estimated by the Evans formula whereas there were progressive increases such that burns of 40% total body surface required the same amount as the Evans formula. This method requires continuous monitoring of the patient on a one to one basis by either a physician or a specially trained nurse. There appears to be little advantage to have the patient repeatedly returned from the brink of disaster if the fluid requirements are no less than those of the Evans or Brooke formula in the more serious burn.

Sørensen, at the Burn Unit in Copenhagen, uses 6% dextran (average molecular weight 75,000) in normal saline as his sole resuscitation fluid,

Table II
Fluid and sodium requirements in burn patients.

	ml**	mEq Na**
Brooke*⁺	4.5	0.39
Evans*⁺	4.5	0.43
Composite solution	5.4	0.41
Sørensen (calculated)⁺*	(2.7)	(0.26)
Sørensen (actual adult)*	5.1	?
Baxter⁺	4.6	0.52
Monafo (hypertonic saline)	4.2	0.74

* Colloid solution given as plasma or dextran will be isotonic in respect to saline.
⁺ Calculated on 50% burn in 70 kg pt. including free water maintenance.
** Units/% burn/kg/48 hours.

but does give additional maintenance water either intravenously or as tolerated by mouth. During a five year period, Dr. Sørensen treated 184 patients with this fluid regimen. His formula implies that considerably less total fluid and sodium is required for resuscitation than the other formulas (Table II). When his actual data are used, however (Wilkinson, 1973), the total fluids given are in line with the rest of the formulas. It is likely that these patients received less sodium than the other formulas require but, with similar urine outputs, the actual weight gain (edema fluid) would be comparable. From his data, 30% of the patients were treated exactly according to the formula with good results following burns averaging 26% TBS. An additional 41% increased their oral intake over the calculated value providing additional resuscitation fluid. These patients also had relatively small burns, averaging 27% TBS. 23% required more dextran or saline than the formula provided. These patients all had larger burns, averaging 44% TBS.

It would thus seem that smaller burns can be resuscitated with smaller quantities of dextran and saline – essentially a composite solution – than the other formulas suggest, provided the patient has a liberal oral intake. On the other hand, larger burns, and the overall average of total fluid intake is similar to that of the other formulas.

Isotonic crystalloid alone

A resuscitation plan using an extracellular fluid mimic (Ringer's lactate) is advocated by Baxter (Baxter, 1970, 1973; Baxter and Shires, 1968) and has been adopted as the official recommendation of the American College of Surgeons Committee on Trauma. The Baxter formula (Table III) was derived from isotope studies of body fluid compartments following burns (Baxter, 1973; Shires et al., 1960). Baxter found decreases in plasma volume 25% below control values and a marked reduction of extracellular fluid volume to 50% of control values. He also found that the quantity of ECF expected to be lost in the first 48 hours post burn had already been sequestered by the 18th hour post-burn. This rate of fluid loss was much faster than previously anticipated by clinical or experimental studies. His experiments indicated that untreated animals sequestered 2 ml of isotonic fluid per kilogram of body weight per percent burn during the first 12 hours post burn. Treatment with this quantity of fluid in the first 24 hours failed to replenish the functional extracellular fluid. He then used various combinations of resuscitative fluids in a 50% flame burn model and found the optimal regimen necessary to maintain a near normal functional extracellular fluid averaged 4 ml/% burn/kg

Table III
Baxter formula.

First 24 hr	
Colloid – 0	
Ringer's lactate – 4 ml/kg/% burn	
Free water – 0	
Second 24 hr	
Colloid – 4–7 ml/kg	
Ringer's lactate – 0	
Free water – 50 ml/kg	

Rate of administration

1 st 8 hours	2nd 8 hours	3rd 8 hours
1/2	1/4	1/4

of lactated Ringer solution given during the first 24 hours. He also found that plasma or other colloid did not improve the plasma volume during the first 24 hours but, in the second 24 hours, increased the plasma volume by the amount given. Based on these animal data a series of 100 burn patients with burns above 35% TBS were evaluated in a similar fashion. Results were similar to those found in dogs and the resuscitation program was then adopted at the Burn Unit of Parkland Memorial Hospital at Dallas. It was found that the treatment not only restored extracellular volume to near normal levels, but that cardiac outputs in nearly all patients returned to the normal range during the first 24 hours. Cardiac output responses were sometimes less than optimal in elderly patients with severe burns and in young patients with more than 65% TBS involved in deep third degree burns. This finding is similar to those with other resuscitation programs and may be due to the presence of a circulating 'myocardial depressant factor' that limits the circulatory response to fluid volume therapy no matter what the resuscitation regimen (Baxter et al., 1966; Heimbach et al., 1973; Lefer, 1970). This treatment plan has now been used in more than 600 patients in Parkland Hospital with results comparable to those of other resuscitation plans.

No one contests the efficacy, ease of administration, and diminished cost of this formula. Critics feel that edema formation is greater and that the chance of precipitating pulmonary edema is somewhat higher if colloid is not used in more abundance. Data for this are not convincing, however, and a comparison of the various formulas (Table II) shows no significant differences in either total volume of fluid for 48 hours or in actual milliequivalents of sodium given. The basic difference of the Baxter formula is that crystalloid is given more rapidly and earlier with the colloid being given after the 'capillary leak' has sealed.

Hypertonic saline

In attempts to diminish edema formation, several investigators have studied hypertonic saline solution as prime therapy for burn shock (Caldwell et al., 1971; Casali et al., 1972; Markley et al., 1965; Monafo, 1970, 1973; Monafo et al., 1973; Moylan et al., 1973). Interest was generated in hypertonic saline following Monafo's report on the successful treatment of ten patients with significant body burns using only hypertonic lactated saline solution containing 300 mEq/l sodium. His follow-up report now includes forty patients (Monafo, 1973b). His results of resuscitation are similar to those with other methods but when the actual fluid requirement is tabulated during the entire 48 hour resuscitation period, 4.2 ml per kilogram per percent body burn are required; this value does not differ significantly from the other formulas (Table II). Although the clinical response was quite satisfactory, moderate hypernatremia occurred and demanded careful following of serum electrolytes. Manafo's patients' burn wounds are treated with 0.5% silver nitrate solution which leaches sodium from the blood at a rapid rate. Large amounts of salt must be replaced in such patients during their chronic care, and it is possible that this ancillary treatment may affect the outcome of resuscitation. A theoretical disadvantage of hypertonic resuscitation is that the circulating hypertonic extracellular fluid may produce intracellular dehydration to provide the mandatory edema fluid. This has been suggested by measurement of intracellular membrane potentials in muscle tissue during hypertonic burn resuscitation (Baxter, unpublished data).

Conclusion

It is hoped that the above discussion will put fluid resuscitation in some orderly perspective. With so many excellent means of resuscitation, the whole issue becomes something of a clinical tempest in a tea pot. Formulas that cut off fluid requirements at 50% TBS frequently require additional fluid administration in larger burns (Reckler and Mason, 1971). As can be seen from Table II, which was compiled from formula calculations and actual patient data, there is very little difference in either the total volume of fluid administered or in the amount of sodium. The controversy cannot be resolved by objective data and is thereby highly charged with clinical impressions and personal preferences. The dispassionate observer would choose a method based on familiarity, accessibility, ease of administration, expense, and need for complicated monitoring equipment or excessive personnel required for treatment. While the chronic care of the seriously burned patient should take place in specialized facilities, the patient is usually first seen by a physician without a special interest in burns and in a hospital without specialized monitoring equipment. Even in these circumstances the airways should be checked and resuscitation begun immediately, since the sooner fluids are given the lower the mortality and incidence of renal failure (Leape, 1971). In this setting, the dispassionate observer's criteria become important. The main advantage of the lactated Ringer's resuscitation is its availability and ease of administration. Electrolyte abnormalities are not produced, urinary output is easily measured, and no decisions of 'which bottle to hang next' are required. It is for these reasons that the American College of Surgeons Committee on Trauma has recommended its use and is providing each Emergency Room in the United States a copy of the treatment plan to be hung on the Emergency Room wall. Once resuscitation is well under way, the patient can leisurely be transferred to a specialized burn center. If the resuscitation plan is easy, it is likely to be started by the untrained physician; but if it is complicated, he is more likely to attempt rapid transfer to a burn center with the net result of several hours elapsing before resuscitation is started at all.

Anesthetic Problems in the Early Burn Period

Fortunately for the anesthesiologist, uncomplicated burned patients rarely need surgery in the early post-burn phase. In fact, anesthesia in the 'burn shock' phase is hazardous as the contracted vascular volume may accentuate the problems discussed below. Debridement and wound cleansing is done under mild sedation, escharotomies do not require anesthesia, and tracheostomies can generally be done with local anesthesia. If surgery is required, there are several problems unique to the burn patient making his anesthetic hazardous. Because the skin heat barrier has been destroyed, patients, especially children, become poikilothermic under anesthesia. Use of a warming blanket and an overhead heater and using only warmed i.v. fluids and warmed saline for irrigation is mandatory to prevent the patient's core temperature from falling to 90°F or below. Monitoring of blood pressure and EKG is frequently difficult and may be inaccurate. It is the policy at Parkland Hospital to avoid inhalation agents, such as halothane and enflurane, that might cause hypotension. Because of the transient hypotension sometimes seen with curare, the relaxant of choice at the Burn Unit at Parkland Hospital is pancuronium. In acutely ill patients with facial swelling, it is wise to do an awake naso-tracheo intubation rather than risk losing the airway in a patient who has become paralyzed. This is equally important in patients with severe neck contractures in the later stages of burn care. Deaths have been reported from sudden cardiac arrhythmias following the use of depolarizing muscle relaxants in acute burns. This presumably results from sudden hyperkalemia following potassium release in damaged muscle tissue (Schaner et al., 1969). For this reason it is probably wise to avoid the use of all depolarizing agents in the acutely burned patient.

Summary

Burn shock is a complex problem and its pathophysiology is not yet fully understood. The injured tissue serves as a sponge for plasma and extracellular fluid leading to severe plasma and extracellular fluid defects in untreated patients. The end result is a markedly diminished cardiac output, hemoconcentration, and the other manifestations of hypovolemic shock. Many resuscitation programs have been devised and most are successful in terms of patient survival. All serve only as guidelines and actual fluid requirements may vary as much as 25%, especially in small and large burns. The practitioner should choose one plan, become familiar with its use, and stick to it until a new plan has documented superiority over all others. His choice should be based on availability, expense, and ease of application using a minimum of personnel, monitoring equipment, and laboratory tests. Resuscitation should be started at the first hospital encountering the patient, and should not be delayed until transfer to a burn center has been arranged. Over 50% of burn deaths occur within the first week. While some of these deaths are related to associated injuries, carbon monoxide poisoning, and inhalation injury, many are related to inadequate or delayed resuscitation. Resuscitation is the easiest part of burn care and the advances in wound care, control of burn wound sepsis, hyperalimentation, and rehabilitation will be of little use to the patient who dies or develops non-reversible renal failure in the first few post-burn days.

References

Achauer, B.M., Allyn, P.A., Furnas, D.W. and Bartlett, R.H. (1973): Pulmonary complications of burns: the major threat to the burn patient. *Ann. Surg., 177*, 311.

Baxter, C.R. (1970): Early resuscitation of patients with burns. In: *Advances in Surgery, Vol. 4*. Editor: C.E. Welch. Year Book Medical Publishers, Chicago, Illinois.

Baxter, C.R. (1973): Crystalloid resuscitation of burn shock. In: *Contemporary Burn Management*, pp. 7–32. Editors: H.C. Polk, Jr. and H.H. Stone. Little, Brown and Company, Boston, Mass.

Baxter, C.R., Cook, W.A. and Shires, G.T. (1966): Serum myocardial depressant factor of burn shock. *Surg. Forum, 17*, 1.

Baxter, C.R., Frenkel, E.L., Shires, G.T. and Crenshaw, C.A. (1967): Rheologic changes in acute thermal burns: research in burns. In: *Transactions of the Third International Congress on Research in Burns*, p. 609. Hans Huber Publication.

Baxter, C.R. and Shires, G.T. (1968): Physiologic response to crystalloid resuscitation of severe burns. *Ann. N. Y. Acad. Sci., 150*, 874.

Brooks, S., Dragstedt, L.R., Warner, L. and Knisley, M.H. (1950): Sludged blood following severe thermal burns. *Arch. Surg. (Chicago), 61*, 387.

Caldwell, F.T., Casali, R.E., Flanigan, W.J. and Bowser, B. (1971): What constitutes the proper solution for resuscitation of the severely burned patient? *Amer. J. Surg., 122*, 655.

Casali, R.E., Bowser, B.H., Smith, V., Enloe, J., Caldwell, F.T. and Flanigan, W.J. (1972): Critical factors in resuscitation of the severely burned rat: the relative merit of volume, tonicity, sodium load, and concentration of the solution used. *Ann. Surg., 175*, 138.

Davies, J.W.L. and Topley, E. (1956): The disappearance of red cells in patients with burns. *Clin. Sci., 15*, 135.

Dressler, D.P. and Skornik, W.A. (1972): Effect of antimicrobial therapy on lung bacterial clearance in the burned rat. *Ann. Surg., 175*, 241.

Epstein, B.S., Hardy, D.L., Harrison, H.N., Teplitz, C., Villarreal, Y. and Mason, A.D. Jr. (1963): Hypoxemia in the burned patient: a clinical–pathologic study. *Ann. Surg., 158*, 924.

Evans, E.I., Purnell, O.J., Robinett, P.W. et al. (1952): Fluid and electrolyte requirements in severe burns. *Ann. Surg., 135*, 804.

Foley, F.D., Moncrief, J.A. and Mason, A.D. Jr. (1968): Pathology of the lung in fatally burned patients. *Ann. Surg., 167*, 251.

Gehrke, C.F., Penner, J.A., Niederhuber, J..and Feller, I. (1971): Coagulation defects in burned patients. *Surg. Gynec. Obstet., 133*, 613.

Gilmore, J.P. and Fozzard, H.A. (1960): Mechanism of acute erythrocyte loss following burn. *Amer. J. Physiol., 198, 3*, 487.

Heimbach, D.M., Fisher, W.D., Hutton, I., McArdle, C.S. and Ledingham, I.McA. (1973): Myocardial blood flow and metabolism during and after hemorrhagic shock in the dog. *Surg. Gynec. Obstet., 137*, 243.

Hutcher, N. and Haynes, B.W. Jr. (1972): The Evans formula revisited. *J. Trauma, 12*, 453.

Jelenko, C., III (1967): Studies in burns. I. Water loss from the body surface. *Ann. Surg., 165*, 83.

Jelenko, C., III, Smulyan, W.I. and Wheeler, M.L. (1967): Studies in burns. IV. The relationship of eschar water content to eschar water transmissivity. *Ann. Surg., 166*, 278.

Jelenko, C., III, Smulyan, W.I. and Wheeler, M.L. (1968): Studies in burns. VI. The role of lipids in the transmissivity of membranes. *Ann. Surg., 167*, 521.

Jelenko, C., III, Ginsburg, J.M., Wheeler, M.L. and Anderson, A.P. (1971): Studies in burns. VIII. The role of cutaneous water-holding lipid in post-burn thermoregulation. *Ann. Surg., 174*, 109.

Jones, D.M., Alpen, E.L. and Davis, A.K. (1956): Acute erythrocyte destruction in severe thermal injury. *Amer. J. Physiol., 184*, 147.

Leape, L.L. (1971): Urgency of fluid administration in resuscitation of burn shock. *J. surg. Res., 11*, 513.

Lefer, A.M. (1970): Role of a myocardial depressant factor in the pathogenesis of circulatory shock. *Fed. Proc., 29*, 1836.

Loebl, E.C., Baxter, C.R. and Curreri, P.W. (1973): The mechanism of erythrocyte destruction in the early post-burn period. *Ann. Surg., 178*, 681.

Loebl, E.C., Marvin, J.A., Curreri, P.W. and Baxter, C.R. (1974): Erythrocyte survival following thermal injury. *J. surg. Res., 16*, 96.

Markley, K., Smallman, E. and Millican, R.C. (1965): The efficacy and toxicity of iso-, hypo-, and hypertonic sodium solutions in the treatment of burn shock in mice. *Surgery, 57*, 698.

Michie, D.D., Goldsmith, R.S., Mason, A.D. Jr. and Moncrief, J.A. (1963): Hemodynamics of the immediate postburn period. Part I. Hemodynamic alterations produced by thermal burns. *J. Trauma, 3*, 111.

Monafo, W.W. (1970): The treatment of burn shock by the intravenous and oral administration of hypertonic lactated saline solution. *J. Trauma, 10*, 575.

Monafo, W.W. (1973): Hypertonic sodium solutions for the treatment of burn shock. In: *Contemporary Burn Management*, pp. 33–42. Editors: H.C. Polk, Jr. and H.H. Stone. Little, Brown and Company, Boston, Mass.

Monafo, W.W., Chuntrasakul, C. and Ayvazian, V.H. (1973): Hypertonic sodium solutions in the treatment of burn shock. *Amer. J. Surg., 126*, 778.

Moncrief, J.A. and Mason, A.D. Jr. (1964): Evaporative water loss in the burned patient. *J. Trauma, 4*, 180.

Moore, F.D., Peacock, W.C., Blakely, E. and Cope, O. (1946): The anemia of thermal burns. *Ann. Surg., 124*, 811.

Moritz, A.R., Henriques, F.C. Jr. and McLean, R. (1945): The effects of inhaled heat on the air passages and lungs – an experimental investigation. *Amer. J. Path., 21*, 311.

Moylan, J.A. Jr., Reckler, J.M. and Mason, A.D. Jr. (1973): Resuscitation with hypertonic lactate saline in thermal injury. *Amer. J. Surg., 125*, 580.

Neely, W.A., Petro, A.B., Holloman, G.H. Jr., Rushton, F.W. Jr., Turner, M.D. and Hardy, J.D. (1974): Researches on the cause of burn hypermetabolism. *Ann. Surg., 179*, 291.

Rapaport, F.T., Nemirovsky, M.S., Bachvaroff, R. and Ball, S.K. (1973): Mechanisms of pulmonary damage in severe burns. *Ann. Surg., 177*, 472.

Reckler, J.M. and Mason, A.D. Jr. (1971): A critical evaluation of fluid resuscitation in the burned patient. *Ann. Surg., 174*, 115.

Reiss, E., Stirman, J.A. and Artz, C.P. (1953): Fluid and electrolyte balance in burns. *J. Amer. med. Ass., 152*, 1309.

Robb, H.J. (1967): Dynamics of the microcirculation during a burn. *Arch. Surg. (Chicago), 94*, 776.

Rubin, L.R. and Bongiovi, J. Jr. (1970): Central venous pressure. An unreliable guide to fluid therapy in burns. *Arch. Surg., 100*, 269.

Saliba, M.J. Jr., Dempsey, W.C. and Kruggel, J.L. (1973): Large burns in humans. Treatment with heparin. *J. Amer. med. Ass., 225*, 261.

Schaner, P.J., Brown, R.L. et al. (1969): Succinylocholine-induced hyperkalemia in burned patients. I. *Anesth. Analg. Curr. Res., 48*, 764.

Shires, G.T., Williams, J. and Brown, F. (1960): Simultaneous measurement of plasma volume, extracellular fluid volume, and red blood cell mass in utilizing I^{131}, $S^{35}{}_{04}$, and CR^{51}. *J. Lab. clin. Med., 55*, 776.

Skornik, W.A. and Dressler, D.P. (1970): Lung bacterial clearance in the burned rat. *Ann. Surg., 172*, 838.

Sørensen, B. (1973): Fluid therapy with dextran. In: *Contemporary Burn Management*, pp. 71–92. Editors: H.C. Polk, Jr. and H.H. Stone. Little, Brown and Company, Boston, Mass.

Sørensen, B., Sejrfen, P. and Thomsen, M. (1967): Dextran solutions in the treatment of burn shock. *Scand. J. plast. Surg., 1*, 68.

Sørensen, B. and Thomsen, M. (1968): The burns unit in Copenhagen. I. Principles of treatment. *Scand. J. plast. reconstr. Surg., 2*, 3.

Stone, H.H. and Martin, J.D. Jr. (1969): Pulmonary injury associated with thermal burns. *Surg. Gynec. Obstet., 129*, 1242.

Stone, H.H. (1973): The composite burn solution. In: *Contemporary Burn Management*, pp. 93–104. Editors: H.C. Polk, Jr. and H.H. Stone. Little, Brown and Company, Boston, Mass.

Stone, H.H., Rhame, D.W., Corbitt, J.D., Given, K.S. and Martin, J.D. Jr. (1967): Respiratory burns: a correlation of clinical and laboratory results. *Ann. Surg., 165*, 157.

Stone, H.H., Rhame, D.W., Black, W.F. and Martin, J.D. Jr. (1969): A universal burn solution. Evaluation of initial intravenous fluid resuscitation. *Arch. Surg. (Chicago), 99*, 464.

Vaught, M., Illner, H., Curreri, P.W. and Baxter, C.R. (1974): Mechanisms of Fluid Losses in the Immediate Post Burn Period in Primates. Presented at the Meeting of the American Burn Association in Cincinnati, Ohio.

Wilkinson, A.W. (1973): Limited volume therapy with colloid. In: *Contemporary Burn Management*, pp. 53–70. Editors: H.C. Polk, Jr. and H.H. Stone. Little, Brown and Company, Boston, Mass.

Wilson, J.S. and Moncrief, J.A. (1965): Vapor pressure of normal and burned skin. *Ann. Surg., 162*, 130.

Zawacki, B.E., Spitzer, K.W., Mason, A.D. Jr. and Johns, L.A. (1970): Does increased evaporative water loss cause hypermetabolism in burned patients? *Ann. Surg., 171*, 236.

Ledingham (ed.). Shock

Fluid replacement in shock

U.F. GRUBER, Verena STURM and K. MESSMER

Introduction

Shock is characterised by an acute reduction in the nutritive blood supply to vital tissues, associated with a disproportion between oxygen supply and demand, and with inadequate elimination of acid metabolites from the tissues. As a result of the haemodynamic disturbance, functional and structural changes occur in some organs.

Fluid replacement is one of the most important steps in the treatment of all forms of shock since few shocked patients fail to show an absolute or relative hypovolaemia. In the acute treatment of hypovolaemia, success is likely to depend more on the speed and volume of fluid administration than on the nature of fluid given. Complications and the ultimate prognosis may, however, be affected by the pharmacological properties and side effects of the therapeutic regimen used. Recent concepts in the treatment of hypovolaemia have been described by Messmer and Sunder-Plassmann (1974).

The Aims of Fluid Administration

The treatment of hypovolaemia in shock is directed not only at the restoration of blood volume but also at the normalisation of impaired tissue perfusion and the optimal oxygenation of organs. An understanding of the effects of hypovolaemia in the microcirculation enables treatment to be more carefully planned.

Pathophysiology

Figure 1 shows the structures which influence capillary pressure and thus plasma volume. Normally capillary hydrostatic pressure plus tissue oncotic pressure, and plasma oncotic pressure (plasma colloid osmotic pressure) plus tissue hydrostatic pressure are equal but acting in opposite directions (Fig. 2). For simplicity tissue pressures are neglected because they are relatively minor. It is important to note that plasma oncotic pressure is the only force which can draw water into the circulation. When plasma is lost there is an initial transcapillary movement of water and salt, but the body is unable to replace plasma proteins immediately and cannot return plasma oncotic pressure to

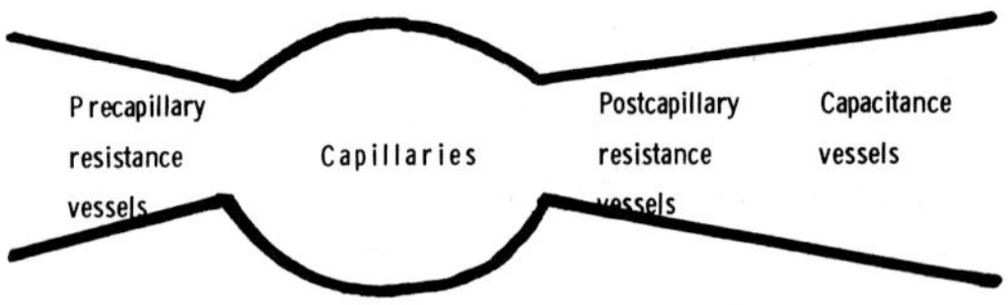

Fig. 1. Pre- and postcapillary resistance vessels influence capillary pressure and thus plasma volume.

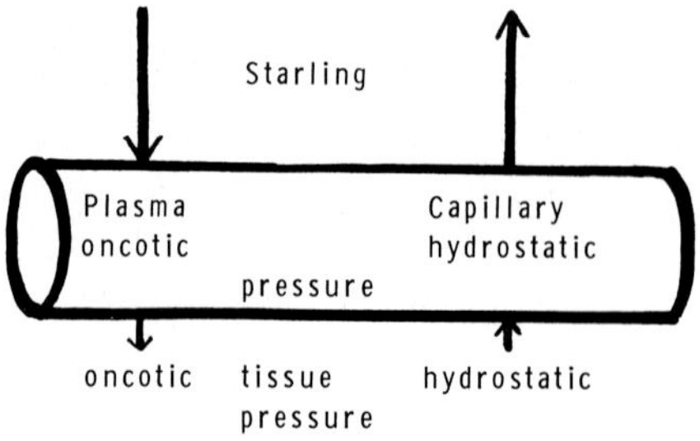

Fig. 2. Normally capillary hydrostatic pressure and plasma oncotic pressure are equal.

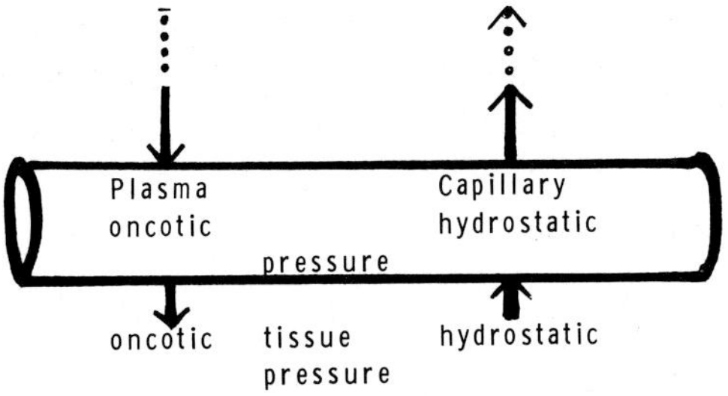

Fig. 3. When no colloid infusion is given, the body can only restore equilibrium by lowering capillary hydrostatic pressure.

normal in the short term. The only mechanism by which the body can increase plasma volume, in the absence of an infusion of colloid, is by lowering capillary hydrostatic pressure (see Fig. 3 and formula below) and thus increasing transcapillary movement of salt and water. There is a change in the ratio of pre- to postcapillary resistance (see Fig. 1 and formula below) resulting in decreased microcirculatory flow and thus in impaired nutritive flow.

$$P_c = \frac{\left(\frac{r_v}{r_a} \times P_a\right) + P_v}{1 + \frac{r_v}{r_a}}$$

P_c = hydrostatic capillary pressure
P_a = arterial inflow pressure
P_v = venous outflow pressure
r_v = postcapillary resistance
r_a = precapillary resistance

These theoretical concepts have been confirmed experimentally by Grega et al. (1971). In this and numerous other studies (Appelgren and Lewis, 1972; review in Gruber, 1969; Lewis et al., 1973) it has been shown that infusion of a colloid solution is able to normalise blood flow and peripheral resistance immediately.

Flow improving properties of volume substitutes

Volume expansion. Lasting volume expansion effects resulting from colloid infusions will only occur if most of the colloid molecules have a size greater than the renal threshold and are thus not excreted by the kidney. Solutions of pasteurised plasma protein and albumin are in this category and yield a volume expansion which roughly equals the amount of isoncotic (i.e. about 5%) volume infused. Of all artificial colloids a 6% solution of dextran 70 in normal saline (Macrodex, Pharmacia) is best fractionated and provides a lasting volume expansion which is initially somewhat greater than the volume infused (Gruber, 1969) and corresponds to the infusion of an equal volume of 5% albumin. In Germany Macrodex has an average molecular weight of 60,000 (dextran 60). The renal threshold for dextran is at a molecular weight of around 50,000.

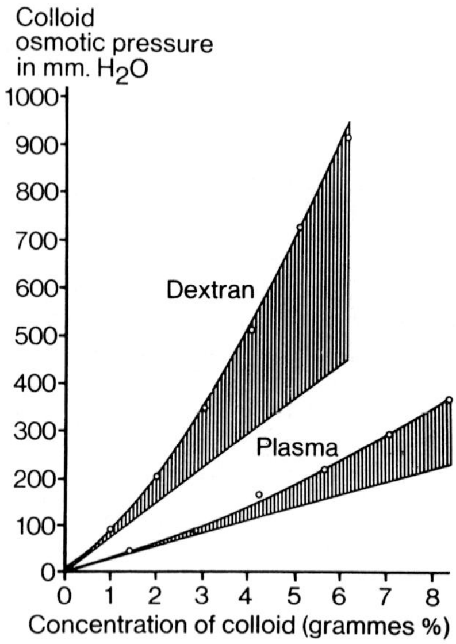

Fig. 4. The relationship between colloid concentration and colloid osmotic pressure for dextran (average molecular weight 70,000) and normal plasma. Straight lines: oncotic pressure calculated from Van 't Hoff's law; shaded area: colloid osmotic pressure resulting from molecular interaction (Gruber, 1969).

Colloid osmotic effect. The gain in circulating volume (Fig. 4) after infusion of 6% dextran 70 is caused by its slightly hyperoncotic properties which result in an initial absorption of fluid from the extravascular space. The colloid osmotic effect of dextran (Fig. 5), expressed as water retaining capacity per gram of the non-diffusing polymer, is slightly greater than that of albumin or plasma proteins (Gruber, 1969; Hint, 1973).

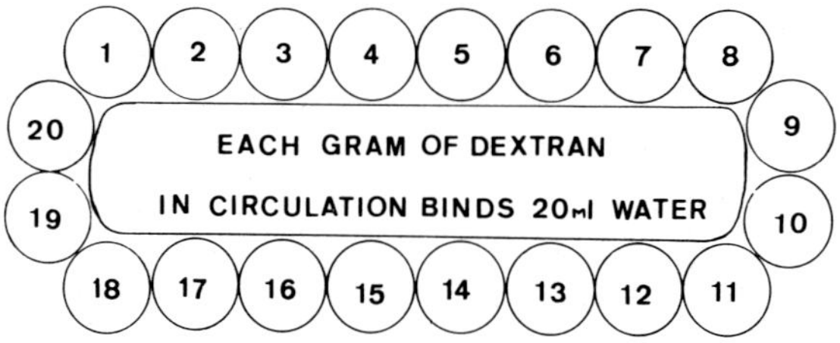

Fig. 5. The water retaining capacity of albumin is around 14 ml/g, that of dextran about 20 ml/g.

Dextran with an average molecular weight of 40,000 is available as a 10% solution (dextran 40) in normal saline or 5% dextrose. Both solutions are strongly hyperoncotic but more rapidly excreted by the kidney. Because of the high oncotic pressure of dextran 40, which corresponds to the colloid osmotic pressure exerted by a 17% albumin solution, water is absorbed from the interstitial space into the capillaries and causes an initial dilution

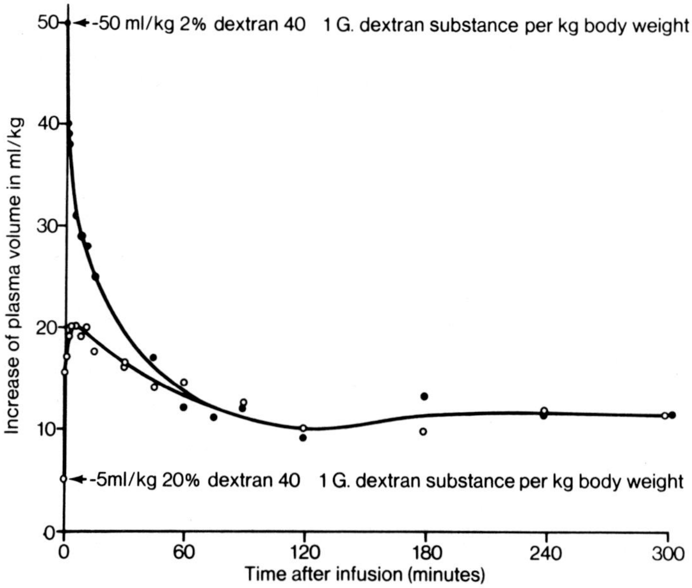

Fig. 6. Experiments in rabbits show that the in vivo water-binding capacity of dextran is relatively independent of the concentration of infused dextran solution. Because 1 g of dextran 40 is capable of retaining only 20–25 ml of water in circulation, the excess water in the hypotonic solution is rapidly filtered out into the tissues or excreted and the plasma volume decreased until the maximum water-retaining capacity of the circulating dextran is reached. It can be seen that only a few minutes after the injection of the hypertonic solution the plasma expansion amounts to about 20 ml/kg and therefore water must have been rapidly absorbed from the tissues into the circulation (Hint, 1973).

in the venous part of the microcirculation. This initial dilution depends only on the oncotic gradient across the vascular walls and is not specific for dextran 40 (Messmer and Schmid-Schönbein, 1972). Figure 6 illustrates the effect of infusion of a colloid hypo- or hypertonic solution on plasma volume. Dextran 40 (Rheomacrodex, Pharmacia) is indicated in cases of long-standing shock where profound changes have already occurred in the microcirculation.

Rheological effects on blood. A characteristic feature of shock is the decreased fluidity of blood due to the exponential increase in its viscosity at low flow rates (Chien, 1972; Messmer and Schmid-Schönbein, 1972; Sunder-Plassmann et al., 1973) shown in Figure 7. A volume substitute used in shock therapy should therefore not further increase and ideally should decrease blood viscosity and thus improve small vessel flow (Chien et al., 1970; Gruber, 1969; Sunder-Plassmann et al., 1972a). Of all colloids that are used, albumin raises blood viscosity least because of its low solution viscosity (Chien et al., 1970). Recent studies have shown, however, that the in vivo effects of a colloid solution cannot necessarily be inferred from in vitro studies. Thus 6 or 10% dextran, as colloid osmotically active solutions, cause a fluid shift in vivo with a resulting dilution of blood which is greater than a simple volume effect.

This difference in the viscosity effects in vivo and in vitro is illustrated in Figure 8, where blood viscosity is plotted against actual haematocrit. It can be seen that the dilution of blood by dextran 60 in vitro decreases whole blood viscosity although the viscosity of plasma alone is significantly increased because of the raised colloid concentration. If, in contrast, haemodilution is

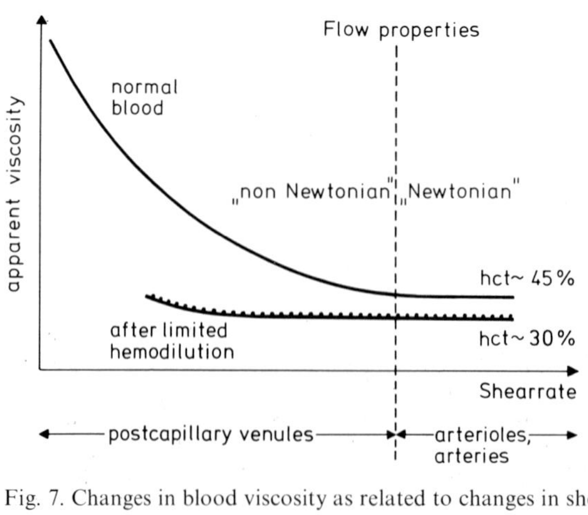

Fig. 7. Changes in blood viscosity as related to changes in shear rate in vivo in different vascular compartments (according to Sunder-Plassmann et al., 1972b, 1973).

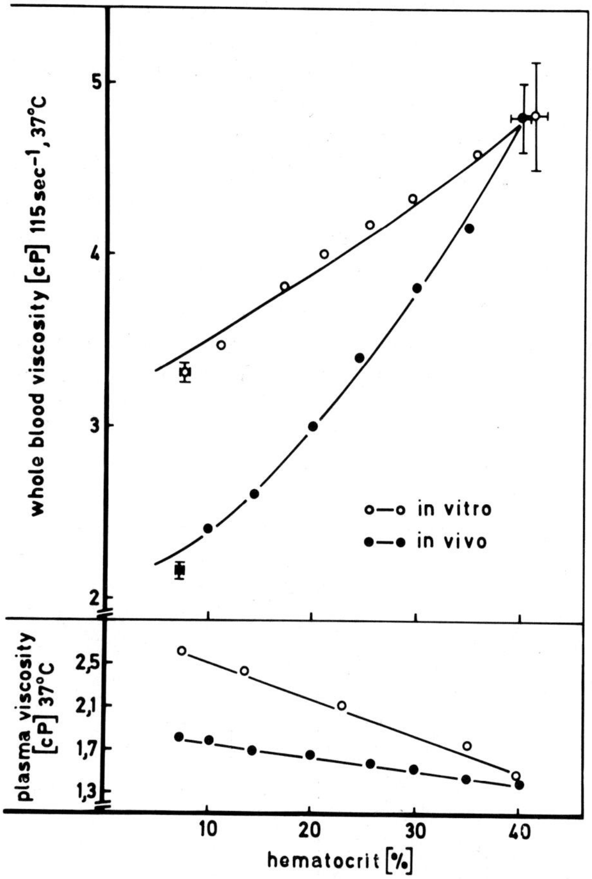

Fig. 8. Whole blood viscosity (upper part) and plasma viscosity in relation to haematocrit during haemodilution in vitro and in vivo with dextran 60. Note the significant effect of dextran 60 on whole blood viscosity in presence of a slightly increased plasma viscosity in vivo (according to Messmer et al., 1972b).

performed in vivo and blood viscosity determined at haematocrits corresponding to the red cell concentration in vitro, whole blood viscosity is decreased significantly more at each haematocrit, although the viscosity of plasma alone is slightly increased. This rise in plasma viscosity does not increase whole blood viscosity but causes it to fall by enhancing the fluidity of the cell phase (Chien, 1972; Sunder-Plassmann et al., 1972b).

Haemodynamic relevance of viscosity changes

The haemodynamic advantages of viscosity changes which occur with colloid solutions have been emphasized in recent years (Hint, 1968; Messmer et al., 1972a, 1974; Replogle, 1972; Sunder-Plassmann et al., 1971, 1973). Messmer's group in Munich has compared dextran, gelatin and starch solutions in a standardized model of isovolaemic haemodilution, and concluded that dextran 60 or 70 was preferable as it provided not only a lasting volume effect and an improvement in flow, but also a well documented antithrombotic effect (see below). In these haemodilution studies it was shown that the decrease in haematocrit was accompanied by an exponential decrease in whole blood viscosity, resulting in a rise in cardiac output as well as in nutritional tissue flow.

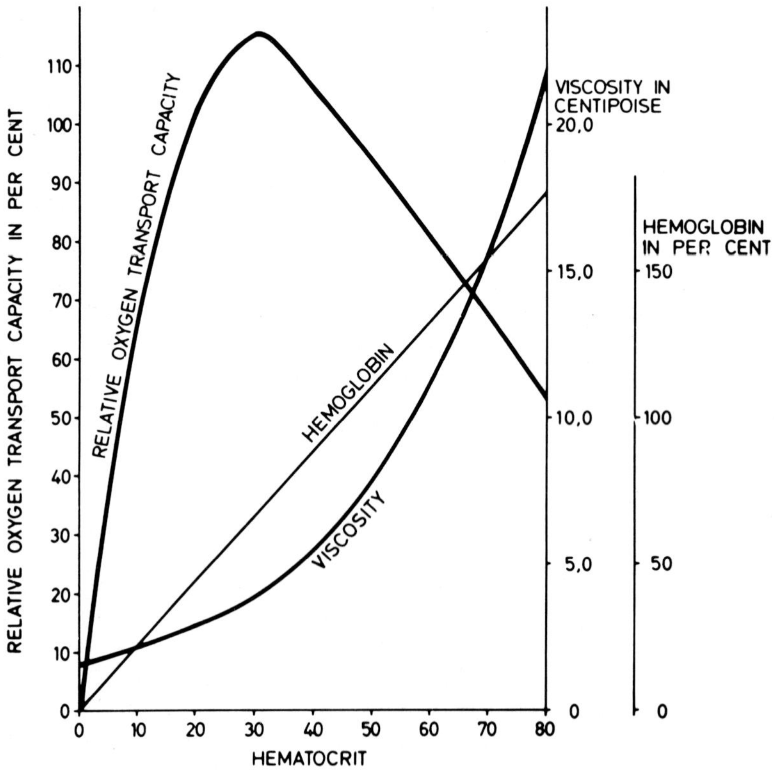

Fig. 9. Calculated relative oxygen transport capacity in dependence of haematocrit (or haemoglobin), based on viscosity data of human blood (Hint, 1968).

Haemodynamic compensation for acute dilutional anaemia

The infusion of colloids is associated with a decrease in the oxygen carrying capacity of the blood. Does the increase in total and nutritional blood flow, induced by its lowered viscosity, compensate for the decrease in haemoglobin concentration? In a first approach to this problem Hint (1968) calculated the relative systemic oxygen transport capacity (O_2TC, the product of cardiac output and O_2 capacity) for the haematocrit range from 0–80% for normal human blood. A bell-shaped curve resulted for the viscosity data for human blood with maximum oxygen transport at a haematocrit of 30% (Fig. 9). Sunder-Plassmann et al. (1971) have been able to confirm this shape for the

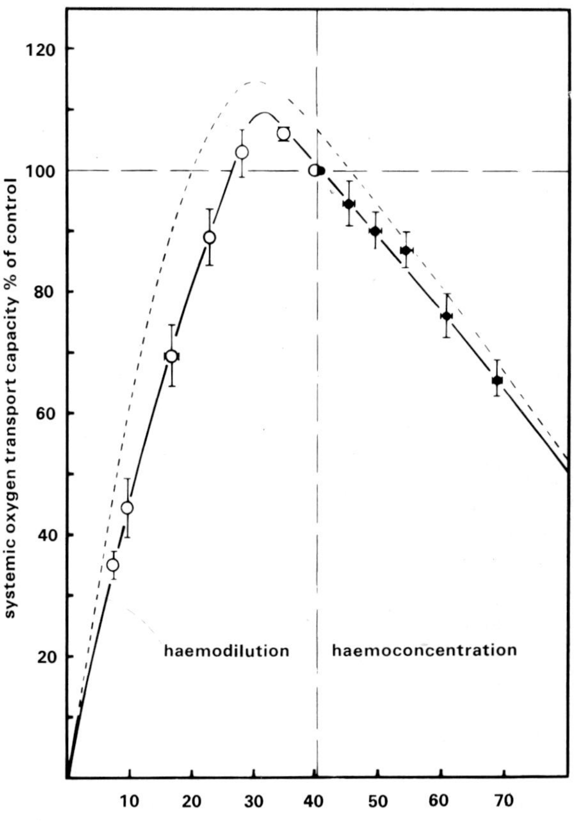

Fig. 10. Relative oxygen transport capacity plotted against arterial haematocrit during acute isovolaemic haemodilution with dextran 60 (open circles) and isovolaemic haemoconcentration with packed RBC's (black circles). Dotted line: theoretical assumption for human blood (Hint, 1968). (From Sunder-Plassmann et al., 1971.)

oxygen transport capacity curve in animal experiments with acutely induced normovolaemic haemodilution as well as normovolaemic haemoconcentration (Fig. 10). Optimal oxygen transport therefore coincides with a haematocrit of 30% and the oxygen transport capacity will not fall below normal values when normovolaemia is maintained unless the haematocrit is less than 25%. O_2TC will, however, immediately decrease with decreasing haematocrit when hypovolaemia occurs (Messmer et al., 1972b).

Since oxygen transport capacity only reflects the carriage of oxygen it conveys no information about its availability to the tissues and makes essential the study of tissue oxygenation during haemodilution in the haematocrit range of clinical interest from 45 to about 20%.

In recent experiments Messmer et al. (1973, 1974) have studied local tissue PO_2 in different organs during normovolaemic haemodilution with dextran 60 using multiwire platinum electrodes. From Figure 11 it is evident that the rise in cardiac output caused by dilution is adequate to compensate fully for the reduction in haemoglobin concentration. This is confirmed by the mean PO_2 values measured in skeletal muscle, liver, pancreas, small intestine and kidney which improve rather than deteriorate with progressive dilution. Precise information on the oxygen tension of tissues was obtained from evaluation of

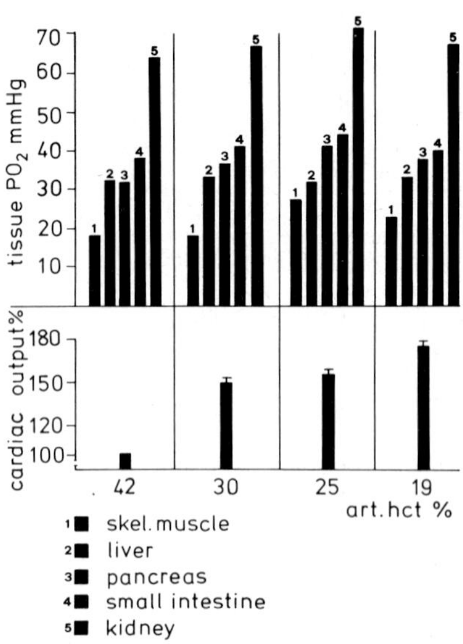

Fig. 11. Changes in local tissue PO_2 of different organs and cardiac output in relation to arterial haematocrit during acute normovolaemic haemodilution with dextran 60 in dogs. Despite a decrease in haematocrit to 19%, the mean tissue PO_2 is maintained or slightly increased in all five organs studied. (From Messmer et al., 1974.)

the spatial PO_2 distribution, and histograms of tissue PO_2 showed no tissue hypoxia even at haematocrit levels as low as 20%; moreover the PO_2 data obtained suggest a more homogenous distribution of nutritive flow with decreasing haematocrit and lowered blood viscosity (Fig. 12).

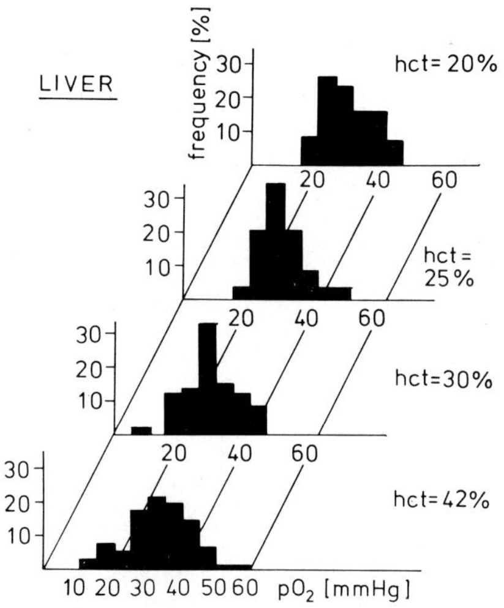

Fig. 12. Frequency distribution of local tissue PO_2 values in the liver at normal haematocrit (bottom) and at different degrees of normovolaemic haemodilution with dextran 60 in dogs. Note that even at the haematocrit of 20% the frequency of low PO_2 values is not higher when compared with controls, but the PO_2 distribution curve is shifted to the right. These findings clearly indicate the absence of local tissue hypoxia. (From Messmer et al., 1973.)

The importance of normovolaemia

Haemodilution improves oxygen supply as long as the haematocrit does not fall below 30% and as long as pulmonary and circulatory compensation for the reduction in oxygen capacity occur. Normovolaemia, however, is the critical requirement (Messmer et al., 1972b). Colloids should be regarded as the volume substitutes of choice, as volume replacement with colloid-free solutions involves not only the risk of hypovolaemic episodes but also of fluid overloading, when significant degrees of dilution are achieved. Heughan et al. (1972) have shown that the administration of large amounts of saline can impair oxygen delivery to tissues, because of oedema formation. It seems, therefore, rational to use colloids with a long intravascular persistence not only for volume replacement in shock, but whenever therapeutic haemodilution is desirable. Limited normovolaemic haemodilution can thus be considered as a valuable method of promoting nutritional flow which avoids the risks of blood transfusion.

Haemodilution studies in man

The results of animal experiments have been confirmed in man (Bauer et al., 1974; Beall et al., 1967; Laks et al., 1973; Messmer and Sunder-Plassmann, 1974). It is important to note that in Laks' study there were no changes in lung water content.

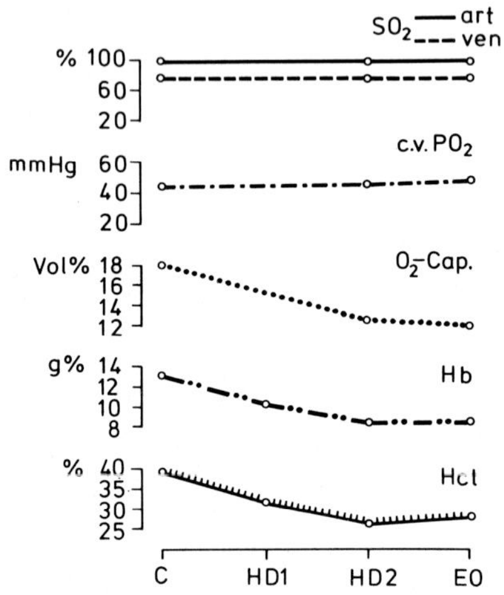

Fig. 13. Acute preoperative haemodilution in patients. Changes in haematocrit, haemoglobin concentration, oxygen capacity, central-venous PO_2 and arteriovenous oxygen saturation difference (see legend to Fig. 14). (From Bauer et al., 1974.)

Recently the results of a study of haemodilution in 34 patients were published by Bauer et al. (1974) who showed normal arteriovenous oxygen saturation differences and normal central venous PO_2 despite decreasing O_2 capacity (but not transport capacity) and decreasing Hb and haematocrit levels (Fig. 13). Acute preoperative haemodilution in these patients shortly after the induction of anaesthesia reduced the haematocrit to 27%, but the blood pressure, CVP and heart rate remained unchanged (Fig. 14).

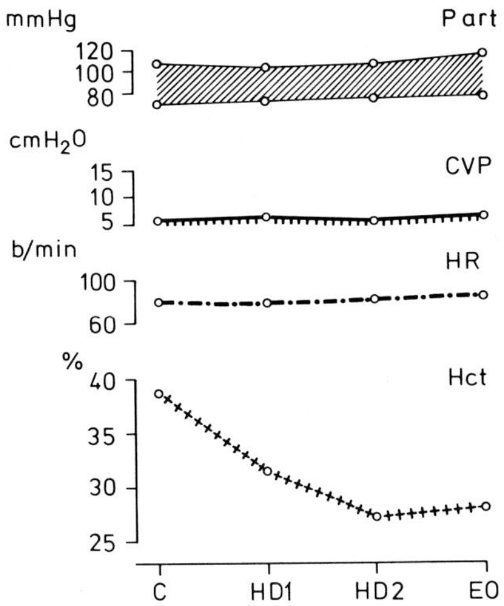

Fig. 14. Acute preoperative haemodilution in patients shortly after induction of anaesthesia. Despite the reduction in the haematocrit to 27%, the arterial, central venous pressure and heart rate remained unchanged. C, control state; HD1, after exchange of 1000 ml blood for 5% albumin; HD2, after the end of dilution; EO, at the end of operation. In the time interval between HD2 and EO intraoperative blood losses were replaced with autologous blood; increases in haematocrit above 30% were avoided. (From Bauer et al., 1974.)

Comparative Advantages of Fluid Replacement Solutions

Blood

The greatest danger in blood transfusion remains the transmission of viral hepatitis. As Grindon et al. (1967) stated: "a reasonable conclusion is that of 1000 patients receiving one unit of blood, approximately 100 patients will develop hepatitis, 10 will become jaundiced and one will die of this disease"; 90 patients will develop anicteric jaundice, by no means a harmless disease. Bacterial contamination, incompatibility and its immunological sequelae, and impairment of blood flow in the capillary and postcapillary bed are further known risks of blood transfusion.

Recently there has been more interest in the effects of blood transfusion on oxygen delivery to the tissues. The position of the oxyhaemoglobin dissociation curve and thus oxygen delivery to the tissues is partly dependent on erythrocyte 2.3-DPG content (*D*-glyceric acid-2.3-diphosphate) and during the storage of blood this decreases. In patients suffering from septic shock extremely low 2,3-DPG levels have been measured. Reduction in 2,3-DPG causes an increased affinity of haemoglobin for oxygen, shifting the dissociation curve to the left (Fig. 15) and in a critically ill patient this change may be crucial. It is one of the reasons for the replacement of ACD solution by CPD-stabiliser (citrate–phosphate–dextrose) in which the 2,3-DPG content of erythrocytes falls less rapidly. Patients needing more than five units in 24 hours should receive fresh blood to avoid problems with decreased oxygen delivery and coagulation disturbances.

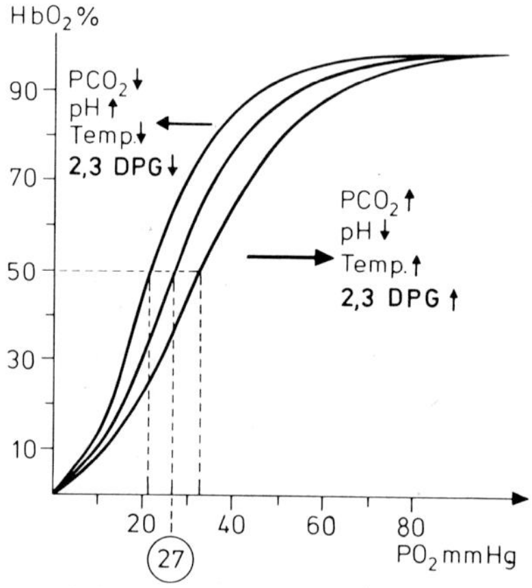

Fig. 15. The influence of the 2,3-DPG content of the erythrocytes on the oxyhaemoglobin dissociation curve. Other important factors are temperature, pH and PCO_2 value.

Washed, deep frozen red cells

The administration of blood in this way reduces the risk of transmitting hepatitis and the cells show no decrease in 2,3-DPG content. Where such preparations are not available, repeatedly washed, packed red cells should be used as there is evidence that they carry a smaller risk of hepatitis.

Plasma

The incidence of hepatitis after administration of fresh, stored or dried plasma is about the same as after whole blood, so these preparations are better not used.

Pasteurised plasma protein and albumin do not transmit hepatitis but are available only in limited amounts and are very expensive. They do not contain gamma-globulins and have no anti-thrombotic properties.

Electrolyte solutions

It has been shown that initial volume replacement can be carried out safely with large amounts of Ringer's lactate solution, using 3–4 times the volume lost, but such treatment may have disadvantages. First, all patients treated in this way will eventually need blood transfusion, with its associated dangers, if they are not to relapse into shock again. Second, Ringer's lactate and whole blood have no anti-thrombotic properties. Third, patients with impaired cardiac, pulmonary or renal function may develop pulmonary oedema quite rapidly after the infusion of large amounts of water and electrolytes. Fourth, there is no proof that the use of large amounts of Ringer's lactate has the advantages of combined treatment with water, electrolytes and colloids.

Plasma substitutes

Gelatin. The use of gelatin cannot be recommended for the following reasons: commercially available preparations of gelatin contain only about 20% of molecules above the renal threshold so that only a short and minimal volume expansion is achieved, unlike that of a plasma infusion (Gruber, 1969). If no volume effect is required a balanced electrolyte solution is as effective as gelatin and much cheaper. Gelatin infusions cause histamine release in man (Messmer et al., 1970) and have no specific flow-improving or anti-thrombotic effect.

Dextran. Dextran is an artificial colloid which is completely metabolised in the human body. Clinically available preparations of dextran have the following properties of importance to the clinician: a) plasma volume expansion; b) blood flow improvement; c) anti-thrombotic properties (see below).

Other plasma substitutes. These include hydroxyethyl starch, purified haemoglobin solution and fluorocarbons and are still under experimental and clinical investigation. They cannot yet be recommended for use in patients. A review of the literature regarding blood substitutes is given by Gruber (1969).

Conclusions

Because of availability and cost, dextran solutions are preferred to pasteurised plasma protein solution and albumin for initial volume replacement in shocked patients and during surgical operations. An important additional reason is that dextrans have well documented anti-thrombotic effects. Thus with the same agent it is possible to increase blood volume and flow and to prevent the complications which commonly occur in patients requiring volume substitution.

Prevention of thromboembolic complications

The problem. By phlebography and radioactive fibrinogen tests it can be shown that postoperative and posttraumatic deep venous thrombosis (DVT) occurs much more frequently than has been thought until now. About 30% of all patients in a general surgical unit develop a postoperative DVT (Becker and Schampi, 1972; Browse et al., 1974; Daniel et al., 1972; Gruber et al., 1973; Korvald et al., 1973; Stephenson et al., 1973). In special groups, for example patients with hip fractures, a frequency of up to 80% has been found (Bronge et al., 1971; Eskeland et al., 1966; Hamilton et al., 1970; Myhre and Holen, 1969; Pinto, 1970; Sevitt, 1962; Sevitt and Gallagher, 1959). Unfortunately pulmonary embolism is far too frequently the first sign of a DVT and Sevitt and Gallagher (1961) state that half of all fatal pulmonary emboli occur without any clinical prodrome. With a fatal embolism death occurs in 50% of patients within 15 minutes of the event and in another 10% within 60 minutes (Coon and Willis, 1959). Thus with a massive pulmonary embolism there is insufficient time for therapy.

Prophylaxis against pulmonary embolism following surgery or trauma is therefore likely to be more satisfactory than the treatment of developed complications. Prophylaxis should start as soon as possible and should be in progress during elective surgical procedures. Following trauma prophylaxis should be instituted immediately after admission to hospital. Prophylaxis should be started early because most postoperative DVT's can be diagnosed within the first 48 hours following an operation (Flanc et al., 1968; Gruber et al., 1973; Negus et al., 1968).

There is no doubt that one of the most important factors leading to thrombus formation is the release of tissue thrombokinase following tissue damage due to trauma or surgery. Premedication, anaesthesia, immobilisation and other conditions leading to impaired blood flow, such as blood loss and positive pressure respiration, are also important.

The anti-thrombotic effects of dextran. The anti-thrombotic properties of dextran may lead to the belief that following its use there will be an increased risk of bleeding complications. It is true that improved microcirculatory blood flow results in increased oozing, but this is only a serious problem in special situations such as liver resection and neurosurgery; it has been shown that the dextran preparations available today used in doses of up to 1.5 g/kg body weight do not produce measurable changes in the clotting mechanisms (Gruber, 1969).

Dextran's anti-thrombotic effects are due to: reduced platelet activity (see Bygdeman, 1969), changed fibrin structure (Muzaffar et al., 1972; Tangen et al., 1972), changes in the mechanical properties of the fibrin clot (Muzaffar

Table I
Review of prospective, randomised studies on the value of dextran 70 in the prevention of deep vein thrombosis. The papers included are those in which objective diagnostic methods were used.

Author	Year	Diagnosis	Surgery
Ahlberg	1968	Phlebography	Orthopedics
Ahlberg	1969	Phlebography	Orthopedics
Becker	1973	Phlebography and fibrinogen test	General
Bergqvist	1972	Phlebography	Orthopedics
Bergqvist	1973	Fibrinogen test	Orthopedics
Bonnar	1972	Phlebography and fibrinogen test	Gynecology
Bronge	1971	Phlebography	Orthopedics
Carter	1973	Fibrinogen test	General
Daniel	1972	Fibrinogen test	Orthopedics
Davidson	1972	Fibrinogen test	Gynecology
Harper	1973	Phlebography	Leg amputation
Johnson	1968	Phlebography	Orthopedics
Kline	1974	Fibrinogen test and phlebography	General
Korvald	1973	Phlebography	Orthopedics
Lambie	1970	Fibrinogen test	Gynecology
Myhre	1969	Fibrinogen test*	Orthopedics
Myrvold	1973	Phlebography	Orthopedics
Sjögren	1971	Fibrinogen test	Urology
Stephenson	1973	Fibrinogen test	General
Vasilescu	1974	Fibrinogen test	General/gynecology

* 53 of the 94 patients were controlled by means of fibrinogen test and phlebography.

Table II
Review of studies documenting the value of dextran 70 in the prevention of deep venous thrombosis in orthopedic surgery.

		Number of patients				Patients with DVT in %				
Author	Year	Controls	Dextran 70	Cumarin	Heparin	Controls	Dextran 70	Cumarin	Heparin	Significance
Ahlberg	1968	45	39			35.5	12.8			$P < 0.05$
Ahlberg	1969	95	70			42.1	18.5			$P < 0.05$
Bergqvist	1972		75	63			33.3	30.2		none
Bergqvist	1973		43	32			44.2	50		none***
Bronge	1971		74	61			36.5	34.4		$P = 0.3$
Daniel	1972	31	35			61.3	60*			none
Harper	1973	15	12			66.6	0			yes
Johnson	1968	25	27			52.0	4.0			$P < 0.05$
Korvald	1973		43	39**			34.9	10.2**		$0.01 < P < 0.05$
Myhre	1969	55	55	50		40	20	18		$0.025 > P > 0.005$
Myrvold	1973		55		39		36		41	none

* From the abstract it is not evident after what time interval the patients were operated upon (fractured femoral neck). This might explain the negative result, since dextran was started during operation only.
** Combined use of cumarins and dextran.
*** There were significantly more large thrombi in the cumarin group.

Table III
Review of studies documenting the value of dextran 70 in the prevention of deep venous thrombosis in gynecological surgery.

Author	Year	Number of patients				Patients with DVT in %				Significance
		Controls	Dextran 70	Cumarin	Heparin	Controls	Dextran 70	Cumarin	Heparin	
Bonnar	1972	140	120			10.7	0.8			$P < 0.01$
Davidson	1972		30	30			10	13		none
Lambie	1970		40	40			10	30		$P < 0.01$
Vasilescu*	1974	93	91		92	37	20**		14**	$P = 0.025$ D $P = 0.005$ H

* It is not clear how many patients belong to which group of surgery, this paper appears therefore in Table IV as well.
** The difference between dextran and heparin is not significant.

Table IV
Review of studies documenting the value of dextran 70 in the prevention of deep venous thrombosis in general surgery.

		Number of patients				Patients with DVT in %				
Author	Year	Controls	Dextran 70	Cumarin	Heparin	Controls	Dextran 70	Cumarin	Heparin	Significance
Becker	1973	35	42			31.4	30.9*			none
Carter	1973	101	106			9.9	0.9			$P < 0.005$
Kline	1974	~ 415	~ 415			11.1	6.3			?**
Stephenson***	1973	46	34			35	29			none
Vasilescu	1974	93	91		92	37	20		14	$P = 0.025$ D $P = 0.005$ H

* The figures given here are based on the fibrinogen test. 7 days after operation patients had phlebography and 1/3 of the thrombi in the dextran group had disappeared by that time. The discrepancy was especially marked in females where the DVT frequency dropped to 9.5%.
** The important finding in this study is that there were 5 fatal pulmonary emboli in the control group and none in the dextran group.
*** Dextran 70 was started postoperatively only which would explain the negative result.

Table V
Review of studies documenting the value of dextran 70 in the prevention of deep venous thrombosis in urology.

		Number of patients				Patients with DVT in %				
Author	Year	Controls	Dextran	Cumarin	Heparin	Controls	Dextran 70	Cumarin	Heparin	Significance
Sjögren*	1971	40	37	–	38	45	27	–	37	D: $P = 0.08$ H: $P = 0.23$

* Data from personal communication, August 1974.

et al., 1972), facilitated fibrinolysis (Tangen et al., 1972; Åberg et al., 1974), and blood flow improvement (see Gruber, 1969).

A large number of prospective and controlled clinical trials have shown the effectiveness of prophylaxis against thromboembolic complications with dextran 70. Good results are obtained in orthopedic and in gynecological surgery; no conclusions can be made yet in general surgery and in urology. In all these studies the presence of a venous thrombus was proven by objective diagnostic methods and it was evident that dextran prophylaxis was as effective as prophylaxis with coumarins or low-dose heparin. Tables I–V summarise the studies. The finding that the occasional thrombus formed in the presence of dextran is more rapidly removed by the body's own fibrinolytic system (Becker and Schampi, 1973) may well be responsible for the effectiveness of dextran prophylaxis in reducing the number of pulmonary emboli (Table VI), and there is no doubt that dextran 40 also has these anti-thrombotic properties (Evarts and Feil, 1971; Gruber et al., 1973).

Table VI
Review of controlled studies on the value of dextran 70 in the prevention of postoperative fatal pulmonary embolism (FPE), verified at autopsy.

		Number of patients			
		Controls		Dextran	
Author	Year	Total	FPE	Total	FPE
Ahlberg	1968	47	2	39	0
Ahlberg	1969	52	2	32	1
Atik	1970	77	5	49	1
Hartshorn	1969	104	2	99	0
Huttunen	1971	100	4	100	1
Jansen	1972	301	4	304	1
Koekenberg	1962	105	1	94	0
Myhre	1969	55	2	55	0
Stadil	1970	397	5	424	1
Total		1238	27	1196	5

The effect of dextran 70 is highly significant ($P < 0.001$).

Clinical management with dextran

Initial volume replacement in hypovolaemic patients. Replacement therapy is instituted by infusing 1000–1500 ml 6% dextran in 0.9% saline. Further volume is given preferably as washed, packed red cells or with pasteurised plasma protein or albumin if this is not available. Normovolaemia is the most important factor apart from oxygen administration.

Correct therapy in shock must take account of the fluid balance of the whole body; it is a mistake to think only in terms of intravascular volume and to neglect the intracellular space. In therapy the time factor is important; if the volume lost can be replaced promptly it is sufficient to infuse the normal daily requirement of water (2500 ml in a man of 75 kg) and electrolytes (100 mEq Na^+, 50 mEq K^+) in addition to volume replacement. In practice, however, this obvious measure is often forgotten and emphasises the importance of hourly measurements of urine output. When treatment is started late, intravascular volume loss must be replaced, the deficits due to fluid shift into the third space made up and the daily requirements covered.

Prevention of thromboembolic complications. Patients in shock who receive dextran 70 for initial volume replacement should be given an additional 500 ml on the first day after trauma and 500 ml every other day until mobilisation. It is also reasonable to begin oral anticoagulant therapy if it is clear that bed rest will be prolonged. During elective surgery, 500 ml dextran should be given shortly after induction of anaesthesia. In this way so-called anaphylactoid reactions may be minimised. These, although very rare, may occur after the infusion of only a small amount of dextran. Their occurrence is even more infrequent in shocked or anaesthetised patients. Treatment of the reaction is by rapid volume replacement, with pasteurised plasma or albumin solution, i.v. steroids (250 mg hydrocortisone), antihistamines and adrenaline (0.1–0.5 ml 1 : 1000 epinephrine).

Summary

1. The purpose of fluid administration in shock is not only the restoration of blood volume but also the normalisation of impaired nutritive flow.

2. Plasma oncotic (≡ colloid osmotic) pressure is the only force which can draw water back into the circulation. In shock the infusion of colloid solutions is able to normalise nutritive flow and peripheral resistance almost at once.

3. 5% solutions of pasteurised plasma protein or albumin and 6% dextran 70 yield a volume expansion corresponding to the amount infused.

4. The decrease in haematocrit produced by the infusion of these three

colloidal solutions is accompanied by a decrease in whole blood viscosity resulting in a rise in cardiac output as well as in nutritional tissue flow.

5. Haemodilution improves oxygen supply as long as the haematocrit does not fall below 30%, although normovolaemia is the critical requirement.

6. Transmission of viral hepatitis is still the greatest danger of blood transfusion.

7. Compared to ACD blood the decrease in erythrocyte-2,3-DPG content can be temporarily counteracted by using CPD-stabilisers instead. Fresh blood should be given to patients who need more than five units in 24 hours.

8. The use of washed, deep frozen or packed red cells is recommended.

9. The use of large amounts of Ringer's lactate is not advised as this solution does not reduce the total number of units of blood which need to be given. Pulmonary oedema may become a problem.

10. Gelatin solutions produce only a short lasting minimal volume expansion and carry the risk of histamine liberation. They have no anti-thrombotic properties.

11. Dextrans are best suited to initial volume replacement in shock. They increase plasma volume, improve blood flow, have antithrombotic properties, are easily available and relatively cheap. Anaphylactoid reactions are rare.

12. Every third patient undergoing general surgery develops a deep venous thrombosis. Widespread prophylaxis to prevent thromboembolic complications is mandatory.

13. The anti-thrombotic properties of dextran are due to reduction in platelet adhesiveness, a change in fibrin clot structure and to the increased lysability of thrombi and the improvement of blood flow.

References

Åberg, M., Bergentz, S.E., Hedner, U. and Nilsson, I.M.S. (1974): The mechanism of action for the anti-thrombotic effect of dextran. *Europ. surg. Res., 6, Suppl. 1*, 29.

Ahlberg, A. (1969): Trombosprofylax med macrodex i ett collumfrakturmaterial. *Studentlitt. Lund*, 89.

Ahlberg, A., Göran, N., Robertson, B., Cronberg, S. and Nilsson, I. (1968): Dextran in prophylaxis of thrombosis in fractures of the hip. *Acta chir. scand., Suppl. 387*, 83.

Appelgren, K.L. and Lewis, D.H. (1972): Capillary flow and capillary transport in dog skeletal muscle in hemorrhagic shock. *Europ. surg. Res., 4*, 29.

Atik, M., Harkess, J.W. and Wichman, H. (1970): Prevention of fatal pulmonary embolism. *Surg. Gynec. Obstet., 130*, 403.

Bauer, H., Pichlmaier, H., Ott, E., Klövekorn, W.P., Sunder-Plassmann, L. and Messmer, K. (1974): Autotransfusion durch akute, präoperative Hämodilution – erste klinische Erfahrungen. *Langenbecks Arch. klin. Chir., Suppl. Forum*, 185.

Beall, A.C. Jr., Yow, E.M., Bloodwell, R.D., Hallmann, G.L. and Cooley, D.A. (1967): Open heart surgery without blood transfusion. *Arch. Surg. (Chicago), 94*, 567.

Becker, J. and Schampi, B. (1973): The incidence of postoperative venous thrombosis of the legs. A comparative study on the prophylactic effect of dextran 70 and electrical calf-muscle stimulation. *Acta chir. scand., 139*, 357.

Bergqvist, E., Bergqvist, D., Bronge, A., Dahlgren, S. and Lindquist, B. (1972): An evaluation of early thrombosis prophylaxis following fracture of the femoral neck. *Acta chir. scand., 138*, 689.

Bergqvist, D. and Dahlgren, S. (1973): Leg vein thrombosis diagnosed by ^{125}I-fibrinogen test in patients with fracture of the hip: a study of the effect of early prophylaxis with dicoumarol or dextran 70. *Vasa, 2*, 121.

Bonnar, J. and Walsh, J. (1972): Prevention of thrombosis after pelvic surgery by British dextran 70. *Lancet, 1*, 614.

Bronge, A., Dahlgren, S. and Lindquist, B. (1971): Prophylaxis against thrombosis in femoral neck fractures – a comparison between dextran 70 and dicumarol. *Acta chir. scand., 137*, 29.

Browse, N.L., Clemenson, G. and Croft, D.N. (1974): Fibrinogen-detectable thrombosis in the legs and pulmonary embolism. *Brit. med. J., 1*, 603.

Bygdeman, S. (1969): Prevention and therapy of thromboembolic complications with dextran. *Progr. Surg., 7*, 114.

Carter, A.E. and Eban, R. (1973): The prevention of postoperative deep venous thrombosis with dextran 70. *Brit. J. Surg., 60*, 681.

Chien, S. (1972): Present state of blood rheology. In: *Hemodilution*, pp. 1–40. Editors: K. Messmer and H. Schmid-Schönbein. Karger, Basel–New York.

Chien, S., Usami, S. and Gregersen, M. (1970): Effects of plasma expanders on blood viscosity. In: *Body Fluid Replacement in the Surgical Patient*, p. 138. Editors: Ch.L. Fox and G.G. Nahas. Grune and Stratton, New York–London.

Coon, W.W. and Willis, P.W. (1959): Deep venous thrombosis and pulmonary embolism. *Amer. J. Cardiol., 4*, 611.

Daniel, W.J., Moore, A.R. and Flanc, C. (1972): Prophylaxis of deep vein thrombosis (DVT) with dextran 70 in patients with a fractured neck of the femur. *Austr. N. Z. J. Surg., 41*, 289.

Davidson, A.I., Brunt, M.E.A. and Matheson, N.A. (1972): A further trial comparing dextran 70 with warfarin in the prophylaxis of postoperative venous thrombosis. *Brit. J. Surg., 59*, 314.

Eskeland, G., Solheim, K. and Skjørten, F. (1966): Anticoagulant prophylaxis, thromboembolism and mortality in elderly patients with hip fractures. A controlled trial. *Acta chir. scand., 131*, 16.

Evarts, C.M. and Feil, E.J. (1971): Prevention of thromboembolic disease after elective surgery of the hip. *J. Bone Jt Surg., 53*, 1271.

Flanc, C., Kakkar, V.V. and Clarke, M.B. (1968): The detection of venous thrombosis of the legs using ^{125}I-labelled fibrinogen. *Brit. J. Surg., 55*, 742.

Grega, G.J., Schwinghamer, J.M. and Haddy, F.J. (1971): Changes in forelimb weight and segmental vascular resistances following severe hemorrhage. *Circulat. Res., XXIX*, 691.

Grindon, A.J., Holland, P.V. and Schmidt, P.J. (1967): Posttransfusion hepatitis. *Amer. Heart J., 74*, 591.

Gruber, U.F. (1969): *Blood Replacement*. Springer, Berlin–Heidelberg–New York.

Gruber, U.F., Rem, J., Altorfer, R., Schaub, N., Frede, K.E., Fridrich, R. and Duckert, F. (1973): Efficacy of dextran 40 or heparin in prevention of deep vein thrombosis after major surgery. *Europ. surg. Res., 5, Suppl. 2*, 15.

Hamilton, H.W., Crawford, J.S., Gardiner, J.H. and Wiley, A.M. (1970): Venous thrombosis in patients with fracture of the upper end of the femur. A phlebographic study of the effect of prophylactic anticoagulation. *J. Bone Jt Surg., 52B*, 268.

Harper, D.R., Dhall, D.P. and Woodruff, P.W.H. (1973): Prophylaxis in iliofemoral venous thrombosis. The major amputee as a clinical research model. *Brit. J. Surg., 60*, 831.

Hartshorn, J.W.S., Teale, S.N. and Faiz, M. (1969): Dextran 75 and postoperative phlebitis.

Evaluation of dextran 75 in the prophylaxis of postoperative thrombophlebitis, pulmonary embolism and myocardial infarction. *Arch. Surg. (Chicago)*, *98*, 694.

Heughan, Ch., Niinikoski, J. and Hunt, T.K. (1972): Effect of excessive infusion of saline solution on tissue oxygen transport. *Surg. Gynec. Obstet.*, *135*, 257.

Hint, H. (1968): The pharmacology of dextran and the pathophysiological background for the clinical use of Rheomacrodex and Macrodex. *Acta anaesth. belg.*, *19*, 119.

Hint, H. (1973): Vor- und Nachteile der Infusionstherapie mit kolloidalen Lösungen: theoretische und experimentelle Gesichtspunkte. *Infusionstherapie*, *1*, 32.

Huttunen, H.J., Mattila, M.A.K., Hakalehto, J., Kettunen, K., Rehnberg, V. and Babinsky, M. (1971): Single infusion of dextran 70 in the prophylaxis of postoperative deep vein thrombosis. *Ann. Chir. Gynaec. Fenn.*, *60*, 119.

Jansen, H. (1972): Postoperative thromboembolism and its prevention with 500 ml dextran given during operation. *Acta chir. scand., Suppl. 427.*

Johnson, S.R., Bygdeman, S. and Eliasson, R. (1968): Effect of dextran on postoperative thrombosis. *Acta chir. scand., Suppl. 387*, 80.

Kline, A.L., Hughes, L.E. and Campbell, H. (1974): Dextran prophylaxis of deep vein thrombosis: organization of a clinical trial. *Brit. J. Surg.*, *61*, 332.

Koekenberg, L.J.L. (1962): Experimental use of Macrodex as a prophylaxis against postoperative thromboembolism. *Bull. Soc. int. Chir.* *21*, 501.

Korvald, E., Stoeren, E.J. and Ongre, A. (1973): Simultaneous use of warfarin-sodium and dextran 70 to prevent post-operative venous thrombosis in patients with hip fractures. A controlled trial. *J. Oslo Cy Hosp.*, *23*, 25.

Laks, H., O'Connor, N.E., Pilon, R.N., Anderson, W., MacCallum, J.R., Klövekorn, W.P. and Moore, F.D. (1973): Acute normovolemic hemodilution. Effects on hemodynamics, oxygen transport and lung water in anaesthetized man. *Surg. Forum*, *24*, 201.

Lambie, J.M., Barber, D.C., Dhall, D.P. and Matheson, N.A. (1970): Dextran 70 in prophylaxis of postoperative venous thrombosis. A controlled trial. *Brit. med. J.*, *I*, 144.

Lewis, D.H., Jansen, H. and Matheson, N. (1973): The effect of dextran 40 on venous flow changes in the leg induced by abdominal operations. *Brit. J. Surg.*, *60*, 312.

Mellander, St. and Johansson, B. (1968): Control of resistance, exchange and capacitance functions in the peripheral circulation. *Pharmacol. Rev.*, *20*, 117.

Messmer, K., Görnandt, L., Jesch, F., Sinagowitz, E., Sunder-Plassmann, L. and Kessler, M. (1974): Oxygen transport and tissue oxygenation during hemodilution with dextran. *Advanc. exp. Med. Biol.*, in press.

Messmer, K., Lewis, D.H., Sunder-Plassmann, L., Klövekorn, W.P., Mendler, N. and Holper, K. (1972a): Acute normovolemic hemodilution: changes of central hemodynamics and microcirculatory flow in skeletal muscle. *Europ. surg., Res.*, *4*, 55.

Messmer, K., Lorenz, W., Sunder-Plassmann, L., Klövekorn, W.P. and Hutzel, M. (1970): Histamine release as cause of acute hypotension following rapid colloid infusion. *Naunyn-Schmiedeberg's Arch. exp. Path. Pharmak.*, *267*, 433.

Messmer, K. and Schmid-Schönbein, H. (1972): *Hemodilution: Theoretical Basis and Clinical Application.* Karger, Basel–New York.

Messmer, K. and Sunder-Plassmann, L. (1974): Hemodilution. *Progr. Surg.*, *13*, 216.

Messmer, K., Sunder-Plassmann, L., Jesch, F., Görnandt, L., Sinagowitz, E. and Kessler, M. (1973): Oxygen supply of the tissues during limited normovolemic hemodilution. *Res. exp. Med.*, *159*, 152.

Messmer, K., Sunder-Plassmann, L., Klövekorn, W.P. and Holper, K. (1972b): Circulatory significance of hemodilution: rheological changes and limitations. *Advanc. Microcirculat.*, *4*, 1.

Muzaffar, T.Z., Stalker, A.L., Bryce, W.A.J. and Dhall, D.P. (1972): Dextrans and fibrin morphology. *Nature (Lond.)*, *238*, 288.

Myhre, H.O. och Holen, A. (1969): Tromboseprofylakse. Dextran eller warfarin-natrium? *Nord. Med.*, *82*, 1534.

Myrvold, H.E., Persson, J.-E., Svensson, B., Wallenstein, S. and Vikterloef, K.J. (1973):

Prevention of thromboembolism with dextran 70 and heparin in patients with femoral neck fractures. *Acta chir. scand., 139*, 609.

Negus, D., Pinto, D.J., LeQuesne, L.P., Brown, N. and Chapman, M. (1968): ^{125}I-labelled fibrinogen in the diagnosis of deep-vein thrombosis and its correlation with phlebography. *Brit. J. Surg., 55*, 835.

Pinto, D.J. (1970): Controlled trial of an anticoagulant (warfarin-sodium) in the prevention of venous thrombosis following hip surgery. *Brit. J. Surg., 57*, 349.

Replogle, R. (1972): Hemodynamic compensation of acute changes of the hemoglobin concentration. In: *Hemodilution: Theoretical Basis and Clinical Application*. Editors: K. Messmer and H. Schmid-Schönbein. Karger, Basel–New York.

Sevitt, S. (1962): Venous thrombosis and pulmonary embolism: their prevention by oral anticoagulants. *Amer. J. Med., 33*, 703.

Sevitt, S. and Gallagher, N. (1959): Prevention of venous thrombosis and pulmonary embolism in injured patients. A trial of anticoagulant prophylaxis with phenindione in middle-aged and elderly patients with fractured necks of femur. *Lancet, 2*, 981.

Sevitt, S. and Gallagher, N. (1961): Venous thrombosis and pulmonary embolism. *Brit. J. Surg., 48*, 475.

Sjögren, S., Hedlund, P.O. and Palmlöv, A. (1971): Trombosstudier vid prostataoperationer (preliminär rapport). *Nord. Med., 86*, 1163.

Stadil, F. (1970): Prevention of venous thrombosis. *Lancet, 2*, 50.

Stephenson, C.B.S., Wallace, J.C. and Vaughan, J.V. (1973): Dextran 70 in the prevention of post-operative deep vein thrombosis with observations on pulmonary embolism: Report on a pilot study. *N. Z. med. J., 77*, 302.

Sunder-Plassmann, L., Jesch, F., Klövekorn, W.P. and Messmer, K. (1973): Limited hemodilution in hemorrhagic shock in dogs: effects on central hemodynamics and the microcirculation in skeletal muscle. *Res. exp. Med., 159*, 167.

Sunder-Plassmann, L., Klövekorn, W.P., Holper, K., Hase, U. and Messmer, K. (1971): The physiological significance of acutely induced hemodilution. In: *Proceedings of the 6th European Conference on Microcirculation, Aalborg 1970*, p. 23. Editors: Ditzel/Lewis. Karger, Basel–New York.

Sunder-Plassmann, L., Klövekorn, W.P., Messmer, K. and Brendel, W. (1972a): Microcirculatory patterns in hemorrhagic shock in dogs. In: *New Aspects on Trasylol Therapy 5*, p. 33. Editors: W. Brendel and G.L. Haberland. Schattauer, Stuttgart–New York.

Sunder-Plassmann, L., Klövekorn, W.P. and Messmer, K. (1972b): Hemodynamic and rheological changes induced by hemodilution with colloids. In: *Hemodilution: Theoretical Basis and Clinical Application*, p. 184. Editors: K. Messmer and H. Schmid-Schönbein. Karger, Basel–New York.

Tangen, O., Wik, O., Almqvist, J.A.M., Arfors, K.E. and Hint, H.C. (1972): Effects of dextran on the structure and plasmin-induced lysis of human fibrin. *Thrombos. Res., 1*, 487.

Vasilescu, C. (1974): A multi-unit trial of dextran and heparin in the prophylaxis of deep vein thrombosis. *Brit. J. Surg., 61*, 320.

Ledingham (ed.). Shock

Vasoactive agents in the treatment of shock

H.S. LOEB and R.M. GUNNAR

The shock syndrome should be considered present when a patient develops circulatory inadequacy sufficient to result in progressive multiorgan dysfunction, lactic acidemia and progressive cellular injury and death. Associated signs include mental obtundation, oliguria, hypotension, decreased pulse volume, increased capillary filling time, peripheral cyanosis and cold extremities. Signs of compensatory mechanisms such as tachypnea, tachycardia and diaphoresis are also frequently present as may be signs related to the underlying illness.

Principles to be followed in the management of the patient with shock include: 1) stabilization of vital functions; 2) identification and correction of the specific hemodynamic and metabolic derangements present; 3) identification and correction of the underlying disease process or other factors contributing to the shock syndrome.

Before discussing the role of specific vasoactive agents used in the treatment of shock certain 'ground rules' should be laid. Whether due to hypovolemia, sepsis, cardiac disease, or to multiple or unidentified factors, shock should be considered a true medical emergency. Patients developing this syndrome should therefore be placed in an intensive care area equipped and staffed for continuous on line monitoring of the following parameters:

Supported in part by National Institutes of Health Grant HL15040.

1. Cardiac rate and rhythm (EKG).
2. Ventricular filling pressure (pulmonary artery diastolic or wedge, or central venous).
3. Arterial pressure (preferably by direct intraarterial line).
4. Arterial pH, PO_2, PCO_2.
5. Urine output (usually by indwelling bladder catheter).

In addition to the above parameters, frequent clinical observations of mental status, respiratory rate and depth, core and peripheral skin temperature, are necessary. Measurement of cardiac output and total circulating blood volume may be helpful under certain circumstances, but are often not available.

The drugs to be discussed in this chapter can be grouped in the following manner: 1) plasma volume expanders, 2) vasoconstrictors, 3) inotropic agents, 4) vasodilators.

Plasma Volume Expanders

Expansion of the intravascular volume is indicated when the shock syndrome is due, at least in part, to suboptimal ventricular filling resulting in an inadequate cardiac output. Common causes of hypovolemic shock are acute hemorrhage, burns, peritonitis, and dehydration. Under these circumstances the nature of the problem is often apparent. Hypovolemia may also occur under less obvious conditions such as drug overdosage, sepsis, or following acute myocardial infarction. With insufficient intravascular volume ventricular filling is inadequate and the stroke output falls. Unless compensated for by an increase in heart rate, cardiac output and systemic perfusion may become inadequate and the shock syndrome will result. Insufficient ventricular filling implies a less than optimal end-diastolic fiber length and a shift downward along the Frank–Starling curve. This may result from either an absolute reduction in intravascular volume or an increase in venous capacitance leading to a relative hypovolemia. For this reason measurement of the blood volume cannot be depended upon as a means of identifying hypovolemia in patients with shock. Since decreased ventricular filling is usually associated with a reduced filling pressure, hypovolemia should be suspected whenever a patient with the shock syndrome is found to have a normal or low ventricular filling pressure. In patients without cardiac disease, the central venous pressure (CVP) can be used as a guide to fluid therapy. When central venous pressure is 10 cm of water or less, plasma volume expansion should be attempted. A favorable response will be recognized by improvement in urine flow, arterial pressure, pulse volume and reduction in the clinical manifestations of shock. During volume expansion, the CVP should be monitored continuously. When hypovolemia is at fault the CVP will usually increase only slightly as volume is given (Loeb et al., 1969c). In patients with acute myocardial infarction (AMI) or with preexisting cardiac disease, the CVP may not accurately reflect the filling pressure in the left ventricle (Loeb et al., 1973). In such patients measurement of the pulmonary artery diastolic (PADP) or wedge (PWP) pressure using the Swan–Ganz balloon tipped catheter will more accurately reflect left sided filling pressures. In some patients because of abnormal left ventricular function and/or reduced compliance, optimal stroke volume will require a higher than normal PADP or PWP (Crexells et al., 1973). A similar situation may exist with regard to the CVP in patients with right ventricular dysfunction secondary to chronic pulmonary disease, recurrent pulmonary emboli or long standing left ventricular failure. It must also be pointed out that both right and left ventricular filling pressures can be significantly altered by concomitant administration of vasoactive drugs (Loeb et al., 1969a), most of which alter ventricular contractility and/or venous capacitance. Therefore, when using the filling pressure as a guide during volume expansion, the infusion rate of vasoactive agents given at the same time should be held constant.

When treating shock patients with plasma volume expanders, we usually prefer to begin with a colloid solution rather than a crystalloid solution. Plasma, reconstituted serum albumin and low molecular weight dextran may remain in the intravascular compartment longer and can rapidly restore circulating blood volume. If significant anemia or acute blood loss is present, packed red blood cells can also be administered. By infusion of colloid solution at rates of 100 ml every 10 minutes, the response to plasma volume expansion can usually be determined within 30 to 60 minutes, and if no improvement has occurred, other modes of therapy can be instituted. Avoidance of acute pulmonary edema during rapid volume expansion is best accomplished by closely monitoring filling pressures during the infusion and stopping the infusion if the PADP or PWP exceed 20 mmHg or CVP exceeds 15 cm of water. If acute pulmonary edema does develop it can be immediately reversed by removal of blood through the central venous or pulmonary artery catheter.

Vasoconstrictors

These agents are used to increase the arterial pressure, by a direct vasoconstricting effect on resistance vessels. It should be remembered however, that arterial pressure is the product of cardiac output and vascular resistance. The commonly used term vasopressor agent should, therefore, not be used synonymous with the term vasoconstrictor agent since a *vasopressor effect* may occur in the absence of vasoconstriction. It would seem wise, therefore, to avoid using the term vasopressor agent since this says nothing about the mode of action of the particular drug.

In addition to arteriolar constriction, vasoconstrictor drugs may also cause venoconstriction and temporarily augment ventricular filling. During administration of these agents arteriolar constriction may not be the same in all vascular beds and, therefore, their effects on perfusion of regional vascular beds may not be uniform. Currently available vasoconstrictor agents which have been used for the treatment of shock patients include the alpha-adrenergic agonists, phenylephrine and methoxamine and the non-adrenergic drug, angiotensin. Norepinephrine, metaraminol and dopamine, although also having alpha-adrenergic vasoconstricting properties, have direct cardiac effects and thus are considered with the inotropic agents.

Although some differences exist regarding methoxamine, phenylephrine and angiotensin, the three drugs are considered together because their major effect is to increase arterial pressure by constricting arteriolar smooth muscle. Bradycardia, which occurs when normo-tensive patients are given these drugs, is the result of a reflex increase in vagal tone mediated by baroreceptor mechanisms.

Theoretically, vasoconstrictor drugs could be of value when the shock syndrome develops as the result of generalized vasodilatation. The use of vasoconstrictors temporarily to reverse hypotension induced by drugs or anesthetics is probably indicated for patients with preexisting cerebral or coronary artery disease, because perfusion beyond areas of partial obstruction is often dependent upon the arterial pressure. An additional use of these agents is in the treatment of certain supraventricular tachycardias, which may respond to the increased vagal tone secondary to the baroreceptor reflex. However, for established shock, the value of these relatively pure vasoconstrictor agents is questionable, and at present they are infrequently used.

Inotropic Drugs

This group of drugs can be subdivided into those which act by direct or indirect stimulation of cardiac beta-adrenergic receptors, and those which exert their cardiac effects by other mechanisms. The beta-adrenergic active drugs which are frequently used in the treatment of shock include norepinephrine, metaraminol, dopamine and isoproterenol. An additional agent, dobutamine, is currently under investigation and has not yet been approved for clinical use in the USA. Each of these drugs has cardiac effects which can be inhibited by administration of beta-adrenergic blocking agents. They each increase the rate and force of myocardial fiber shorting (inotropic effect), and may increase sinus node automaticity (chronotropic effect). Increased automaticity of ectopic foci may also occur and result in arrhythmias. Although these agents are qualitatively similar in their cardiac action they differ markedly from each other with regard to their effects on peripheral blood vessels.

Norepinephrine. This is the natural neuro-transmitter of the post-ganglionic sympathetic fibers and is stored in nerve terminals throughout the myocardium and elsewhere. Exogenous administration of norepinephrine to normotensive individuals results in elevation of the arterial pressure due to alpha-adrenergic induced peripheral vasoconstriction. Bradycardia occurs secondary to baroreceptor reflexes and cardiac output is reduced. A similar effect may occur in patients with shock if norepinephrine is given in excessive amounts in an attempt to restore arterial pressure to 'normal' levels (Shubin and Weil, 1965). The direct inotropic and chronotropic effects of norepinephrine become unmasked when the drug is given in modest amounts to shock patients who are markedly hypotensive. Out of a total group of 122 patients with shock of various etiologies treated with norepinephrine we observed average increases in cardiac output and heart rate of 32% and 15% respectively in those patients whose control mean arterial pressure (MAP) was under 50 mmHg (Gunnar and Loeb, 1972). When control MAP was 50 to 70 mmHg cardiac output increased by 16% and heart rate by 6% and in patients whose MAP was 70 mmHg or above, norepinephrine infusion did not consistently increase either cardiac output or heart rate.

Thus when norepinephrine is given to shock patients in amounts to bring MAP to between 70 and 80 mmHg (but not higher), hemodynamic improvement is the rule. Since excessive elevation of arterial pressure is contraindicated, direct measurement of intraarterial pressure may be necessary when using norepinephrine since pressures measured by the cuff method may be falsely reduced or unobtainable as the result of vasoconstriction (Cohn, 1967). In patients with cardiogenic shock following acute myocardial infarction, temporary improvement of arterial pressure and cardiac output can usually be achieved with norepinephrine (Gunnar et al., 1970), and although myocardial oxygen demand is increased, myocardial oxygen delivery is similarly improved and myocardial lactate production does not worsen (Mueller et al., 1972). Although generally contraindicated in patients with hypovolemic shock, norepinephrine may be used under desperate circumstances to stabilize arterial pressure long enough to permit volume expansion. Under these circumstances venoconstriction induced by norepinephrine may temporarily improve ventricular filling and cardiac output.

Metaraminol. This agent has essentially the same hemodynamic effects as norepinephrine and acts in part by liberating norepinephrine stores from nerve terminal endings. Its time of onset and dissipation of action is longer than that of norepinephrine and it may be administered intramuscularly. Metaraminol is frequently ineffective however in patients who are catecholamine depleted due to prior therapy with reserpine.

At the present time norepinephrine or metaraminol appear to be the agents of choice for temporary pharmacologic support of the circulation in patients with shock of any etiology who are severely hypotensive and in whom rapid plasma volume expansion is either impossible or is ineffective in reversing the manifestations of shock.

Dopamine. Dopamine is a derivative of norepinephrine and has recently been approved for clinical use in the USA. Like norepinephrine it increases contractility and heart rate by direct stimulation of cardiac beta-adrenergic receptors (McNay and Goldberg, 1966). At higher doses dopamine causes alpha-adrenergic mediated vasoconstriction. Unlike norepinephrine, dopamine causes selective, nonadrenergic vasodilatation in the renal and splanchnic (McNay et al., 1965). This unique property of dopamine would tend to selectively favor flow to these regions thus preventing ischemic damage to the kidney and gut which frequently complicates shock. In animals, dopamine improves the hemodynamic derangements of endotoxemic and cardiogenic shock (MacCannell et al., 1966). Dopamine has also been found useful in the treatment of patients with bacteremic shock and shock following acute myocardial infarction. When compared to norepinephrine however dopamine is less reliable an agent for reversing severe hypotension. Since cardiac output tends to be greater during dopamine infusion than during norepinephrine infusion, it may however be preferred over norepinephrine in shock patients who are only mildly hypotensive. The effects of dopamine on renal blood flow although established in animals are difficult to document in clinical shock. In our own studies (Loeb et al., 1971), we found improved urine flow in as many patients during norepinephrine infusion as during dopamine infusion. Side effects during dopamine infusion include supraventricular tachycardia, ventricular irritability, and occasional nausea and vomiting. We have recently observed a marked increase in left ventricular filling pressure associated with acute arterial oxygen desaturation during dopamine administration to patients with chronic low output cardiac failure who were not in clinical shock. Tissue necrosis at the site of extravasation apparently does not occur with dopamine as it does with norepinephrine. Dopamine must be given by continuous intravenous infusion, and although its time of onset and duration of action are slightly longer than norepinephrine, the infusion rate must be titrated closely to achieve optimal hemodynamic effects. Very high infusion rates of dopamine may cause excessive vasoconstriction by stimulation of alpha-adrenergic receptors and thereby limit its effectiveness.

Isoproterenol. This agent is a potent inotropic and chronotropic drug which has a rapid onset and dissipation of action. Its major peripheral vascular effect is vasodilatation, mediated through stimulation of beta-adrenergic receptors. Isoproterenol can be considered a nearly pure beta-adrenergic agent and thus differs from norepinephrine, metaraminol and dopamine, each of which exert alpha-receptor mediated vasoconstriction. Because it consistently improves cardiac output isoproterenol has been advocated for shock patients with reduced cardiac output who are not responsive to volume expansion. Clinical experience, however, suggests that its usefulness is limited because it also causes widespread vasodilatation in skin and skeletal muscle. The increased cardiac output thus tends to be directed away from vital areas (brain, myocardium and kidneys). Arterial mean pressure may be unchanged or fall during infusion of isoproterenol and therefore it should rarely be given to hypotensive patients who need restoration of an adequate perfusion pressure. Isoproterenol is particularly dangerous in patients with shock following acute myocardial infarction or in elderly patients likely to have diffuse obstructive coronary artery disease (Gunnar et al., 1967), since in such patients myocardial blood flow in areas distal to the obstruction is likely to be dependent upon arterial diastolic pressure. Like all inotropic agents, isoproterenol will increase myocardial oxygen demands, however, unlike norepinephrine, metaraminol or dopamine, isoproterenol usually does not improve arterial perfusion pressure and thus myocardial oxygen delivery may fail to keep up with oxygen need

(Mueller et al., 1970), thereby resulting in more ischemia or cell necrosis.

Isoproterenol may be of benefit in an occasional shock patient if the increased cardiac output following its administration exceeds the reduction in vascular resistance resulting from its peripheral vasodilatation effect. Under these circumstances the mean arterial pressure will be increased, or if not initially low, will remain adequate. In our experience patients responding well to small amounts of isoproterenol are usually those with very high ventricular filling pressures, very low cardiac outputs and fairly normal mean arterial pressures when measured directly. Isoproterenol may also be of benefit when shock is associated with sinus bradycardia and/or heart block. Improved heart rate may occur by acceleration of sinus rate, by improved AV conduction, or by increasing the rate of an escape focus. When in such patients stroke output is limited because of poor ventricular function, the dual effect of isoproterenol in increasing both the rate and extent of myocardial contraction can dramatically improve cardiac output. Because of its arrhythmogenic effects and its effects on myocardial oxygen consumption we favor temporary cardiac pacing for the management of bradyarrhythmias in such patients. However, isoproterenol may be necessary for stabilization of the patient in preparation for emergency pacing. Isoproterenol may be of value in patients with cardiogenic shock secondary to severe aortic or mitral regurgitation. By reducing impedance to left ventricular ejection the amount of blood regurgitated can be diminished and forward flow improved.

Dobutamine. This agent is still under investigation and has not been approved for clinical use. Dobutamine is a synthetic catecholamine drug, developed to retain the direct inotropic effects but to eliminate the peripheral vascular, chronotropic and arrhythmogenic properties shared by the drugs discussed above. Experimental studies on a variety of catecholamine agents suggested that such was possible by molecular manipulation and after testing many compounds dobutamine appeared to fulfill the desired goal. Animal (McRitchie et al., 1973) and limited clinical studies have shown dobutamine to be a potent inotropic agent which acts by cardiac beta-receptor stimulation. Although carefully controlled studies have demonstrated that dobutamine does possess both alpha (vasoconstriction) and beta (vasodilatation) effects on peripheral blood vessels (Robie et al., 1974), it seems that these effects are small relative to its inotropic effect. Unlike dopamine, dobutamine does not appear selectively to vasodilate renal or splanchnic vascular beds. Like the other inotropic agents discussed, dobutamine does increase the heart rate, apparently by directly increasing sinus node automaticity (Loeb et al., 1974). This effect may however be less than that which occurs with isoproterenol when the two drugs are given in dosages having similar effects on cardiac output (Fig. 1). Although dobutamine has been shown to consistantly improve cardiac output in patients with chronic congestive cardiac failure (Loeb et al., in press), its efficacy in patients with shock has not been tested.

Digitalis. The digitalis preparations are used primarily to improve myocardial contraction by exerting inotropism through nonadrenergic mechanisms. Although digitalis does exert a direct vasoconstrictor effect, this effect appears to be rather short lived and is of doubtful clinical significance. Digitalis will also impede AV nodal conduction and thus is of value in slowing the ventricular response to certain supraventricular tachycardias. Unlike the catecholamines, digitalis does not increase cardiac output or alter heart rate when administered to patients without heart disease or to patients with acute myocardial infarction who do not have heart failure. Its inotropic effects, however, are well demonstrated by its effects on other indices of contractility such as left ventricular dp/dt or V_{max} (Rahimtoola et al., 1972). Since digitalis reduces the elevated left ventricular end-diastolic pressure associated with

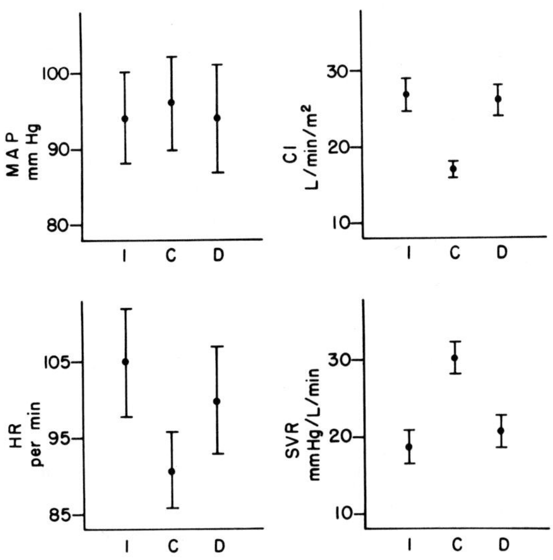

Fig. 1. Hemodynamic comparison between isoproterenol (I) and dobutamine (D) in 10 patients with chronic low output cardiac failure. The mean values and standard errors are shown for mean arterial pressure (MAP), cardiac index (CI), heart rate (HR) and systemic vascular resistance (SVR) during the control period (C) and during infusion of I and D. For each patient the dosage ratio was 500 D to 1 I. The actual dosages used were 0.014 + 0.001 μg/kg/min for I and 7.3 ± 0.3 μg/kg/min for D. Five patients received I as the first drug studied and five received D first. HR rate was significantly faster during I infusion than during D infusion. However, MAP, CI and SVR were not significantly different between the two drugs.

acute myocardial infarction while stroke work is unchanged improvement in ventricular function is implied. Although it is well established that digitalis can improve the circulatory status of patients with various types of chronic heart failure, its efficacy in shock remains unproven. In patients with shock following acute myocardial infarction, digitalis is rarely effective in reversing the shock state (Gunnar et al., 1970). Occasionally, however, significant clinical hemodynamic improvement does occur. At present the indications for administration of digitalis to patients with cardiac failure and/or cardiogenic shock following acute myocardial infarction are ill defined and controversial. If digitalis is to be used it should be given in small amounts since patients with acute myocardial infarction are probably at increased risk for the development of digitalis-induced arrhythmias (Morrison and Killip, 1971). It also seems prudent to stabilize the arterial pressure with norepinephrine or dopamine before administration of digitalis glycosides. An exception to this might be in the treatment of very rapid ventricular rates in patients with atrial flutter or fibrillation.

Digitalis is more often effective in reversing the manifestations of shock when they occur in patients with primary valvular heart disease or cardiomyopathy. Severe hypotension may not be present in such patients and the hemodynamic derangement is often characterized by a marked reduction in cardiac output and elevation of ventricular filling pressures. It is frequently unclear as to what precipitates the shock state in such patients. Unfortunately, the state of prior digitalization is often unknown and administration of additional digitalis under these circumstances carries significant risk of inducing serious digitalis intoxication in patients already critically ill. When in doubt it is probably advisable to use alternative measures until results of a blood digitalis level can be obtained. The use of digitalis in patients with septic shock unresponsive to volume expansion is based on the premise that abnormal cardiac function may be contributing to the shock state. Although cardiac output may be normal or increased in such patients, a significant number show evidence of impaired cardiac function when challenged with a volume load (Winslow et al., 1973). There are several possible mechanisms for impaired cardiac function in patients with sepsis some of which are preexisting heart disease, reduced coronary perfusion during protracted hypotension and release from the pancreas of a myocardial depressant factor. The routine use of digitalis in the treatment of septic shock although advocated by some, does not, however, seem justified from available data, and if digitalis is to be used the same precautions should be taken as suggested for patients with shock following acute myocardial infarction.

Glucagon. A few years ago glucagon was advanced as a promising inotropic agent for treatment of cardiogenic shock and related low output states. Its inotropic effects have been well established in both animal and man. Its mode of action is different from the catecholamines and from digitalis, and glucagon appears to act by activating adenyl cyclase to convert adenosine triphosphate to cyclic AMP, thereby activating the contractile mechanism (Epstein et al., 1971). Glucagon appears to have diminished inotropic effects on the chronically failing myocardium (Goldstein et al., 1970) and its clinical efficacy has been limited both by the rather high incidence of side effects (nausea and vomiting) and by its relative lack of potency when compared to other available inotropic agents (Armstrong et al., 1971).

Ionophores. These compounds are mostly metabolites of microbes which act by transporting various cations across cell membranes. A calcium ionophore has recently been shown by DeGuzman and Pressman (1974) to have striking inotropic activity when given to normal anesthetized dogs. The unique mode of action and potency of the ionophores suggest their potential for use in clinical shock, however, no clinical studies have been reported to date.

Vasodilators

The final group of vasoactive drugs to be discussed, although not new, are currently receiving renewed attention. The concept of vasodilator therapy for treating shock states was advocated by Nickerson (1963) and has been a subject of controversy during the past decade. Since the shock state is one of inadequate organ perfusion, it seemed reasonable that vasodilators might result in improved organ perfusion, particularly if post-capillary vasoconstriction was responsible for stasis of the microcirculation and loss of effective intravascular volume. The early advocates of vasodilator therapy were primarily concerned with the effects of vasodilators on the peripheral circulation, since inappropriate vasoconstriction was considered to be a primary factor in the genesis of refractory shock. These concepts, based largely upon animal models of endotoxemic and hemorrhagic shock, although important failed to take into consideration the role of perfusion pressure, which as indicated earlier, is of particular clinical importance when shock occurs in patients with preexisting arteriosclerosis. Furthermore, in the primate the significance of post-capillary vasoconstriction in the pathophysiology of shock remains unsettled (Buckberg et al., 1971). Recently the focus of attention with regard to vasodilator therapy has shifted from the microcirculation to the heart. Thus although vasodilators were originally advocated primarily for the treatment of septic or hemorrhagic shock, their role in cardiogenic shock is currently of major interest. When the shock syndrome is associated with adequate or increased ventricular filling pressures and reduced cardiac output, abnormal cardiac function is present either as a primary problem as in AMI or as a secondary factor complicating shock of various etiologies. Under either circumstance, efforts to improve cardiac function seem worthwhile as a means of reversing the shock state. Although inotropic agents are often at least temporarily effective in improving cardiac output and peripheral perfusion, they also increase myocardial oxygen consumption and thus can result in ischemic damage to the heart when myocardial oxygen delivery or utilization is limited. In addition to the frequency (heart rate) and velocity of myocardial fiber shortening (contractility) both of which are increased by most inotropic agents, an important determinent to myocardial oxygen requirement is the intramyocardial wall tension developed during each systole. Wall tension (T) is in turn related to the pressure (P) developed within the ventricle, the internal radius (r) of the ventricle and the thickness of the myocardium (h) according to the LaPlace equation where $T = Pr/h$. Since for a given stroke volume pressure is determined largely by the systemic arteriolar resistance (afterload) drugs which vasodilate these arterioles will lower myocardial wall tension and oxygen requirements if heart rate and contractility remain constant. In addition to their effect on systemic arterioles most vasodilator drugs also increase venous capacitance and reduce the size (i.e. radius) of the ventricular chamber which will also reduce myocardial wall tension and oxygen requirements.

Vasodilators may therefore improve peripheral perfusion by 1) acting directly to reverse inappropriate pre- or post-capillary vasoconstriction, and 2) improving myocardial performance by reducing afterload and preload thus favorably influencing the relationship between myocardial oxygen delivery and requirements.

The vasodilator drugs available for use in clinical shock are a heterogenous group. The alpha-adrenergic receptor blocking agents include phenoxybenzamine, phentolamine and chlorpromazine, the latter also having significant central nervous system effects at higher dosages. Recently two antihypertensive agents, nitroprusside (Guiha et al., 1974) and trimetaphan (Shell and Sobel, 1974) have been evaluated as a means of improving myocardial function or reducing infarct size following acute myocardial infarction. Nitroglycerine has also been shown to improve cardiac function in patients with acute myocardial infarction complicated by left ventricular failure.

Corticosteroids in massive dosages have also been advocated for their vasodilator effect; however our own studies suggest that even when given in massive amounts, corticosteroids do not consistently reduce peripheral vascular resistance in shock patients (Winslow et al., 1973).

Specific indications for vasodilator therapy in patients with shock are yet to be defined. We found moderate hemodynamic improvement following administration of 5 to 10 mg of chlorpromazine as a single i.v. bolus in a group of patients who had clinical manifestations of shock associated with an elevated central venous pressure and mean arterial pressure above 70 mmHg (Loeb et al., 1969b). On the other hand, patients who were markedly hypotensive or who had a central venous pressure under 12 mmHg, did not show hemodynamic improvement following chlorpromazine. In elderly patients or in patients with coronary artery disease vasodilator drugs should be used with caution since a fall in arterial pressure can result in diminished perfusion of the brain or myocardium. Vasodilator drugs should also not be given to patients likely to be hypovolemic since venodilatation can further reduce ventricular filling pressure and result in a precipitous fall in cardiac output and arterial pressure. Administration of vasodilator drugs to patients with significant arterial hypotension (confirmed by intraarterial measurement) is probably rarely indicated.

Vasodilators may be of particular value in patients with shock associated with mitral or aortic regurgitation. Under these circumstances reduction in systemic arterial resistance will tend to favor forward flow and reduce the excessive volume load placed on the heart by valvular regurgitation. They may also be of value in shock patients who are markedly vasoconstricted and not responsive to volume expansion, particularly under conditions when inotropic agents might induce myocardial ischemia or cause excessive tachycardia.

In summary, selection of the appropriate vasoactive agent for temporary support of the patient with shock depends upon identification of the hemodynamic derangement present, the specific cause of shock, and the preexisting condition of the patient. Accurate monitoring of ventricular filling and systemic arterial pressure is necessary, and frequent reassessment of cardiac, pulmonary, renal and cerebral function is mandatory as a guide to optimal therapy. Hypovolemia must be searched for and corrected. In hypotensive patients the arterial pressure must be increased to a level which permits perfusion of vital organs, and this is usually best accomplished with norepinephrine, metaraminol or dopamine. Vasodilator drugs should not be used until correction of hypovolemia and then only if arterial pressure can be maintained at a satisfactory level. Ability to reverse the underlying problem which caused shock to develop is nevertheless usually necessary in order to achieve long term survival and drug support must always be considered as a temporary means of buying time to accomplish this more difficult goal.

References

Armstrong, P.W., Gold, H.K., Daggett, W.M., Austen, W.G. and Sanders, C.A. (1971): Hemodynamic evaluation of glucagon in symptomatic heart disease. *Circulation, 44*, 67.

Buckberg, G., Cohn, J. and Darling, C. (1971): *Escherichia coli* bacteremic shock in conscious baboons. *Ann. Surg., 173*, 122.

Cohn, J.N. (1967): Blood pressure measurement in shock. *J. Amer. med. Ass., 199*, 972.

Crexells, C., Chatterjee, K., Forrester, J.S., Dikshit, K. and Swan, J.J.C. (1973): Optimal level of filling pressure in the left side of the heart in acute myocardial infarction. *New Engl. J. Med., 289*, 1263.

DeGuzman, N.J. and Pressman, B. (1974): The inotropic effects of the calcium ionophore X-537A in the anesthetized dog. *Circulation, 49*, 1072.

Epstein, S.E., Levey, G.S. and Skelton, C.L. (1971): Adenyl cyclase and cyclic AMP: biochemical links in the regulation of myocardial contractility. *Circulation, 43*, 437.

Goldstein, R.E., Skelton, C.L., Levey, G.S., Glancey, D.L., Beiser, G.D. and Epstein, S.E. (1970): Effects of glucagon on contractility and adenyl cyclase activity of human papillary muscle. *Circulation, 42, Suppl. III*, 111-158.

Guiha, N.H., Cohn, J.N., Mikulic, E., Franciosa, J.A. and Limas, C.J. (1974): Treatment of refractory heart failure with infusion of nitroprusside. *New Engl. J. Med., 291*, 587.

Gunnar, R.M. and Loeb, H.S. (1972): The use of drugs in cardiogenic shock due to acute myocardial infarction. *Circulation, 45*, 1111.

Gunnar, R.M., Loeb, H.S., Pietras, R.J. and Tobin Jr., J.R. (1967): Ineffectiveness of isoproterenol in the treatment of shock due to acute myocardial infarction. *J. Amer. med. Ass., 202*, 1124.

Gunnar, R.M., Loeb, H.S., Pietras, R.J. and Tobin Jr., J.R. (1970): The hemodynamic effects of myocardial infarction and results of therapy. *Med. Clin. N. Amer., 54*, 235.

Loeb, H.S., Gunnar, R.M., Pietras, R.J. and Tobin Jr., J.R. (1969a): Relationships between central venous and left ventricular filling pressures prior to and during treatment of shock. *Amer. J. Cardiol., 23*, 125.

Loeb, H.S., Khan, M., Klodnycky, M.L., Sinno, M.Z., Towne, W.D. and Gunnar, R.M. (in press): Hemodynamic effects of dobutamine in man. *Circulat. Shock*.

Loeb, H.S., Pietras, R.J., Ninos, N., Tobin Jr., J.R. and Gunnar, R.M. (1969b): Hemodynamic responses to chlorpromazine in patients in shock. *Arch. intern. Med., 24*, 354.

Loeb, H.S., Pietras, R.J., Tobin Jr., J.R. and Gunnar, R.M. (1969c): Hypovolemia in shock due to acute myocardial infarction. *Circulation, 40*, 653.

Loeb, H.S., Rahimtoola, S.H., Rosen, K.M., Sinno, M.Z., Chuquimia, R. and Gunnar, R.M. (1973): Assessment of ventricular function after acute myocardial infarction by plasma volume expansion. *Circulation, 47*, 720.

Loeb, H.S., Sinno, M.Z., Saudye, A., Towne, W.D. and Gunnar, R.M. (1974): Electrophysiologic properties of dobutamine. *Circulat. Shock, 1*, 217.

Loeb, H.S., Winslow, E.B.J., Rahimtoola, S.H., Rosen, K.M. and Gunnar, R.M. (1971): Acute hemodynamic effects of dopamine in patients with shock. *Circulation, 44*, 163.

MacCannell, K.L., McNay, J.L., Meyer, M.B. and Goldberg, L.I. (1966): Dopamine in the treatment of hypotension and shock. *New Engl. J. Med., 275*, 1389.

McNay, J.L. and Goldberg, L.I. (1966): Hemodynamic effects of dopamine in the dog before and after alpha adrenergic blockade. *Circulat. Res., 18, Suppl. I*, 1–110.

McNay, J.L., McDonald Jr., R.H. and Goldberg, L.I. (1965): Direct renal vasodilation produced by dopamine in the dog. *Circulat. Res., 16*, 510.

McRitchie, R.J., Vatner, S.F., Tuttle, R. and Braunwald, E. (1973): Cardiovascular effects of dobutamine, a cardiospecific β-adrenergic stimulant, in conscious dogs. *Circulation, 47 and 48, Suppl. IV*, 132.

Morrison, J. and Killip, T. (1971): Serial serum digitalis levels in patients with acute myocardial infarction. *Clin. Res., 19*, 353.

Mueller, H., Ayres, S.M., Giannelli Jr., S., Conklin, E.F., Mazzara, J.T. and Grace, W.J. (1972): Effect of isoproterenol, l-norepinephrine and intraaortic counter pulsation on hemodynamics and myocardial metabolism in shock following acute myocardial infarction. *Circulation, 45*, 335.

Mueller, H., Ayres, S.M., Mazzara, J.T., Giannelli, S., Conklin, E.F., Grace, W.J. and Nealon, T. (1970): Coronary flow-pressure relation and its role for myocardial metabolism in human coronary shock. *Amer. J. Cardiol., 26*, 651.

Nickerson, M. (1963): Sympathetic blockade in the therapy of shock. *Amer. J. Cardiol., 12*, 619.

Rahimtoola, S.H., Sinno, M.Z., Chuquimia, R., Loeb, H.S., Rosen, K.M. and Gunnar, R.M. (1972): Effects of ouabain on impaired left ventricular function in acute myocardial infarction. *New Engl. J. Med., 287*, 527.

Robie, N.W., Nutter, D.O., Moody, C. and McNay, J. (1974): In vivo analysis of adrenergic receptor activity of dobutamine. *Circulat. Res., 34*, 663.

Shell, W.E. and Sobel, B.E. (1974): Protection of ischemic myocardium by reduced ventricular afterload. *New Engl. J. Med., 291*, 481.

Shubin, H. and Weil, M.H. (1965): Hemodynamic alterations in patients after acute myocardial infarction. In: *Shock and Hypotension*, p. 499. Editors: Mills and Moyer. Grune and Stratton, New York, N.Y.

Winslow, E.J., Loeb, H.S., Rahimtoola, S.H., Kamath, S. and Gunnar, R.M. (1973): Hemodynamic studies and results of therapy in 50 patients with bacteremic shock. *Amer. J. Med., 54*, 421.

Ledingham (ed.). Shock

Management of septic shock

I.McA. LEDINGHAM and J.D. SLEIGH

Although sharing many of the clinical features of other forms of shock, septic shock presents problems which are sufficiently distinctive to merit separate mention. Treatment is often protracted and mortality remains high even in centres with specialised facilities. There are probably two main explanations for these facts – delay in diagnosis until after the onset of the refractory stage of the syndrome and uncertainty as to the precise mechanisms whereby bacteria (or bacterial products) produce shock.

Septic shock is readily diagnosed when a previously healthy patient develops a high fever and prostration after, for example, some form of instrumentation but the diagnosis may not be so obvious in the elderly, dehydrated, atherosclerotic patient during the postoperative period, or in the leukaemic or chronic renal failure patient in relapse.

During recent years there has been a tendency to attribute the clinical features of septic shock to circulating endotoxin presumably, in part, because of the high incidence of gram-negative septicaemia. However, by no means all patients with gram-negative septicaemia develop shock, and furthermore, shock secondary to gram-positive septicaemia is clinically indistinguishable from endotoxin shock. The development of the shock syndrome, therefore, requires a combination of factors including a major source of infection, bacterial invasion of the blood stream and some unusual form of host response.

The site of origin of the infection influences the severity and outcome of the associated shock state. Baue (1969) recorded that the urinary tract was the most frequent site of infection; the respiratory tract was second and the gastrointestinal tract joint third equal with skin (which included burns). In Altemeier's series (1967) over 75% of the patients developed septic shock while in hospital. Neely and his colleagues (1971) found that in a series of 152 patients there was an overall mortality of 66% but this represented a scatter from 36% in sepsis of urological origin to 84% in sepsis after various general surgical manoeuvres. It is therefore important to define the clinical background when presenting data on septic shock.

Bacteriology

It is something of a surprise and disappointment to learn that the possession of a whole range of powerful antimicrobial drugs has not resulted in a decline in the incidence of septicaemia; in fact the converse is true (*British medical Journal*, 1974a). Septicaemia is on the increase and its profile is changing. Nowadays the organisms most often isolated from the blood are aerobic gram-negative bacilli (*Escherichia, Klebsiella, Proteus, Pseudomonas* species and the like) and a number of different hospitals have reported a two to four fold rise in the incidence of septicaemia due to these bacteria during the last fifteen years.

The wide-spread, even indiscriminate, use of antibiotics has resulted in resistant strains of these gram-negative organisms becoming established in the hospital environment and in the intestinal tract of patients (*Lancet*, 1971). As a result, these bacteria, often disregarded in past years, are recognised as opportunistic pathogens in susceptible patients found in hospital wards today. Many of the patients are elderly and have been subjected to radical surgical procedures that would not have been undertaken a generation ago; in others the host defences have been compromised either by the nature of the primary disease (e.g., malignancies, especially the leukaemias and reticuloses) or by treatment with cytotoxic, immunosuppressive or corticosteroid drugs. Although the source of infection is often endogenous from the patient's own intestinal tract, cross-infection may occur and portals of entry created by intravenous lines, intubation of the respiratory tract and in-dwelling catheterisation of the urinary tract may allow the 'unfair introduction' of these bacteria.

Bacteroides species have been the subject of much recent attention and these organisms are now incriminated as an important cause of septicaemia. The clinical significance of these gram-negative non-sporing anaerobic bacilli has been underestimated in the past. Improvements in bacteriological techniques have facilitated their isolation but, nevertheless, it is easy to acquire an out-of-sight/out-of-mind attitude to these anaerobes which comprise more than 99% of the human faecal bacteria (*Lancet*, 1973).

The pathogens involved in serious infection include not only the bacteria already mentioned but also nocardia, yeasts and true fungi such as phycomycetes and aspergilli, viruses, in particular the herpes viruses varicella-zoster and cytomegalovirus, and the protozoa, *Toxoplasma gondii* and *Pneumocystis carinii*. The manifestations of the resultant disease may be bizarre and difficult to recognise. In this country the most common problem encountered in the intensive care situation is superinfection with the yeast *Candida albicans*. The principal predisposing factor is repeated courses of different antibiotics which alter the normal commensal microflora of the patient to allow colonisation of the respiratory, alimentary and urinary tracts, the skin and buccal mucosa with candida. This course of events is common and as a rule has no serious consequences but in a minority of patients systemic, usually fatal, candidiasis results.

Each year, the Western Infirmary, Glasgow admits some 21,000 patients and the Diagnostic Bacteriology Laboratory handles 1000 sets of blood cultures. The incidence of septicaemia in a 3 year period (1971–1973) was approximately 3 per 1000 admissions and this is similar to the findings reported from other general hospitals (Murdoch et al., 1968). Therefore, some 70 patients annually are found to have a septicaemia either on admission or subsequently during their hospital stay. In approximately 50% of patients with a positive blood culture the causal organism is an aerobic gram-negative bacillus and the *Bacteroides* species account for a further 10%.

The cornerstone of bacteriological diagnosis and, therefore, rational treatment is the examination of a series of blood cultures taken from the patient. There is no uniformity of opinion regarding either the number of cultures it is necessary to take or the best time of sampling. A laboratory swamped with excessive numbers of blood broths is unable to give proper attention to those that really matter and it has been reported that a subsequent positive culture is unlikely when two samples have been found to be sterile (Crowley, 1970). When septicaemia is suspected, a reasonable plan is to take three separate sets of cultures before any kind of therapy is given. If the patient has a swinging fever with intervening afebrile periods the usual instruction is to take the samples as the temperature begins to rise and when the patient may suffer a rigor but the time of maximal opportunity cannot be predicted with certainty (Association of Clinical Pathologists, 1974). The blood, collected using careful aseptic precautions, should be inoculated into the appropriate bottles at the bedside and information about the media provided and the amount of blood to be placed in each bottle should be clearly indicated by the laboratory.

Endotoxin

Not all patients with septicaemia become shocked but when this is the outcome, gram-negative bacteria are responsible for two-thirds of cases and gram-positive bacteria for the remainder. As many as half of the patients with septicaemia due to aerobic gram-negative bacilli and one-third of those with *Bacteroides* species as the infecting organism develops shock (*Lancet*, 1963) whereas this complication occurs in only one patient out of ten suffering from septicaemia due to *Staphylococcus aureus*. When septicaemia is accompanied by shock the disturbance is attributed to endotoxin or other microbial products. Endotoxin is the lipopolysaccharide present in the cell walls of gram-negative bacteria and its toxic properties are believed to reside in the phospholipid part of the molecule – the so-called 'lipid A'. Endotoxin from the lumen of the intestinal tract is normally removed by the cells of the reticulo-endothelial system in the liver, but if this mechanism fails either because of an overwhelming endotoxaemia initiated from a septic focus (e.g., in faecal peritonitis) or liver failure (e.g., in hepatic cirrhosis) the uncleared endotoxin increases the permeability of the intestinal wall and mobilises more endotoxin from the intra-intestinal flora. In this way, endotoxaemia, once established, can become self-sustaining and so produce fatal shock (Fine, 1972).

It is possible to estimate the level of circulating endotoxin by employing the limulus lysate coagulation test. In this test, the patient's plasma is added to a lysate prepared from the disintegrated amoebocytes (blood cells) of *Limulus polyphemus* (the horse-shoe crab); endotoxin produces gel formation in the lysate. It is claimed to be an accurate, reproducible, specific and sensitive test with the ability to detect endotoxin in picogram amounts (Fossard et al., 1974). Despite its extreme sensitivity it has been recorded that patients apparently suffering from shock consequent upon gram-negative infection may have no evidence of circulating endotoxin as demonstrated by the limulus test (*British medical Journal*, 1974b).

There has been much speculation about the method whereby endotoxin produces its profound physiological effects in man and experimental animals. It has been noted that the effects of endotoxin are similar to those that can following antigen–antibody reactions in vivo and it has been postulated that there might be a common mediator. Many antigen–antibody reactions activate complement, an enzymatic system of serum proteins composed of nine components. The activated system utilises the components in the following sequence, C1, 4, 2, 3, 5, 6, 7, 8, 9, with the liberation of biologically active substances. Endotoxins are very efficient at activating the complement system both in vitro and in animals, and the complement consumption induced involves the latter part of the cascade C3–C9 with minimal utilisation of the components C1, 4 and 2. It is not known whether this phenomenon is the result of very efficient utilisation of the first components or to the triggering of the system via an alternative pathway starting at C3. Whatever the mechanism, pharmacologically active substances are generated which may be responsible for certain of the effects observed in septic shock, mainly changes in the clotting system, vascular permeability, smooth muscle reactivity and neutrophil chemotaxis. Confirmation that this mechanism may be of clinical importance has come from a study of patients with gram-negative septicaemia where it was shown that those with reduced levels of the third component of complement (C3) were more likely to become shocked than those patients with normal values (McCabe, 1973). However, apart from this report there has been no study on carefully diagnosed patients although there is much information on animal models and in vitro systems. It appears very likely that although not all the effects of endotoxin upon the host can be explained by complement system activation, endotoxin–complement interaction is of major importance in mediating certain host reactions to endotoxin in vivo.

Clinical Comments

The recommendations made in this section are largely based on experience arising from a detailed study of patients with septic shock over the past eight years in the Western Infirmary, Glasgow (Ledingham et al., 1974b; McArdle et al., 1975). The majority of the patients presented with some form of post-operative complication, frequently intra-abdominal sepsis, but other sources of infection were not uncommon and included gynaecological, urological and respiratory sepsis. Very few transplant or leukaemic patients are included although septicaemia and septic shock are recognised problems in these patients. During the early years of the study the mortality was high – 70–75% – particularly amongst patients with faecal peritonitis (Ledingham et al., 1974a).

Presenting features

Part of the problem of establishing the diagnosis of septic shock is the variety of ways in which this form of shock presents. The mode of presentation is influenced by the type of infection, by the nature of the underlying clinical condition and by the duration of shock. In the otherwise healthy patient the earliest features may be those of the so-called hyperdynamic stage of the syndrome in which although hypotension may be present, the peripheral tissues are warm and urine output may appear adequate. In many patients this stage may be transient or non-existent and the more classical features of hypovolaemic shock are present from the outset.

In a group of postoperative patients with septic shock (McArdle et al., 1975), the commonest features on initial referral were dehydration (associated with oliguria, uraemia and a high haematocrit), hypoxaemia, hyperventilation, non-respiratory acidosis and cardiac arrhythmias. The conscious level was variable. Less than one-third of these patients had warm extremities. An assessment was made of those factors which were considered to have most significantly contributed to death. The duration of shock was clearly important (more than one-third had been shocked for periods exceeding 12 hours). Elimination of sepsis was a fundamental aim of treatment and failure to achieve this aim either because of inadequate surgery or an inappropriate antibiotic regimen led to irreversible shock on a number of occasions. The onset of cardiac arrhythmias (most frequently atrial fibrillation) during the course of resuscitation carried a grave prognosis. Finally, an insidious process principally affecting the respiratory system was observed among some of the patients surviving the initial period of resuscitation.

During the early stages of septic shock arterial oxygen tension (PaO_2) is often normal but if PaO_2 begins to fall, especially if associated either with an increase in the work of breathing or in the arterial carbon dioxide tension ($PaCO_2$), death from respiratory failure is the usual outcome. In the post-operative situation this sequence of events is often attributed to primary respiratory infection. The more likely explanation is that there is some underlying vascular disturbance resulting from a combination of factors including left ventricular failure, increased pulmonary capillary pressure or permeability, and disseminated intravascular coagulation, all of which may be ascribed to the effects of either circulating endotoxin or a period of severe hypotension.

If treatment of septic shock is not prompt and adequate the result is failure to resuscitate or early recurrence of the shock state. Resuscitation in some patients, however, is protracted, and long-term complications are more frequent and refractory to treatment after septic shock than after hypovolaemic or haemorrhagic shock.

Treatment

Successful treatment of the shock syndrome demands a level of continuous monitoring found only rarely outside Intensive Therapy Units. In septic shock a mixture of underlying disturbances may be present. Thus the middle-aged patient with a ruptured colonic diverticulum who becomes shocked after surgical intervention may very well have evidence of frank dehydration and cardiac failure in addition to major sepsis.

The various haemodynamic and respiratory monitoring techniques used in the shock state have been described elsewhere in the monograph. Some of these may be regarded as essential, e.g., measurement of arterial blood pressure, central venous pressure, core and peripheral temperatures, fluid input and output, and blood gases, in addition to the usual electrocardiographic, biochemical, bacteriological and haematological measurements. Others of these techniques may not be regarded as essential but significantly improve understanding of the clinical condition and help to facilitate treatment e.g., cardiac output, pulmonary arterial pressures, colloid osmotic pressure (Da Luz et al., 1975) and various measurements of ventilation. From the practical point of view the extent and frequency of monitoring and measurement is determined largely by the need to achieve adequate and complete resuscitation in as short a time as possible. An important limiting factor in this connection is the number of available experienced personnel.

Fluid and electrolytes

Intravenous fluids are an essential primary component of treatment. Opinion varies as to the optimal fluid regimen but, in general, it is logical to begin with some form of colloid solution – plasma (hepatitis-screened), plasma protein fraction (PPF) or dextran-70 – adding crystalloid solutions after the first 1.5–2 litres. Thereafter the nature of the fluid administered will be determined by measurement of serum electrolytes, plasma proteins, plasma osmolality, colloid osmotic pressure and haematocrit. The amount of fluid required is generally considered to be that which will restore adequate peripheral perfusion and urine output; blood volume measurement has not proved very helpful in practice (Szabo, 1973). It is usual to give some whole blood or red cell suspension during resuscitation although a normal haematocrit need not be achieved for optimal perfusion (see chapter 12). If these general principles of fluid administration are pursued it will be found that cardiac output and central venous pressure is often considerably above normal, and the latter may contribute to the onset of pulmonary oedema which tends to develop during resuscitation unless the patient is being ventilated. Nevertheless, there is reasonable evidence that to settle for less than an adequate urine output is to increase the risk of late renal failure which is often an intractable complication in septic shock (Lucas et al., 1973). The intravenous administration of mannitol (not exceeding 60 g) may be of value in reducing the incidence of the renal complications but there is a growing awareness of the dangers of other diuretics e.g., frusemide, particularly if used in large doses and in combination with certain antibiotics e.g. cephaloridine.

It goes without saying that any acid-base abnormality should be corrected although the restoration of a normal blood pH may have little immediate effect on the haemodynamic and respiratory pattern. Electrolyte disturbances should also receive prompt attention after the acute fluid deficit has been corrected when the true extent of these disturbances will be more easily assessed. Hyperkalaemia is common in shock but hypokalaemia may rapidly occur if large volumes of intravenous fluids are administered. Such disturbances in serum potassium concentrations complicate resuscitation, especially in the presence of cardiac failure when digitalisation may be considered necessary. Hypocalcaemia is a common finding in major sepsis and in the past, intravenous calcium has been recommended with the aim of improving myocardial contractility. The changes in calcium balance in response to shock are, however, complex (Barry, 1971) and there is no real indication that calcium administration is of any value in this situation. Indeed exogenous calcium may be contra-indicated if, as seems likely, this ion is involved in the process of disseminated intravascular coagulation.

Oxygenation and ventilation

The beneficial effect of fluid repletion will be attenuated if hypoxaemia is present. Thus rapid restoration to normal of the oxygen capacity of the blood is imperative. In the first instance this aim may be achieved by an increase in the inspired oxygen concentration but, as explained previously, more often than not there will be a progressive deterioration in pulmonary gas exchange with a substantial increase in the work of breathing. Perhaps one of the more important recent advances in the treatment of septic shock has been the realisation of the importance of early intermittent positive pressure ventilation. In a group of 21 consecutive patients with septic shock (Milligan et al., 1974) 17 were subjected to intermittent positive pressure ventilation (IPPV). In 10 of these, the indications for ventilation were a steadily falling arterial oxygen tension with increasing hyperventilation; in 7, ventilation was instituted at a stage when the arterial oxygen tension was still adequate, that is, as an elective procedure. In the former category, the alveolar arterial oxygen tension gradient immediately prior to IPPV was 330 ± 21 mmHg; immediately after the start of IPPV it was 434 ± 44 mmHg, and the highest value after 12 hours of IPPV was 448 ± 53 mmHg. The average duration of continuous IPPV in this group was 8 ± 2 days. The corresponding data for the second group were 180 ± 21 mmHg, 207 ± 30 mmHg and 185 ± 34 mmHg. The average duration of continuous IPPV in this group was 7 ± 3 days. IPPV, therefore, prevents further deterioration of pulmonary gas exchange and, when instituted early, reduces the need for high concentrations of inspired oxygen. Positive end-expiratory pressure (10–15 cm of water) is of additional value in the treatment of the pulmonary complications of shock (Falke et al., 1972; Sugerman et al., 1972), but not all shocked patients require this sophistication and high end-expiratory pressure can cause a reduction in cardiac output and oxygen transport (Harken et al., 1974).

The association between the pulmonary and haematological disturbances of septic shock has given rise to the possibility of a cause and effect relationship. An example of this relationship is illustrated in Figure 1 and the following clinical history.

A 44 year old woman developed gram-negative septic shock as a result of faecal peritonitis. A sharp rise in alveolar arterial oxygen tension gradient during the first 24 hours coincided with a platelet count of less than 60,000 per cu.mm and elevation in the prothrombin and partial thromboplastin time. In association with elevated fibrinogen degradation products this haematological syndrome is recognised as being consistent with the diagnosis of disseminated intravascular coagulation. IPPV was commenced immediately prior to the maximum alveolar arterial oxygen tension gradient with a steady improvement thereafter. The haematological values deteriorated for 4 to 5 days, then improved spontaneously. The chest radiograph which was normal on the first day, showed evidence of pulmonary oedema which was at its worst on the third day at a stage when the arterial oxygen tension was already improving, but by the following day the changes were described as minimal.

In this case, which is characteristic of many general surgical septic shock patients, IPPV presumably acted to prevent the progression of pulmonary oedema until such time as the underlying process resolved spontaneously. Whether disseminated intravascular coagulation caused the lung lesion is uncer-

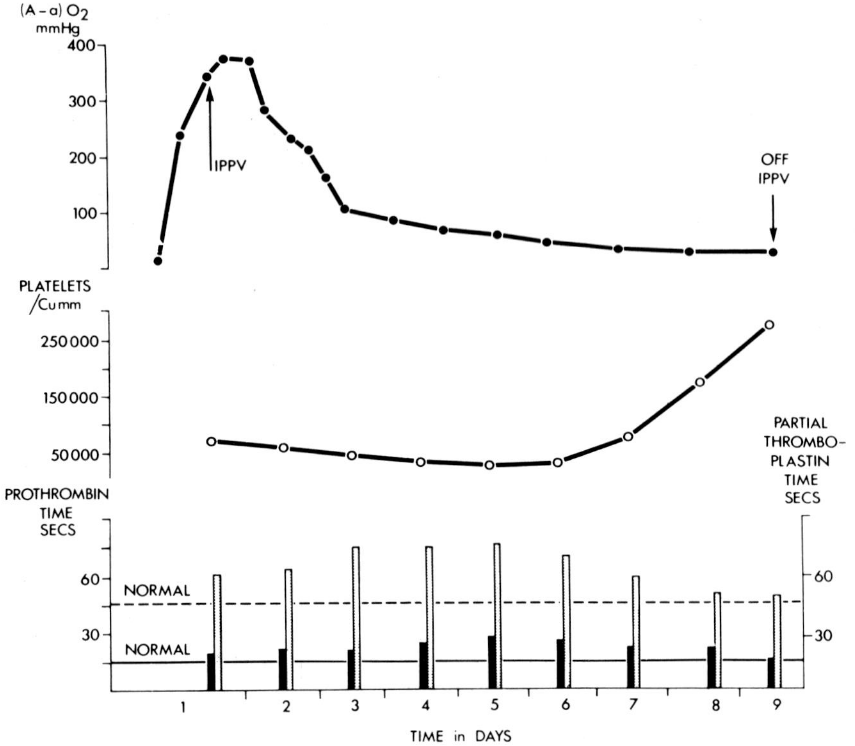

Fig. 1. Changes in alveolar arterial oxygen tension gradient and haematological data in a patient with gram-negative septic shock. Prothrombin time – closed columns; partial thromboplastin time – open columns.

tain but elsewhere in this monograph Olsson (p. 160) indicates that the pulmonary capillary vessels may be specifically susceptible to this condition. From a practical point of view, thrombocytopoenia appears to be related to the presence of endotoxaemia (Beller and Douglas, 1973) and is an important guide to clinical progress. Its persistence after 4–5 days suggests residual sepsis and augurs poorly for an early resumption of adequate spontaneous ventilation. Attemps to discontinue IPPV at this stage may be associated with the re-appearance of pulmonary oedema and experience indicates that it is better to await a progressive rise in the platelet count.

Antibiotics

There is no general agreement as to the best antibiotic combination in the treatment of septic shock. Therapy often requires to be started on a ‘best guess' basis before the bacteriological culture results and antibiotic sensitivity tests are available. The aminoglycoside antibiotic gentamicin is probably the current drug of choice in the treatment of life-threatening infections known to be due to or likely to be caused by aerobic gram-negative bacilli. Gentamicin is bactericidal against a wide range of these organisms including *Pseudomonas aeruginosa*, and the majority of strains of these organisms are inhibited by concentrations of the drug ranging from 0.25 to 4 μg/ml. Streptococci are much less sensitive and *Clostridium* and *Bacteroides* species are resistant. To ensure adequate treatment peak serum concentrations of 5–8 μg/ml should be attained. Resistant strains of normally sensitive species are rarely encountered and resistance to gentamicin is distinct from that of the earlier aminoglycosides. In normal dosage the drug is safe as long as renal function is good and ototoxicity, which usually involves the vestibular branch of the eighth cranial nerve, is almost always associated with renal failure. Toxicity, formerly thought to be related to high peak serum levels of between 12 and 15 μg/ml is now believed to be more closely associated with the maintenance of high trough serum levels. Nephrotoxicity is rare and is usually reversible. Whenever possible, treatment with gentamicin should be controlled by assay of the amount of drug in the patient's serum, not only to avoid possible toxicity but also to ensure that adequate therapeutic concentrations are being attained (Noone et al., 1974).

Other antibiotics employed in the treatment of serious infections with the aerobic gram-negative bacilli are the cephalosporins and carbenicillin. Gaya (1975) in a discussion of the treatment of serious, often septicaemic, infections in patients with acute leukaemia usually caused by gram-negative enteric organisms, recommended the use in combination of two out of three antibiotics, carbenicillin, cephalothin and gentamicin. Three regimens are possible and an international prospective comparative trial is in progress at present. The *Bacteroides* species are uniformly resistant to gentamicin and the other aminoglycosides and the cephalosporin antibiotics are rarely of value in the treatment of infections with these bacteria. Of the drugs mentioned so far, on the basis of in vitro testing only carbenicillin might be useful in the treatment of bacteroides infections and this drug has yet to be tried clinically (Phillips, 1974). Therefore, when treating patients with serious sepsis originating in the gastrointestinal or genital tracts, it is usual to widen the antibiotic spectrum of gentamicin by the addition of lincomycin since this combination will include the *Bacteroides* species, *Clostridium welchii* and some streptococci. Lincomycin is currently the antibiotic of choice for *Bacteroides* infection but the role of parenteral metronidazole requires to be investigated because this drug is the only agent so far identified that is consistently bactericidal in its action against these anaerobic gram-negative bacilli. The drug of choice for systemic candidiasis was formerly amphotericin B; 5-fluorocytosine is a recently introduced alternative which is certainly less toxic but perhaps also less effective.

A summary of the antibiotics mentioned above and their recommended doses is given in Table. I. The practice of giving an initial loading dose of antibiotic to ensure the rapid attainment of a therapeutic blood level is advocated.

Table I
Antibiotic dosage recommended for seriously ill patients.

Drug	Daily dose per kg of body weight	Average adult daily dose*
Gentamicin	5 mg	360 mg
Lincomycin	25 mg	1.8 g
Cephalothin	160 mg	12 g
Carbenicillin	400 mg	30 g
5-Fluorocytosine	200 mg	15 g

* Usually given 3 or 4 divided doses by the intravenous route.

Pharmacological agents

It is unlikely that the programme of treatment so far outlined would be challenged other than in detail. The same cannot be said for the use of pharmacological agents which continues to be a source of controversy. Part of the reason for this may be that, in the absence of sophisticated measurement techniques, precise evaluation of these drugs is difficult. There are four main categories of drugs used in septic shock:

1. Those with a primary effect on cardiac function e.g., digoxin and isoprenaline.

2. Those with a primary effect on tissue perfusion e.g., isoprenaline, dopamine and alpha-blocking agents.

3. Those with anti-coagulant effects e.g., heparin, fibrinolysin and epsilon-aminocaproic acid.

4. Those with multiple effects e.g., steroids and trasylol.

A detailed assessment of the effect of these various drugs is presented by others in this monograph. The following account merely highlights the views of the authors of this chapter with specific reference to septic shock.

1. Digitalisation at an early stage of resuscitation is justified on three main counts. Firstly, atrial fibrillation developing soon after the onset of shock is a common, and often rapidly fatal, complication. Even in the presence of sinus tachycardia, however, an increase in cardiac output frequently follows intravenous digoxin although the shorter acting compound ouabain may be required to produce a convincing demonstration of this effect. Finally there is experimental evidence that digitalisation at an early stage of endotoxin shock

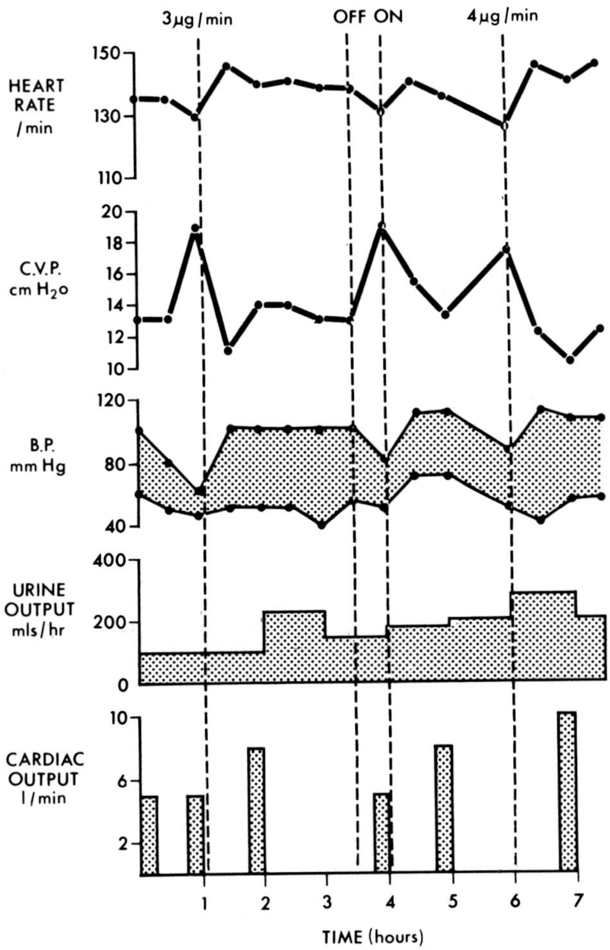

Fig. 2. The effect of isoprenaline infusion in a 26 year old female patient with gram-negative septic shock. Haemodynamic improvement followed initial administration of the drug, with deterioration when the drug was temporarily discontinued at 3.5 hours. Optimal dose was 4 μg/min.

maintains integrity of the myocardial cell although the mechanism of this action remains obscure (Coalson et al., 1972).

It is the practice of the Glasgow group to digitalise all patients suffering from septic shock with the occasional exception of the young, previously healthy individual who is not severely shocked and whose source of infection is known to have been eliminated. The usual precautions relating to the administration of this drug are observed, particularly in the presence of electrolyte disturbance or heart block, and dosage is reduced in the presence of renal failure. Blood levels are helpful if the results are rapidly available.

In the event of a poor response to digitalisation, isoprenaline by intravenous infusion will increase cardiac output and improve peripheral perfusion in most cases. The optimal dose of this drug is determined by continuous haemodynamic measurement (Fig. 2). After a few hours of stable haemodynamic measurement the drug should be discontinued under careful surveillance. Tachydysrhythmias are known to occur with isoprenaline but the patient suffering from septic shock does not appear to be unduly susceptible. Indeed it is not uncommon under these circumstances to note a fall in heart rate and elimination of dysrhythmias during the infusion of isoprenaline, presumably on the basis of increased stroke volume and improved coronary perfusion. When attempts are made to reduce heart rate using drugs which do not produce a simultaneous increase in stroke volume cardiac output falls precipitously. β-blocking drugs fall into this category and their use in isolation during resuscitation from septic shock seems ill-advised.

2. Although the main effect of isoprenaline is on the heart it also produces dilatation of some peripheral blood vessels (Winslow et al., 1973). Dopamine has been extensively investigated on the continent and in the U.S.A., and seems to have a definite beneficial influence on splanchnic perfusion during resuscitation. In the United Kingdom there is more experience of the α-blocking agents which may be short-, medium- or long-acting. An illustrative example of the effect of the medium-acting α-blocker thymoxamine is illustrated in Figure 3. There is no doubt that α-blocking drugs can rapidly improve skin perfusion and it is usual to find that as the peripheral blood vessels dilate there is a substantial increase in the requirement for intravenous fluid which produces a secondary improvement in cardiac output. It seems reasonable, during the initial stage of resuscitation, to concentrate on increasing the circulating blood volume and improving cardiac function but in a few instances when peripheral vasoconstriction persists, elimination of this effect with α-blocking drugs allows rapid return of haemodynamic stability.

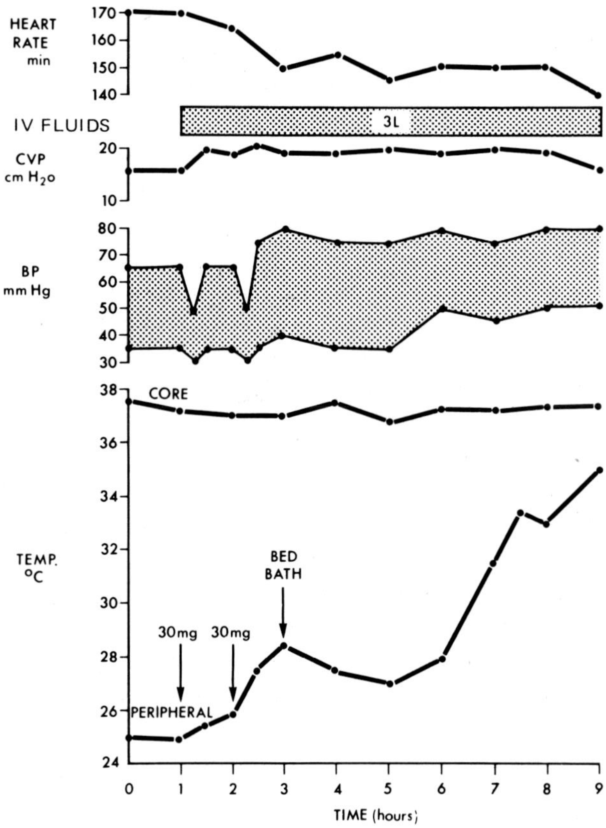

Fig. 3. The effect of thymoxamine by bolus injection in a 30 year old female patient with Bacteroides septic shock. Haemodynamic improvement followed two injections of the drug. Infusion of colloid was necessary to fill the dilated vascular compartment.

3. Corrigan and his colleagues (1968) suggested the use of heparin in patients with septicaemia and disseminated intravascular coagulation. In theory, heparin might ameliorate the severity of disseminated intravascular coagulation but in practice, its value is doubtful except possibly in some obstetric conditions in which low-dose heparin therapy is being evaluated (see chapter 10). The great majority of patients who manifest the haematological disturbances of disseminated intravascular coagulation improve spontaneously. Less than 10% of the general surgical patients with septic shock develop fibrinogen deficiency with the associated risk of frank bleeding. Even in these patients

the first priority should be the administration of fibrinogen, platelet concentrates and coagulation factors. Fibrinolysin is of no proved value and epsilon-aminocaproic acid is contra-indicated, since by blocking endogenous fibrinolysis, intravascular coagulation may proceed unchecked.

4. In spite of the fact that probably more has been written about corticosteroids than any other drug in the treatment of shock, uncertainty about their value remains. There is little doubt that if given to experimental animals coincident with or shortly after the administration of endotoxin, steroids will reduce subsequent mortality (Thomas and Brockman, 1968). This is attributed variously to haemodynamic and metabolic effects, the latter principally associated with membrane stabilisation (Wilson and Fisher, 1968; Schumer, 1969). Nevertheless, no convincing evidence of the value of steroids in a controlled trial in patients with septic shock has been published (Schumer and Nyhus, 1970). Indeed, in the Glasgow study, application of the previously outlined programme of treatment (which does not include corticosteroids) has been associated with a steady improvement in survival which now compares favourably with the best published data in equivalent groups of patients. This observation does not exclude the possibility that corticosteroids may be of some value in the treatment of the shock syndrome but more detailed and critical information is required before such drugs can be recommended for routine clinical use.

Ultimately, success in the treatment of septic shock depends on rapid elimination of the source of infection and resuscitation, particularly if protracted, should be interrupted at intervals to confirm that no residual sepsis remains. In this regard, the possibility should always be considered that systems used in monitoring and in treatment itself e.g., catheters and intravascular shunts, may perpetuate infection.

Mortality and Complications

Mortality amongst high risk patients in the Glasgow study has fallen to 38% during the past 18 months (Fig. 4). The pattern of mortality has also changed (Fig. 5). During the early period the major mortality occurred in the first 24 hours whereas now most patients survive the acute episode. Some die several days later of ill-defined complications, usually involving more than one organ. Invasion by organisms of low pathogenicity has already been

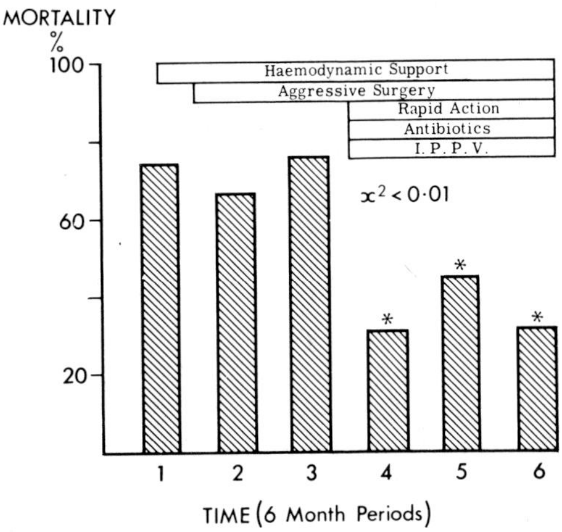

Fig. 4. Western Infirmary Shock Project: septic shock. Overall mortality.

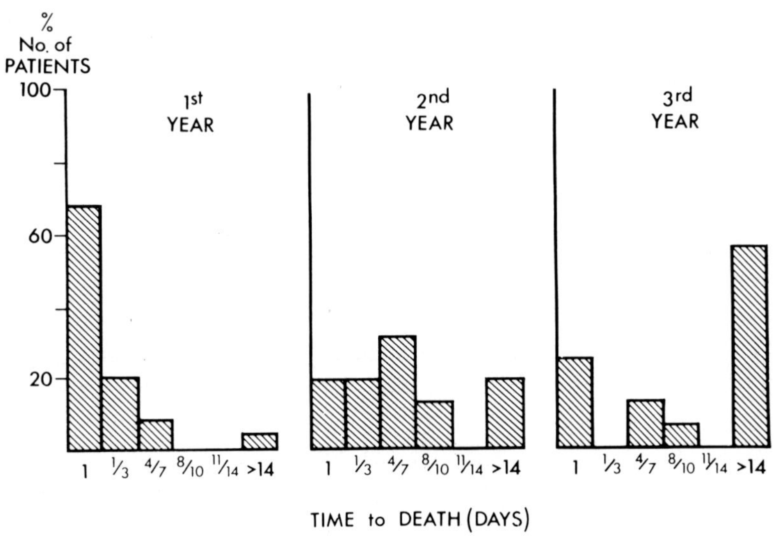

Fig. 5. Western Infirmary Shock Project: septic shock. Pattern of mortality.

described. Of the other complications two may be mentioned in more detail – gastrointestinal bleeding and late renal failure.

Gastrointestinal bleeding occurs only in a small proportion of patients with major sepsis but when it occurs is a source of major concern. The first essential is to identify the source of bleeding. A generalised bleeding diathesis should be excluded by careful haematological screening. In the absence of a haematological disturbance the most likely source of haemorrhage is acute erosive gastritis (Wangensteen and Golden, 1973). Other parts of the intestinal tract may also show diffuse haemorrhagic changes (Lucas et al., 1972) but erosions appear to be limited to the stomach and to the acid-producing mucosa in particular. There are many possible aetiological factors including mucosal ischaemia, acid hypersecretion, diminution of mucosal protective factors, back-diffusion of hydrogen ions with release of vasoactive amines, release of lysosomal enzymes, and sepsis. The incidence of acute erosive gastritis in patients with major sepsis is significantly higher when blood cultures are positive and healing of the gastric lesion has been observed to follow elimination of organisms from the blood stream (J.R. Le Gall, personal communication). Treatment remains uncertain and includes iced saline lavage of the stomach, neutralisation of gastric acid, selective perfusion of the coeliac axis with vasopressin (Athanasoulis et al., 1974), anticholinergic drugs and high doses of vitamin A. Analysis of various surgical manoeuvres suggests that vagotomy and partial gastrectomy carries the lowest incidence of rebleeding and overall mortality (Drapanas et al., 1971). Experience with total gastrectomy, although apparently even more satisfactory, is too limited for comment.

Like the other complications of septic shock late renal failure is likely to occur in those patients whose infections have proved difficult to eradicate. Dysfunction of other organs is often present but even when this is not the case initially, by the time several haemodialyses have been performed progressive cardio-respiratory failure is common (Fig. 6a, b). Haemodialysis in the presence of double or multiple organ failure, particularly if associated with continuing infection, is markedly less successful than when the kidney is the sole organ involved (Robson, 1975; Lewin and Maxwell, 1974). Moreover there is little to support the suggestion that earlier dialysis will significantly improve results. The reasons for these observations are not clear although several explanations may be advanced. Patients with protracted sepsis are often subjected to further surgical operations and given large doses of antibiotics some of which are known to be nephrotoxic, particularly when administered in combination with diuretics. On the other hand, late renal failure after septic shock may represent part of a widespread disruption of cell function for which there is at present no adequate therapy.

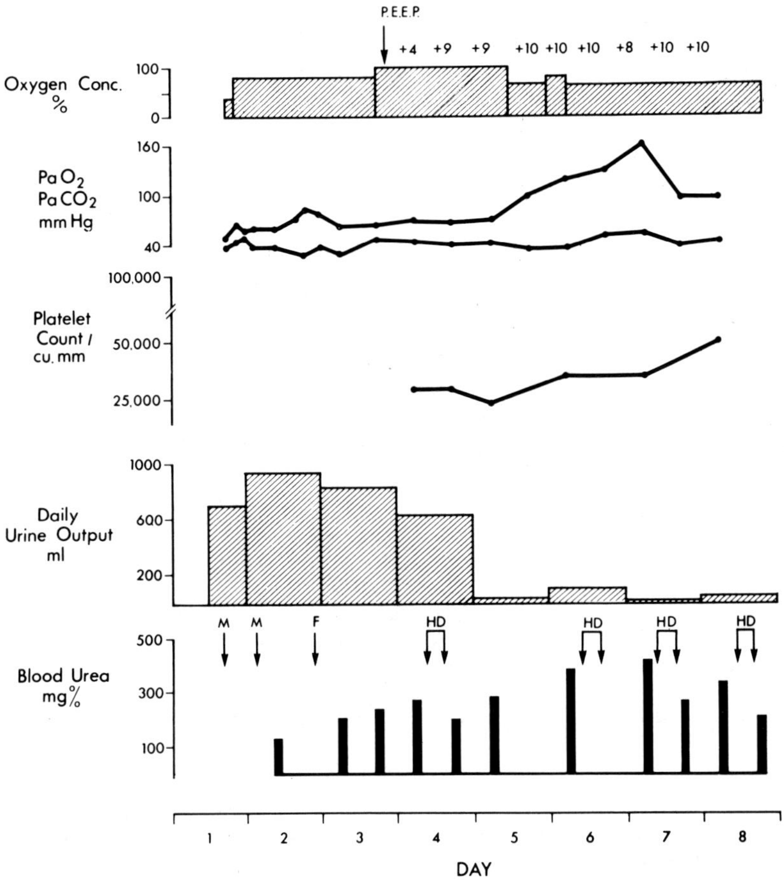

Fig. 6a. Respiratory, haematological and biochemical changes occurring during resuscitation in a 37 year old patient with gram-negative septic shock. M, mannitol; F, frusemide; HD, haemodialysis. Prolonged defective pulmonary and renal function in association with persistent thrombocytopoenia.

Future Developments

The high mortality amongst patients with major sepsis provides a continuous stimulus to the development of new therapeutic techniques. As yet most of those listed below remain confined to the research laboratory but some have begun to be assessed in clinical practice. The relative lack of success of con-

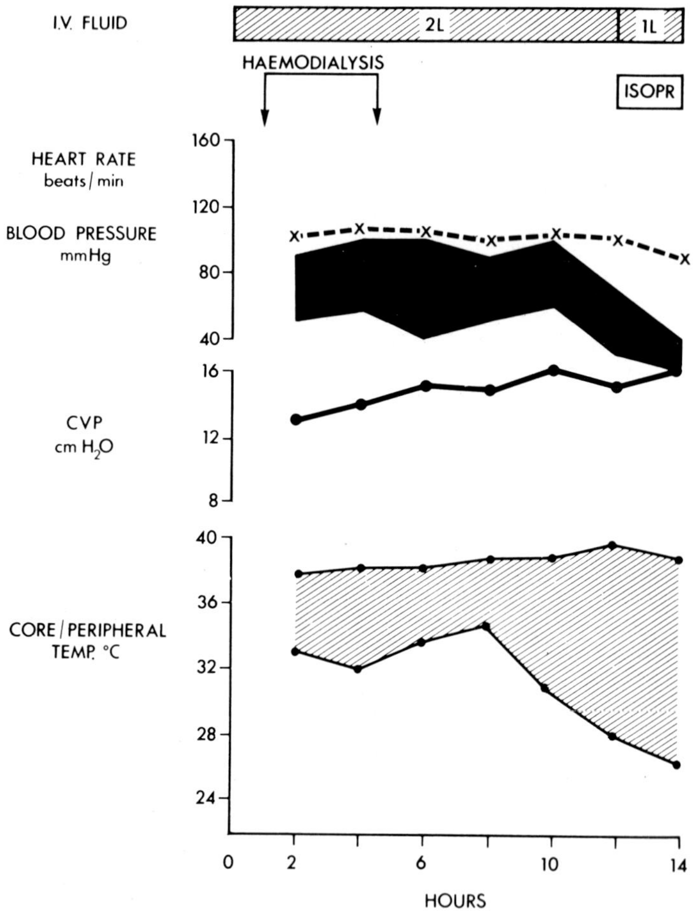

Fig. 6b. Terminal cardiac failure on day 9 in spite of isoprenaline infusion.

ventional therapy once the shock state has become established has prompted exploration of the possibility of inducing resistance to gram-negative bacteria (Cuevas et al., 1974) which might be useful as a prophylactic measure in high risk patients. From the same centre comes the concept of selective perfusion of the splanchnic circulation with corticosteroids and vasodilators in an attempt to minimise absorption of bacteria through ischaemic mucosa. A similar rationale underlies the use of continuous peritoneal lavage in the presence of faecal peritonitis. The frequency of heart failure in septic shock has led to an evaluation of cardiac assist devices, including intra-aortic balloon counter pulsation, more commonly used in other forms of cardiogenic shock (Grossman and Furman, 1971). Other new forms of treatment under investigation include fresh leucocyte transfusions to increase natural resistance to infection, and various pharmacological agents e.g., certain of the prostaglandin series and anti-inflammatory drugs, which are known to have effects on the microcirculation and on the coagulation mechanism (Raflo et al., 1973).

Summary

Septic shock continues to be a source of major clinical concern. Gram-negative bacteria are the principal organisms involved and, in spite of the availability of a wide selection of effective antibiotics, persistent sepsis remains the main cause of death. The precise mechanisms whereby bacteria produce shock are uncertain but the rapid institution of antibiotic therapy and elimination of the source of sepsis are first priorities in treatment. Resuscitation consists of the administration of intravenous fluids with correction of acid base and electrolyte disturbances. Oxygenation and ventilation have also proved to be important components of the treatment programme, particularly in preventing the lung lesion of shock. The use of pharmacological agents remains controversial but those whose action is directed towards sustaining cardiac function and improving regional perfusion appear to be of definite value.

References

Altemeier, W.A., Todd, J.C. and Inge, W.W. (1967): Gram-negative septicemia; a growing threat. *Ann. Surg., 166*, 530.

Association of Clinical Pathologists (1974): *Blood Culture Technique, Broadsheet 81*, published by Journal of Clinical Pathology, B.M.A. House, Tavistock Square, London.

Athanasoulis, C.A., Baum, S., Waltman, A.C., Ring, E.J., Imbembo, A. and Salm, T.J.V. (1974): Control of acute gastric mucosal hemorrhage: intraarterial infusion of posterior pituitary extract. *New Engl. J. Med., 290*, 597.

Barry, G.D. (1971): Plasma calcium concentration changes in hemorrhagic shock. *Amer. J. Physiol., 220*, 874.

Baue, A.E. (1969): The treatment of septic shock; a problem intensified by advancing science. *Surgery, 65*, 850.

Beller, F.K. and Douglas, G.W. (1973): Thrombocytopenia indicating gram-negative infection and endotoxemia. *Obstet. Gynec., 41*, 521.
Brit. med. J. (1974a): Septicaemia on the increase. *4*, 615.
Brit. med. J. (1974b): Endotoxaemia. *4*, 730.
Coalson, J.L., Woodruff, H.K., Greenfield, L.J., Guenter, C.A. and Hinshaw, L.B. (1972): Effects of digoxin on myocardial ultrastructure in endotoxin shock, *Surg. Gynec. Obstet., 135*, 908.
Corrigan, J.J., Ray, W.L. and May, N. (1968): Changes in the blood coagulation system associated with septicemia. *New Engl. J. Med., 279*, 851.
Crowley, N. (1970): Some Bacteraemias encountered in Hospital Practice. *J. clin. Path., 23*, 166.
Cuevas, P., Fine, J. and Monaco, A.P. (1974): Successful induction of increased resistance to gram negative bacteria and to endotoxin in immunosuppressed mice. *Amer. J. Surg., 127*, 460.
Da Luz, P.L., Shubin, H., Weil, M.H., Jacobson, E. and Stein, L. (1975): Pulmonary edema related to changes in colloid osmotic and pulmonary artery wedge pressure in patients after acute myocardial infarction. *Circulation, 51*, 350.
Drapanas, T., Woolverton, W.C., Reeder, J.W., Reed, R.L. and Weichert, R.F. (1971): Experiences with surgical management of acute gastric mucosal haemorrhage; a unified concept in the pathophysiology. *Ann. Surg., 173*, 628.
Falke, K.J., Pontoppidan, H., Kumar, A., Leith, D.E., Geffin, B. and Laver, M.B. (1972): Ventilation with end-expiratory pressure in acute lung disease. *J. clin. Invest., 51*, 2315.
Fine, J. (1972): Endotoxaemia in man. *Lancet, 2*, 181.
Fossard, D.P., Kakkar, V.V. and Elsey, P.A. (1974): Assessment of limulus test for detecting endotoxaemia. *Brit. med. J., 2*, 465.
Gaya, H. (1975): The treatment of infection in acute leukaemia. *Brit. J. Hosp. Med., 13*, 124.
Grossman, J.I. and Furman, S. (1971): Intra-aortic balloon augmentation during drug-induced myocardial depression. *Surgery, 70*, 304.
Harken, A.H., Brennan, M.F., Smith, B. and Barsamian, E.M. (1974): The hemodynamic response to positive end-expiratory ventilation in hypovolemic patients. *Surgery, 76*, 786.
Lancet (1963): Septic shock. *2*, 1265.
Lancet (1971): Epidemiology of Klebsiella infections. *2*, 416.
Lancet (1973): Bacteroides in the blood. *1*, 27.
Ledingham, I.McA., McArdle, C.S., Fisher, W.D. and Maddern, M. (1974a): The incidence of the shock syndrome in a general hospital. *Postgrad. med. J., 50*, 420.
Ledingham, I.McA., McArdle, C.S., Fisher, W.D., Maddern, M., MacDonald, J.A.E., Milligan, G.F., Mellon, A., Waddell, G., Scott, P.D.R. and Lees, N.W. (1974b): A prospective clinical study of septic shock. In: *Scientific Abstracts; First World Congress on Intensive Care*, p. 46. Editor: I.McA. Ledingham. Bell and Bain, Glasgow.
Lewin, A.J. and Maxwell, M.H. (1974): Acute renal failure: diagnostic and therapeutic criteria. *Crit. Care Med., 2*, 305.
Lucas, C.E., Rector, F.E., Werner, M. and Rosenberg, I.K. (1973): Altered renal homeostasis with acute sepsis: clinical significance. *Arch. Surg. (Chicago), 106*, 444.
Lucas, C.E., Sugawa, C., Friend, W. and Walt, A.J. (1972): Therapeutic implications of disturbed gastric physiology in patients with stress ulcerations. *Amer. J. Surg., 123*, 25.
McArdle, C.S., MacDonald, J.A.E. and Ledingham, I.McA. (1975): A three year retrospective analysis of septic shock in a general hospital. *Scot. med. J., 20*, 79.
McCabe, W.R. (1973): Serum complement levels in Bacteraemia due to gram-negative organisms. *New Engl. J. Med., 288*, 21.
Milligan, G.F., MacDonald, J.A.E., Mellon, A. and Ledingham, I.McA. (1974): Pulmonary and hematologic disturbances during septic shock. *Surg. Gynec. Obstet., 138*, 43.
Murdoch, J.C.McC., Speirs, C.F. and Pullen, H. (1968): The Bacteraemic shock syndrome. *Brit. J. Hosp. Med., 1*, 346.
Neely, W.A., Berry, D.W., Rushton, F.W. and Hardy, J.D. (1971): Septic shock: clinical, physiological and pathological survey of 244 patients. *Ann. Surg., 173*, 657.

Noone, P., Parsons, T.M.C., Pattison, J.R., Slack, R.C.B., Garfield-Davies, D. and Hughes, K. (1974): Experience in monitoring gentamicin therapy during treatment of serious gram-negative sepsis. *Brit. med. J., 1*, 477.

Phillips, I. (1974): *Antibiotic Sensitivity of Non-Sporing Anaerobes in Infection with Non-Sporing Anaerobic Bacteria*, p. 37. Editors: Phillips, I. and Sussman, M. Churchill, Livingstone.

Raflo, G.T., Wangensteen, S.L., Glenn, T.M. and Lefer, A.M. (1973): Mechanism of the protective effects of prostaglandin E_1 and $F_{2\alpha}$ in canine endotoxin shock. *Europ. J. Pharmacol., 24*, 86.

Robson, J.S. (1975): Acute renal failure. In: *Intensive Care*, p. 144. Editors: Walker, W.F. and Taylor, D.E.M. Churchill, Livingstone, Edinburgh, London and New York.

Schumer, W. (1969): Physiochemical effect of dexamethasone on the primate in oligemic shock. *Arch. Surg. (Chicago), 98*, 259.

Schumer, W. and Nyhus, L.M. (1970): *Corticosteroids in the Treatment of Shock*. University of Illinois Press, Urbana, Chicago, London.

Sugerman, H.J., Olofsson, K.B., Pollock, T.W., Agnew, R.F., Rogers, R.M. and Miller, L.D. (1972): Continuous positive end-expiratory pressure ventilation (PEEP) for the treatment of diffuse interstitial pulmonary edema. *J. Trauma, 12*, 263.

Szabo, G. (1973): Measurement of circulating blood volume and circulation time. In: *Traumatic Shock*, p. 26. Editors: Szántó, G., Hönig, V. and Székely, O. Akadémiai Kiadó, Budapest.

Thomas, C.S. and Brockman, S.K. (1968): The role of adrenal corticosteroid therapy in Escherichia coli endotoxin shock. *Surg. Gynec. Obstet., 126*, 61.

Wangensteen, S.L. and Golden, G.T. (1973): Acute 'stress' ulcers of the stomach: a review. *Amer. Surg., 39*, 562.

Wilson, R.F. and Fisher, R.R. (1968): Hemodynamic effects of massive steroids in clinical shock. *Surg. Gynec. Obstet., 127*, 769.

Winslow, E.J., Loeb, H.S., Rahimtoola, S.H., Kamath, S. and Gunnar, R.M. (1973): Hemodynamic studies and results of therapy in 50 patients with bacteremic shock. *Amer. J. Med., 54*, 421.

Ledingham (ed.). Shock

The role of the anaesthetist in shock

J.G. MONE

Introduction

Shock is difficult to define though the clinical recognition of this condition is frequently easy. A good working definition is that of McLaughlin et al. (1969) who regard it as a state of tissue underperfusion with cellular hypoxia. Hypoxia of all tissues occurs and this has led to the current concept that shock is associated with multiple organ failure. Shock is usually, but not always, accompanied by arterial hypotension. Compensatory circulatory reflexes tend to divert blood from the peripheral tissues to the vital organs. This results in the well recognised picture of a pale cold, hypotensive patient with a rapid thready pulse of low volume. Sweating due to excessive catecholamine production may be present and metabolic acidosis may lead to disturbances of respiratory rhythm.

Preoperative Assessment

A knowledge of the pathophysiology of the shock state will allow the anaesthetist to assess patients for anaesthesia and surgery. His appreciation of the situation will be aided by consideration of the following signs, symptoms and measurements.

Conscious level. The occurrence of coma in shocked patients in the absence of cerebral trauma is a grave sign.

Pulse. Volume is a better guide to cardiac output than is heart rate. Low pulse pressure and a tachycardia usually co-exist. Arrhythmias are common especially in elderly patients.

Arterial blood pressure. In a previously healthy patient the acute loss of 20% or more of the circulating blood volume is necessary to produce hypotension (Hayes et al., 1973), i.e. before the systolic pressure falls below 100 mmHg. Arterial pressure is thus not a sensitive guide to the severity of shock. At low blood pressure levels, measurements utilising sphygomomanometer cuffs are inaccurate and direct intra-arterial recordings are invaluable though it is realised that often this method is not available.

Central venous pressure (CVP) is measured in centimetres of water by a catheter whose tip is placed in the superior vena cava or right atrium. As changes of 10% in circulating volume may be reflected in alteration in CVP readings, they are thus a more sensitive guide to hypovolaemia than is arterial pressure. Absolute measurements should be considered with caution and never in isolation from other parameters. In the acute treatment of hypovolaemic states the response of CVP measurements to fluid loads is a good guide to adequacy of fluid replacement, especially in conjunction with the clinical response of the patient as judged by adequate perfusion, satisfactory urinary output and arterial pressure. Central venous pressure is a dynamic measurement and does not directly correspond to measurement of blood volume. Less importance can be attached to high readings because of the many factors involved, e.g. cardiac failure and sympathetic venous tone.

The detailed physiological basis of central venous pressure measurements is fully discussed on pages 258 and 259 of this monograph. The technique has been well reviewed by Defalque (1968, 1974), English et al. (1969), Mostert et al. (1970) and Latimer (1971). Our own preference is for the percutaneous cannulation of the median basilic vein, external jugular vein or internal jugular vein utilising the Argyle Intramedicut System. The median basilic vein of either arm may be used. In adults 70 cm 14 or 16 guage catheters are favoured. If the external jugular vein is well filled it may be cannulated with a 14 or 16 guage 30 cm catheter. However, the success rate for the catheter to pass into the superior vena cava is not as high as when the internal jugular vein is utilised. The internal jugular vein is approached essentially as described by English et al. (1969), though this is modified in that a higher point of entry in the neck is selected, which obviates the risk of pneumothorax.

The position of the radio opaque catheter is always checked by chest radiograph. Johnson and Clark (1972) found that despite fluctuations in venous pressure with respiration only 64% of their central venous catheters were in an acceptable position radiologically. Kellner and Smart (1972) have shown that respiratory fluctuations do not necessarily indicate central positioning of the catheter. Despite the theoretical considerations external jugular venous pressure measurements may be clinically acceptable in many cases.

Urine flow. This is an excellent guide to perfusion. A urinary catheter should be inserted in all cases of severe shock and hourly measurements recorded. The secretion of 50–60 ml of urine hourly is indicative of adequate perfusion and therapy is aimed at achieving this.

Fluid losses. Assessments of fluid deficits are frequently only guesses though various workers have suggested that blood loss can be estimated in trauma according to the amount of tissue damaged (Grant and Reeve, 1951) or by measurement of the swelling in closed injuries (Clarke et al., 1955). The measurement of blood volume using radioactive tracers for plasma and red cells would appear to be an ideal method of calculating blood loss but difficulties occur in the presence of active bleeding or where the circulation is unstable (Vickers, 1969). In the clinical management of shocked patients, fluid deficits are corrected on an empirical basis by giving sufficient volume to improve the patient's condition as judged by satisfactory perfusion, CVP, arterial pressure, heart rate and urinary flow.

Temperature. Both core (rectal or oesophageal) and skin temperature should be recorded at frequent intervals. Central temperature may be low, normal or elevated. Haemorrhagic shock may be associated with hypothermia which may be worsened if infusion fluids are not warmed. Septic shock presents usually with an elevated temperature though in severe sepsis the temperature may be sub-normal. Skin temperature measured at the great toe is a helpful prognostic sign. Joly and Weil (1969) have shown that in the absence of acute arterial block the great toe skin temperature is an indirect measure of systemic flow. We now monitor routinely the core/peripheral temperature gradient and in conjunction with other measurements find it a good guide to adequacy of treatment.

Ventilation. Respiratory disturbances in shock are common and hypoxaemia is always present in severe shock. The measurement of blood gases are mandatory. Metabolic acidosis may be profound and require correction. The $PaCO_2$ is usually normal or low in the initial stages and the finding of a high $PaCO_2$ unexplained on the grounds of excessive sedation carries a poor prognosis. Wilson and Krome (1969) found that the acid base balance gave a good overall measure of the severity of the shock state.

Detailed analysis of the respiratory measurements in shock appears on page 111.

Laboratory investigations may help in the preoperative assessment of the shocked patient.

Serum electrolyte values may be normal in the presence of considerable loss of isotonic fluid, although losses from the proximal section of the small bowel may show a grossly abnormal electrolyte pattern. A high level of blood urea may indicate dehydration if it is known that prior to admission the blood urea was normal. Serum creatinine will give some indication of renal status. Serum calcium may be low in septic shock, pancreatitis or hypothermia.

Serum potassium may be elevated in acute renal failure associated with shock or depressed where there has been excessive loss from the high small bowel. Abnormalities of serum potassium levels may affect the action of muscle relaxants.

Serial haematocrit estimations are easily performed and are useful in the management of hypovolaemic shock.

The bacteriological examination of infected material is mandatory in septic shock. Blood cultures should be taken as soon as the diagnosis is considered. Until the appropriate antibiotic is identified, selection is made on a 'best guess' basis, e.g. gentamicin and lincomycin for peritonitis. Numerous other more sophisticated measurements can be made in shock such as cardiac output, pulmonary artery pressure etc., and though desirable are not essential to the assessment and management of the patient.

Resuscitation

The resuscitation of the shocked patient is obligatory before anaesthesia and surgery to correct hypoxaemia and oligaemia. The exception to this is the occasional massive haemorrhage as from a ruptured abdominal aneurysm where delay may lead to death. The dangers of anaesthesia in shock are proportional to the degree of oligaemia. Dinnick (1964) thought that the inadequate recognition of oligaemia contributed to the deaths in more than half of the 400 deaths he reviewed.

The therapeutic crescendo in shock therapy involves the following measures:

1. Rapid intravenous infusion of the appropriate fluid – blood, plasma, colloid and crystalloid.

The most important single measure in the treatment of oligaemic shock is the rapid correction of the fluid deficit. In this respect it should be noted that a) adequate volume is more important than the type of fluid administered, b) the volume of fluid required frequently exceeds estimated fluid losses, and that an adequate volume to achieve haemodynamic stability will often be greater than the calculated normal blood volume.

Obviously the fluid transfused should be appropriate to the loss sustained e.g. blood in haemorrhagic shock, and plasma in addition to crystalloid in many acute abdominal conditions.

It is important that when transfusing large volumes of cold stored blood to avoid precipitating hypothermia, simple blood warmers are readily available and should be used whenever more than two litres of blood are given over a short period of time.

2. Oxygen therapy: by mask, endotracheal tube or positive pressure ventilation.
3. Cardiac support by the use of digoxin and isoprenaline.
4. The use of α-blocking drugs: phentolamine, phenoxybenzamine, and thymoxamine.
5. Antibiotics: to combat sepsis where indicated.
6. The correction of acidosis by 8.4% sodium bicarbonate where indicated, although the hyperosmolarity of this solution is leading to the use of 4.2% or even weaker solutions.
7. Surgery: to combat haemorrhage or sepsis.
8. The use of other drugs is controversial and arguments for and against their use are developed elsewhere in this monograph. Such drugs include:

   Steroids
   Vasoactive agents.

Anaesthesia and Shock – Review of Methods and Agents

Since most anaesthetic agents are myocardial depressants or peripheral vasodilators, ideally anaesthesia should not be undertaken until hypovolaemia has been corrected. On occasions delay may prove fatal – as in a ruptured abdominal aneurysm when immediate surgery is the only life saving measure.

The claims of immediate surgery and the dangers of anaesthesia in a partially resuscitated, shocked patient have to be reconciled on the basis of priorities. In the absence of torrential bleeding there is time for rapid correction of hypovolaemia with blood, plasma or crystalloids. Once the circulation has stabilised further delay is unnecessary. It has been estimated that if the systolic arterial pressure is 100 mmHg systolic then the blood volume is approximately 70% of normal – though it must be remembered that circulating volume in shock may have to be considerably increased to achieve haemodynamic stability (MacLean, 1966).

When the patient becomes warm, exhibits stable readings of blood pressure, central venous pressure, and heart rate, and secretes 50–60 ml of urine hourly, then definitive surgery should be undertaken.

There is no ideal anaesthetic for the shocked patient.

All anaesthetic agents administered to a hypovolaemic patient will produce further hypotension to a greater or lesser extent. Thus it is imperative to err on the side of overtransfusion in preparation for anaesthesia.

Acupuncture: the use of acupuncture in 50 cases of shock with a success rate of 86% has been described (*Chinese medical Journal*, 1973). In cases of massive haemorrhage speedy administration of blood and fluid is recommended. Needling on the nose yielded sufficient muscular relaxation for lower abdominal operations and combined with subcutaneous stimulation elsewhere produced adequate analgesia for skin incision. Obviously no opinion on the efficacy of acupuncture in shock can be given on the basis of this article, but the Chinese approach is of interest. No full English translation of the text is available.

Spinal and epidural blocks are contraindicated in the shocked patient. Kennedy et al. (1968) investigated the cardiovascular and respiratory effects of subarachnoid block during acute blood loss induced in normal human volunteers upon whom no surgical procedures were being performed. Significant reductions in mean arterial pressure, cardiac output, stroke volume and central venous pressure were found. The authors concluded that subarachnoid block should be used with caution in the presence of acute untreated blood loss. They emphasised that in this trial the subjects were young healthy volunteers and that patients in poor physical states might not have compensated as effectively.

If general anaesthesia is to be undertaken in hypovolaemic patients there are two cardinal rules:

1. Adequate oxygen must be given.
2. Minimal doses of anaesthetic agents are sufficient.

Inhalational Induction Agents

Cyclopropane is a suitable agent for the shocked patient as it produces less hypotension than many other agents. Additionally it is rapid in action and may be used with high concentrations of oxygen. It is recommended by Horsey (1968).

Ether is the only volatile agent which produces sympathetic stimulation, but for induction of anaesthesia its action is somewhat slow and irritant.

Both these agents produce explosive mixtures in combination with oxygen so that diathermy cannot be used, though this may be a small price to pay if they are regarded as the agents of choice in any situation.

Halothane. This is probably the most widely used volatile agent in general use under normal circumstances and much has been written regarding its suitability and unsuitability in hypovolaemia. Wolfson (1966) considers that because of its marked hypotensive actions, halothane is contraindicated in hypovolaemia.

Weaver (1971) has studied the effects of 0.75% and 2.5% halothane in haemorrhagic shock in dogs anaesthetised with nitrous oxide and oxygen (2 : 1). The following results were noted:

a) With nitrous oxide and oxygen alone the dogs showed a typical response to haemorrhage, the blood pressure being reasonably maintained with blood losses of 30% of blood volume. With further haemorrhage the blood pressure decreased rapidly and one dog died of ventricular fibrillation.

b) With 0.75% halothane anaesthesia, reductions in cardiac output and blood pressure occurred on bleeding, but recovery occurred on retransfusion.

c) With 2.5% halothane the dogs were deeply depressed initially and bleeding produced no further reductions in blood pressure or cardiac output. There was no significant change in blood pressure throughout bleeding and retransfusion.

Weaver concluded that there might be advantages in light halothane anaesthesia in hypovolaemic shock and suggested that this should be studied further. Deep halothane anaesthesia is contraindicated. He found that the myocardial activity in humans suffered the same degree of depression as the canine heart.

Shimosato and his colleagues (1963) studied ventricular function during halothane anaesthesia in the dog and concluded that the mechanical efficiency of the heart was not altered. The ventricles operated at different functional levels during various concentrations of halothane anaesthesia in the presence of a decrease in myocardial contractility.

Despite the theoretical disadvantages of halothane in hypovolaemia we have used it as an inhalational induction agent usually with 100% oxygen or with at least 50% oxygen and nitrous oxide for the hypovolaemic patient. It must be stressed that only small concentrations are necessary to produce sleep and following intubation with a muscle relaxant, usually suxamethonium, halothane is discontinued and anaesthesia is maintained by controlled ventilation using nitrous oxide, oxygen and pancuronium.

An inhalational induction is particularly applicable to the elderly shocked patient in whom it might be difficult to judge an adequate small dose of sodium thiopentone. It provides a rapid smooth induction and is non-irritant to the respiratory passages.

Methoxyflurane. Though a potent anaesthetic agent, induction with this agent is slow as a result of its low volatility. We have no experience of its use in shock as an induction agent, but it would not appear to be particularly indicated.

Trichlorethylene is a good analgesic but a slow induction agent. Though perhaps useful for maintenance of anaesthesia it is not suitable for induction.

In summary, the best agents for inhalational induction are cyclopropane or halothane used with high concentrations of oxygen. Cyclopropane produces a more rapid induction but halothane is probably more familiar to the majority of anaesthetists. The latter is the personal choice of the author where an inhalational induction is indicated.

Nitrous oxide and oxygen. A 50/50 mixture of nitrous oxide and oxygen has been shown by Thornton and his associates (1973) to cause a fall in cardiac output of about 12% and a rise in peripheral resistance. These changes were attributed to the oxygen in the mixture as they occurred when nitrogen was used in place of nitrous oxide. This is a theoretical disadvantage to the use of such a mixture in hypovolaemic shock and the use of 100% oxygen might cause an even greater fall. Despite these considerations the use of oxygen with cyclopropane or halothane is a most valuable clinical technique.

Intravenous Induction Agents

Sodium thiopentone (Pentothal) is theoretically inferior to methohexitone (Brietal) and hexobarbitone (Evipan) as it causes a greater degree of myocardial depression and hypotension. Sodium thiopentone is much more widely used and thus more familiar to anaesthetists and has stood the test of time in clinical practice. In hypovolaemic shock it should be used in dilute form (not greater than 2.5%) and with great caution as an overdose may be lethal.

In hypovolaemia it should be given slowly and in small increments remembering that a slow circulation time is present. Some experienced anaesthetists estimate the dose and give this as a bolus injection followed by a rapidly acting muscle relaxant for intubation. This so called 'crash induction' requires nice judgement and can be disastrous if the dosage is wrongly estimated. It is not to be recommended particularly in the elderly shocked patient. In general 100 mg or less of sodium thiopentone may be sufficient for induction.

Althesin. The cardiovascular depressant effects of this recently introduced induction agent are similar to those of methohexitone and thiopentone (Savege et al., 1972) and it would appear to offer no advantages in the shocked patient.

Ketamine. An induction dose of ketamine 2 mg/kg produced a marked increase in blood pressure, heart rate, central venous pressure, stroke volume and cardiac output and a small rise in total peripheral resistance in fit unpremedicated patients as described by Savege et al. (1973) though a subsequent dose resulted in only a small increase in blood pressure and a decrease in all the other four variables.

Chasapekis et al. (1973) recommended the use of ketamine intravenously in doses of 2 mg/kg as an induction agent regardless of the degree of shock. They postulated that arterial pressure was increased by a) stimulatory reflex action on the heart though the mechanism was not clear; b) inhibition of baroreceptor activity. In contrast to Savege et al. they considered that peripheral vascular resistance was unchanged or diminished.

Bond and Davies (1974) recommended its use as an induction agent in hypovolaemic shock in doses of 1–3 mg/kg and recorded that in 4 cases the arterial pressure either increased or remained the same. The author of this review has used ketamine 2 mg/kg in hypovolaemic shock for several years and has found it a satisfactory induction agent, though in severe shock the rise in blood pressure was not marked. Chasapekis et al. (1973) and Bond and Davies (1974) recommend the combination of ketamine and pancuronium.

Relaxants

Pancuronium is the drug of choice as it is associated with an increase in arterial pressure and cardiac output in the normal patient (Coleman et al., 1972). In hypovolaemia this increase in arterial pressure may not occur though Chasapekis et al. (1973) found an average increase of 30 mmHg systolic in 13 patients when used with ketamine, and assumed that as peripheral resistance did not rise this change was the result of an increased cardiac output. They concluded that this would produce an increase in tissue perfusion. The anaesthetic sequence recommended was premedication intravenously with

0.5 mg atropine despite the presence of a tachycardia in order to reduce the secretions induced by ketamine and suxamethonium. Ketamine 2 mg/kg was followed by suxamethonium to facilitate intubation and continued relaxation was provided by the use of pancuronium 4 mg. Ventilation was controlled in all patients.

Anaesthesia was supplemented when necessary with small doses of pethidene or 0.3–0.5% halothane.

In patients who were less severely shocked, pethidine 50 mg was used intravenously as premedication 30 minutes prior to induction.

Tubocurarine should be used with caution as its ganglion blocking action will accentuate hypotension. When hypovolaemia is corrected preoperatively with adequate intravenous fluids ganglion blockade might increase tissue perfusion despite the fall in arterial pressure. In acute uncorrected hypovolaemia its use should be avoided.

Suxamethonium. This rapidly acting relaxant is recommended for rapid intubation as the shocked patient should always be considered to be at risk from a 'full stomach' whether or not a stomach tube has been passed. The theoretical dangers of causing increased intraabdominal pressure by abdominal muscle fasciculation leading to regurgitation has probably been exaggerated (Smith, G., 1974, personal communication). It is important to use an adequate dose and it is our custom to give 100 mg intravenously to ensure relaxation.

Gallamine is a relaxant which is less frequently used following the introduction of pancuronium. It causes a tachycardia and its elimination mainly by the renal route would be disadvantageous if the patient had acute renal failure.

In summary on the basis of pharmacological considerations the combination of ketamine and pancuronium would appear to be appropriate for anaesthesia in the shocked patient. Despite the theoretical disadvantages the sequence of sodium thiopentone, suxamethonium and pancuronium or tubocurarine has been used successfully for many years and is the technique preferred by many experienced anaesthetists.

Hazards of General Anaesthesia

The two main dangers are 1) rapid haemodynamic decompensation, and 2) vomiting and regurgitation.

The dangers of oligaemia and anaesthesia have been discussed and the need to correct hypovolaemia by intravenous infusions is obvious.

Vomiting and regurgitation in a shocked patient may be lethal. Anaesthesia removes or diminishes certain protective reflexes, but it is not always appreciated that aspiration into the lungs may occur in a feeble shocked patient even when conscious.

If possible a stomach tube should be passed before induction to remove stomach contents. It should be realised that not all the contents will be removed, but the head of pressure will be relieved.

Vomiting is an active process which may occur during an inhalational induction especially if the patient becomes excited. Regurgitation is a passive process and occurs more readily in the presence of an open or incompetent cardiac sphincter and may occur during an intravenous/relaxant sequence if respiratory obstruction and inadequate relaxation occurs. It is our practice to remove the gastric tube when using an intravenous induction as it is thought that the presence of the gastric tube makes the cardiac sphincter incompetent. Others however insist on leaving the gastric tube in situ ensuring that it is patent to allow the escape of fluid stomach contents during induction.

All shocked patients should be intubated for anaesthetic purposes. If it is thought that the induction of anaesthesia is too hazardous, awake intubation under local analgesia may be practised. By obtunding the reflexes local analgesia may allow aspiration of stomach contents and is thus not without danger.

Aspiration of stomach contents can be minimised by:

1. the use of gravity. A left lateral position with slight head down tilt will encourage contents to flow away from the respiratory passages;
2. the use of cricoid pressure (Sellick, 1961);
3. the avoidance of manual inflation with a mask while waiting for flaccidity to occur following the injection of the muscle relaxant.

Summary of Practical Anaesthetic Procedure

There is no ideal technique nor agent for anaesthetising a shocked patient. Much depends on the skill and preference of the individual anaesthetist. After the patient has been resuscitated as far as is possible the following points should be observed.

1. Premedication with an opiate is to be avoided, especially in the more severe cases.
2. 100% oxygen should be administered for at least 3 minutes prior to induction

to build up an oxygen reserve and so provide a margin of safety when unconsciousness occurs.
3. Induction of anaesthesia should only be performed on a tilting trolley or table.
4. An efficient suction apparatus is immediately to hand.
5. An intravenous infusion is running freely.
6. A competent assistant is available to apply cricoid pressure.
7. All equipment (laryngoscope, endotracheal tube) has been checked.

Intravenous induction

0.6 mg atropine is given intravenously immediately prior to induction though this may be omitted in the presence of a marked tachycardia. The following two regimens are commonly used:
a) Ketamine 2 mg/kg is injected intravenously and when unconsciousness occurs suxamethonium 70–100 mg is given. No inflation takes place. Cricoid pressure is applied at the direction of the anaesthetist and rapid intubation with a cuffed oral tracheal tube takes place. Nitrous oxide and oxygen 50:50 mixture is used for maintenance. When breathing is re-established pancuronium is used for more prolonged relaxation and to allow ventilation to be controlled.
b) Sodium thiopentone (suitably diluted) in a dose of approximately 100 mg is given intravenously at a slow rate of injection, followed by suxamethonium and pancuronium as described above. If preferred, tubocurarine may be used instead of pancuronium.

Inhalational induction

Cyclopropane or halothane with oxygen concentrations varying from 50% to 100% are used followed by suxamethonium and intubation. In severely shocked patients the use of suxamethonium may not be necessary though once intubation has been carried out pancuronium is used for maintenance.

Supplemental doses of analgesic to augment nitrous oxide and oxygen may be necessary and morphine 1–2 mg or fentanyl 0.05 mg may be given intravenously if required. Concentrations of nitrous oxide varying from 30% to 70% are used depending on the degree of shock. In moribund cases 100% oxygen may be required.

It is our practice to paralyse and ventilate all patients in hypovolaemic shock who require anaesthesia.

We are not especially concerned if the reversal of relaxants at the end of anaesthesia presents any difficulty as the majority of our severely shocked patients are ventilated electively for at least the first 24 hours postoperatively. Shocked patients who respond quickly to resuscitation and surgery are reversed easily in the normal way and are not necessarily ventilated in the post-operative phase. This group usually include the previously fit younger patients. It is our experience that elderly shocked patients and those suffering from septic shock invariably benefit from elective postoperative ventilation.

McAslan and Cowley (1974) reported that in order to prevent shock lung they electively ventilated more than 1000 patients admitted with major trauma. All patients requiring more than 20% blood volume replacement were immediately intubated and ventilated using positive and expiratory pressure (PEEP). In a series of 258 patients reported the mortality due to respiratory failure was only 0.4%. Respiratory insufficiency is a frequent complication of major trauma and in its most severe form, frequently termed the 'shock lung' syndrome, is associated with a mortality of 60%.

Intraoperative Shock Arising de Novo

The anaesthetist may be confronted with a shocked patient in the course of local, regional or general anaesthesia.

Local: absolute or relative overdosage of any local anaesthetic agent may result in hypotension which on occasions may become profound and may be accompanied by other clinical features of shock. This should be treated by the administration of oxygen, intravenous fluids and respiratory support if indicated.

Both spinal anaesthetics and massive epidurals may result in apnoea combined with profound hypotension. This should not present any problems if immediate intubation, controlled ventilation with supplemental oxygen, and the rapid infusion of fluids is expeditiously carried out. The use of vasopressors in this situation may be appropriate to counteract the extreme degree of vasodilatation.

Shock may occur at any stage during general anaesthesia. During induction, overdose of an induction agent or true anaphylaxis may result in marked hypotension, tachycardia and perhaps apnoea. The usual supportive measures for the cardiovascular and respiratory systems are indicated. During induction the onset of shock may be associated with the aspiration of a large volume of fluid stomach contents into the lung. Even a small volume of highly acid fluid may cause collapse though typically the onset is described as being delayed.

The stage at which sudden collapse occurs may be helpful in diagnosing the cause. Thus amniotic fluid embolism occurs typically in the second stage of labour and is associated with coagulation defects. Unexplained hypotension occurring after blood transfusion may be due to the administration of mismatched or contaminated blood. Air embolism following the opening of thoracic veins and fat embolism in patients with fractured long bones are well recognised syndromes causing intraoperative shock.

Profound collapse consequent upon the initiation of intermittent positive pressure ventilation (IPPV) in patients suffering from chest injuries may result from an unrecognised pneumothorax. This is such a serious complication that, in patients suffering from major trauma to the thorax in whom pneumothorax cannot be excluded on clinical and radiographic grounds, it is our practice to insert bilateral chest drains before starting IPPV.

The occurrence of a massive pulmonary embolism or myocardial infarction during the course of a general anaesthetic may be suspected from the patient's medical history. Under these circumstances surgery and anaesthesia should be abandoned, if possible, and efforts made to resuscitate the patient from the life threatening haemodynamic decompensation.

Postoperative Phase

The anaesthetist's interest in the management of shock in the postoperative phase may arise in two ways:

a) Consultation may be requested regarding the deterioration of patients in the immediate postoperative period. Hypoxia, haemorrhage, or analgesic overdosages may produce acute collapse which requires urgent treatment.

b) The anaesthetist in the Intensive Care Unit will be involved in the continuing treatment of the shocked patient following surgery. The policy of elective ventilation may be adopted especially in the elderly, severely shocked or septic cases, and may be continued for 1–5 days or perhaps longer. During this time the monitoring of ventilation, haemodynamic performance, and renal function will continue. At any stage recrudescence of the shock process may require the renewal of the resuscitative measures utilised previously.

It is perhaps appropriate here to consider some aspects of impaired renal function and its management.

As both hypoxia and metabolic acidosis adversely affect renal function (Rosen, 1972) the correction of these in the early stages is obligatory. Similarly the use of the appropriate antibiotic in cases of septic shock may prevent continuing renal damage.

The early recognition of renal failure in the shocked patient is important as its onset especially in the elderly carries a considerable mortality. Renal failure can be defined as the production of insufficient urine to prevent rising blood levels of nitrogenous end products (Luke and Kennedy, 1967).

It is of considerable practical importance to differentiate between pre-renal (oligaemic) and renal failure as the former is reversible by correction of volume deficits (blood, plasma or electrolytes) though the dividing line between the two forms of failure is seldom rigid. The most useful measurements in the diagnosis are the urine/plasma osmolality ratio and the urine/plasma urea ratio. Normally the plasma urea is concentrated by a factor of at least 14 in the urine (Kennedy, 1968) (Table I).

Table I
Differentiation of pre-renal from renal oliguria, on basis of urine/plasma (U/P) osmolality and urea ratios.

	U/P osmolality ratio	U/P urea ratio
Pre-renal	> 2:1	> 20:1
Renal (early)	< 1.7:1	< 14:1
Renal (late)	< 1.1:1	< 5:1

Serum creatinine is an additional useful index of renal function easily available from most laboratories. Despite the fact that in shocked patients an hourly urinary secretion of 50 ml is usually regarded as satisfactory, on occasions renal failure may be obscured by the secretion of large quantities of poorly concentrated urine.

Our management of the shocked oliguric patient involves:

1. The correction of fluid deficits by the infusion of the appropriate fluid. If this is unsuccessful:
2. The use of diuretics: a) mannitol; b) frusemide or ethacrynic acid.

The relative value of these agents is controversial (Harrington and Cohen, 1973; *Lancet*, 1973). It is our practice to give mannitol 20 g by intravenous infusion over 20 minutes. If a satisfactory urine output occurs up to three doses are given at two hourly intervals. Persistent oliguria despite 60 g of mannitol indicates acute renal failure which is treated by fluid restriction and haemodialysis where indicated.

If shock and acute renal failure persist the management of shock by intravenous fluids to correct oligaemia takes precedence, despite the danger of precipitating pulmonary oedema.

On occasions the anaesthetist may be presented with a shocked patient in renal failure who requires immediate or early surgery (perforated viscus, ruptured bowel anastomosis or dehiscence of an abdominal wound). The choice of the most suitable anaesthetic sequence is one which requires nice judgement on the part of an experienced anaesthetist. The presence of hyperkalaemia contraindicates the use of suxamethonium.

Prognosis in Clinical Shock

The factors affecting prognosis in clinical shock are well reviewed by Wilson and Krome (1969). The outcome of 203 patients in shock were correlated with the state of consciousness, urinary output, ventilation, hepatic disease, acid base balance and age. Anuria, coma and respiratory difficulty were associated with such a poor prognosis that they were termed 'lethal signs'. No patient with hepatic disease recovered to leave hospital. Acidosis gave a poor prognosis. Peretz and his colleagues (1964) confirmed that a high blood lactate, low pH and low bicarbonate levels early in shock indicated a poor outcome. These authors showed that blood lactate levels correlate well with standard bicarbonate levels which are more easily measured.

The proper management of the shocked patient requires on the part of the anaesthetist a knowledge of the pathophysiology of shock so that he may contribute his expertise in the pre-, intra- and postoperative management of this potentially lethal syndrome.

References

Bond, A.C. and Davies, C.K. (1974): Ketamine and pancuronium for the shocked patient. *Anaesthesia, 29*, 59.

Chasapekis, G., Kekis, V., Sakkalis, C. and Kilios, D. (1973): Use of ketamine and pancuronium for anaesthesia for patients in haemorrhagic shock. *Anesth. Analg. Curr. Res., 52*, 282.

Chinese med. J. (1973): Acupuncture anaesthesia for operations in shock and critical cases. *2*, 24.
Clarke, R., Topley, E. and Flear, C.T.G. (1955): Assessment of blood loss in civilian trauma. *Lancet*, *1*, 629.
Coleman, A.J., Downing, J.W., Leary, W.P., Moyes, D.G. and Styles, M. (1972): The immediate cardiovascular effects of pancuronium, alcuronium and tubocurarine in man. *Anaesthesia, 27*, 415.
Defalque, R.J. (1968): Subclavian venipuncture: a review. *Anesth. Analg. Curr. Res., 47*, 677.
Defalque, R.J. (1974): Percutaneous catheterisation of the internal jugular vein. *Anesth. Analg. Curr. Res., 53*, 116.
Dinnick, O.P. (1964): Deaths associated with anaesthesia observations on 600 cases. *Anaesthesia, 19*, 536.
English, K.W., Frew, R.M., Piggott, J.F.G. and Zaki, M. (1969): Percutaneous catheterisation of the internal jugular vein. *Anaesthesia, 24*, 521.
Grant, R.T. and Reeve, E.B. (1951): *Observations on the General Effects of Injury in Man.* M.R.C. Special Report, p. 277. Her Majesty's Stationary Office, London.
Harrington, J.T. and Cohen, J.J. (1975): Current concepts. Acute oliguria. *New Engl. J. Med., 292*, 89.
Hayes, M.F., Rosenbaum, R. and Matsumoto, T. (1973): Diagnosis and treatment of haemorrhagic and septic shock. *Int. Surg., 58*, 299.
Horsey, P.J. (1968): Shock and the anaesthetist. *Brit. J. Hosp. Med., 1*, 341.
Johnson, A.O.B. and Clark, R.G. (1972): Malpositioning of central venous catheters. *Lancet, 2*, 1395.
Joly, H.R. and Weil, M.H. (1969): Temperature of the great toe as an indication of the severity of shock. *Circulation, 39*, 131.
Kellner, G.A. and Smart, J.F. (1972): Percutaneous placement of catheters to monitor 'central venous pressure'. *Anesthesiology, 36*, 515.
Kennedy, A.C. (1968): Acute renal failure and the anaesthetist. *Proc. roy. Soc. Med., 61*, 1165.
Kennedy, W.F., Bonica, J.J., Adamatsu, T.J., Ward, R.G., Martin, W.E. and Grinstein, A. (1968): Cardiovascular and respiratory effects of subarachnoid block in the presence of acute blood loss. *Anesthesiology, 29*, 29.
Lancet Editorial (1973): Acute renal failure. *2*, 134.
Latimer, R.D. (1971): Central venous catheterisation. *Brit. J. Hosp. Med., 5*, 369.
Leader *Lancet* (1973): Nitrous oxide analgesia. *11*, 881.
Luke, R.G. and Kennedy, A.C. (1967): Prevention and early management of acute renal failure. *Postgrad. med. J., 43*, 280.
McAslan, T.C. and Cowley, R.A. (1974): *Scientific Abstracts of the First World Congress on Intensive Care.* Editor: I.McA. Ledingham. Bell and Bain, Glasgow.
McLaughlin, J.S., Suddhimondala, C., Mech, K., Llacer, R.L., Houston, J., Blide, R., Altar, S. and Cowley, R.A. (1969): Pulmonary gas exchange in shock in humans. *Ann. Surg., 169*, 42.
MacLean, L.D. (1966): The clinical management of shock. *Brit. J. Anaesth., 38*, 255.
Mostert, J.W., Kenny, G.M. and Murphy, G.P. (1970): Safe placement of central venous catheter into internal jugular vein. *Arch. Surg. (Chicago), 101*, 431.
Peretz, D.I., McGregor, M. and Dossetor, J.B. (1964): Lacticacidosis: a clinically significant aspect of shock. *Canad. med. Ass. J., 90*, 673.
Rosen, S.M. (1972): Effects of anaesthesia and surgery on renal haemodynamics. *Brit. J. Anaesth., 44*, 252.
Savege, T.M., Blogg, C.E., Foley, E.I., Ross, L., Lang, M. and Simpson, B.R. (1973): The cardiorespiratory effects of althesin and ketamine. *Anaesthesia, 28*, 391.
Savege, T.M., Foley, E.T., Ross, L. and Maxwell, M.P. (1972): A comparison of the cardiorespiratory effects during induction of anaesthesia of althesin with thiopentane and methohexitone. *Postgrad. med. J., 48, Suppl. 2*, 66.
Sellick, B.A. (1961): Cricoid pressure to control regurgitation of stomach contents during induction of anaesthesia. *Lancet, 2*, 404.

Shimosato, S., Li, T. and Etsten, B. (1963): Ventricular function during halothane anaesthesia in close chest dog. *Circulat. Res., XII*, 63.

Thornton, J.A., Fleming, J.S., Goldberg, A.D. and Baird, D. (1973): Cardiovascular effects of 50% nitrous oxide and 50% oxygen mixture. *Anaesthesia, 28*, 484.

Vickers, M.D.A. (1969): The use and limitations of isotope studies in clinical shock. *Postgrad. med. J., 45*, 503.

Weaver, P.C. (1971): A study of the cardiovascular effects of halothane. *Ann. roy. Coll. Surg. Engl., 49*, 114.

Wilson, R.F. and Krome, R. (1969): Factors affecting prognosis in clinical shock. *Ann. Surg., 169*, 93.

Wolfson, L.J. (1966): The anaesthetists' management of the injured patient. *Brit. J. Anaesth., 38*, 274.

Ledingham (ed.). Shock

Cardiogenic shock

M. THOMAS

Cardiogenic shock is a clinical syndrome characterised by skin pallor, coldness of the extremities, reduced arterial pressure and a generally ill appearance. The clinical features are common to other shock syndromes not primarily caused by heart disease and reflect similar component reactions. There is, however, little point, and some danger, in the unqualified general use of the term shock since important differences particular to each cause may determine specific treatment and survival.

Characteristically, the shock syndrome in disease of the heart and major vessels occurs in relation to acute cardiac disasters. The most common is myocardial infarction, when shock now follows in about 5–10% of cases. Less common, but sometimes more dramatic causes include rupture of the interventricular septum, rupture of a chorda papillae, rupture of the ventricular wall with acute tamponade, coronary embolus, rupture of aortic aneurysm, dissecting aortic aneurysm and direct trauma to the heart. Pulmonary embolus, although not strictly 'cardiogenic' is a common complication of heart disease, leading to states of acute profound cardiovascular collapse and shock. Less abrupt and clinically rather different are states of shock found in acute fulminating valvulitis, endocarditis and myocarditis. Finally, and especially important, there are the shock syndromes found in relation to cardiac surgery especially where poor risk patients are accepted for treatment.

The management of patients with cardiogenic shock falls within the precincts of the specialist cardiologist, general physician, clinical pharmacologist, anaesthetist, surgeon, and those responsible for acute casualty services. The topic should not, therefore, be considered sectarian in terms of language, understanding or therapeutic approach. The therapist should not be burdened with the vast literature of these several disciplines however. Rather, he should develop an outline approach and liaise freely with his specialist colleagues. It is as a guideline for such cooperation that this chapter is written.

Key Mechanisms and Pathophysiology

The most striking clinical feature in cardiogenic shock is skin pallor. Evident on even casual examination the waxy sweating appearance is the hallmark of a very serious clinical problem. The appearance depends on extreme vascular constriction within the skin and is naturally followed by a palpable fall in skin temperature due to the reduction in blood flow. It is generally felt that skin constriction is a part of compensatory homeostasis for systemic hypotension, but there is only a general correlation. Skin pallor is more marked in the presence of severe pain, as in acute myocardial infarction, and in illness with abrupt onset. It is a less striking feature with disease of a more subacute nature.

Not evident clinically, but very well substantiated by measurement is a reduction in cardiac output. As a general phenomenon, reduced cardiac output is more constant and more important than any other haemodynamic parameter in cardiogenic shock. Reduction may be mild – to rather less than half the normal cardiac index – down to as little as 7–800 ml blood/minute in a man of average size. It is generally thought that reduced cardiac output as well as being the most constant haemodynamic feature, is the key causative mechanism in cardiogenic shock (Guyton and Crowell, 1961). Patients with even severe cardiac damage do not develop the shock syndrome in the absence of reduced cardiac output.

Systemic hypotension is the other major haemodynamic change. Blood pressure is maintained by the force of heart contraction and ejection in relation to the resistance to flow in the systemic circulation. For non-pulsatile flow,

$$\frac{\text{Mean arterial BP}}{\text{Cardiac output}} = \text{peripheral vascular resistance.}$$

When central venous pressure is markedly elevated, this has to be taken into account by including the pressure gradient across the systemic bed, divided by cardiac output. Consideration of the same relations in pulsatile flow becomes much more complex; but for practical use, regarding the major part of peripheral vascular impedance as 'resistive', and accepting the pressure flow ratio as 'resistance', carries no therapeutic penalties.

In cardiogenic shock, reduced arterial pressure is, therefore, still the net consequence of reduced cardiac output and a variable peripheral vascular resistance (PVR). Sometimes PVR is comparatively well maintained, in which case blood pressure falls less in relation to a drop in cardiac output; in other patients PVR may be low, when blood pressure may be very low in company with low cardiac output. The latter reaction tends to follow a period of acute vasoconstriction and although apparently bad clinically, the lower arterial pressure may in fact presage an improvement in outlook in those patients who ultimately recover (Thomas et al., 1966).

Consequent on a fall in overall blood flow and systemic arterial pressure, regional perfusion becomes defective; this is a direct result of a generally low flow, and in some areas, regional vasoconstriction. Reduced regional perfusion affects particularly the brain, kidneys and lungs.

The brain normally uses about 20% of the basal overall oxygen consumption (Lassen, 1959). It is largely dependent on aerobic metabolism in adults and is, therefore, particularly susceptible to hypoxia. The usual vascular regulatory mechanisms ensure a constant blood supply over wide ranges of cardiac output and arterial pressure, and this mechanism can maintain adequate blood supply to the brain in the presence of quite severe systemic circulation failure. Thus patients may be alert and sensitive in the presence of serious haemodynamic illness. With the most extreme degrees of circulation failure (cardiac index less than one third normal) mental inattention, confusion and eventually coma become important. Cerebral function is especially concerning after cardiac arrest (Ingvar, 1968), when apart from the defects due to a period of total circulatory failure, cerebral vascular homeostasis becomes ineffective with the result that small falls in systemic arterial pressure are associated with unusually marked deterioration in mental function. This has important implications for the clinical policy to maintain blood pressure.

The kidneys too command a large fraction of the normal cardiac output (20–30%) and are subject to the same haemodynamic risks as the brain when systemic circulation fails (Rosen, 1969). Usually an adequate urine output is maintained until quite low values of cardiac output (one third cardiac index) although increase in blood urea may occur long before this. Patients with long standing systemic hypertension may have dramatic increase in blood urea in the presence of quite good systemic circulation. In such cases prognosis for renal function is good providing further cardiac deterioration does not take place. On the other hand, with severe circulatory failure urine output diminishes and renal failure becomes one of the most important therapeutic problems. Complete anuria is typical of the most severe cases of cardiogenic shock (Thomas et al., 1966).

Although very serious troubles in oxygen transfer may be associated with acute pulmonary oedema secondary to an increase in alveolar dead space the lungs do not suffer severe functional difficulties on account of reduced pulmonary blood flow. Hyperventilation due to left ventricular failure may be combined with reduced perfusion. Ventilation/perfusion defects (Valentine et al., 1966), are marked in association with segmental collapse and chest splinting due to pain. Breathlessness may follow lung complications but the most common 'cause' is left atrial hypertension. At higher levels of left atrial hypertension with pulmonary oedema arterial PO_2 falls and V/Q imbalance may be easily shown. When left atrial pressure is extreme, more than 30 mmHg mean, pulmonary oedema may be gross, rendering the chest radiograph almost opaque and making gas transfer problems critical. Arterial PO_2 may fall to around 50 mmHg notwithstanding endotracheal intubation and positive pressure ventilation with 100% O_2. Such difficulties exaggerate the metabolic consequences of low blood flow and blood lactate rises precipitously with a fall in pH in some patients (MacKenzie et al., 1964).

The multiple organ failure which accompanies marked cardiovascular collapse implies a most complicated metabolic confusion. In its own right the subject commands considerable attention and various regimens for metabolic support have been suggested. More particularly related to haemodynamic events in cardiogenic shock is an extreme activation of adrenergic drive (Valori et al., 1967). Neurosympathetic drive has long been clinically suspected from the associated skin pallor, vasoconstriction, sweating, tachycardia etc. but recently the extent of this has been semi-quantified by measurement of blood and urine catecholamines. Blood and urine adrenaline and noradrenaline rise in general relation to the patients clinical illness, being most elevated in acute gross pulmonary oedema and severe cardiogenic shock (Jewitt et al., 1969). Catecholamine drive implies an increased oxygen requirement and possibly adverse effect for critically perfused myocardium. In company with clinical improvement, catechol output diminishes.

Rational Approach to Practical Therapy

Since overall reduction in blood flow is the sine qua non for the shock state, it seems reasonable to direct therapy towards maintaining blood flow. Most of the means available, including drugs and mechanical devices, have the propensity to become a sledge hammer in a china shop when used uncritically, without continuous care and by the inexperienced. An overriding principle with the large majority of patients with cardiogenic shock is that it is much easier to accelerate their demise than to accelerate their recovery. All therapies should be initiated with delicacy. It is easy to give more drugs. It is impossible to recall, and often impossible to antagonise, a relative excess.

On first assessment of the acutely ill patient the questions are: What is the causative diagnosis? Will the patient improve spontaneously with conservative measures? Are there any causative factors that can and should be easily reversed without risk? Finally, what definitive measures specific to a particular diagnosis need to be undertaken; when, and at what risk?

With some exceptions, cardiac patients arriving in hospital with the appearance of shock show signs of improvement after about two hours in a warm comfortable bed, with administration of high concentrations of oxygen and after careful control of any pain with suitable analgesics. A period of observation allows a full appraisal of the diagnosis, with aid of appropriate clinical examination, radiographs, ECG etc. and gives valuable opportunity to discriminate between those patients with a marked neurosympathetic reaction to sudden illness, and those with the more profound problems of a persisting shock state. Intravenous infusion, continuous ECG monitoring, initiation of fluid balance records, base line blood samples for cardiac enzymes, electrolytes and blood urea, haemoglobin are dealt with. Central venous blood pressure should be monitored and at a later stage, if indicated, direct arterial pressure measurements can be helpful where peripheral arterial pulses are impalpable or sphygmomanometer readings not obtainable.

During the preliminary appraisal, a tentative opinion as to the need for any special measures should be defined. Anaesthetists, surgeons and cardiovascular specialists benefit greatly from their own early assessment of the patient as a guide to later advice. Special measures to be borne in mind are relief of intrapericardial pressure by pericardiocentesis in patients with tamponade, mechanical ventilation in patients unable to naturally oxygenate the blood, through breathing problems or gross pulmonary oedema; possibility of angiography in suspected dissecting aortic aneurysm, catheterisation and angiography prior to urgent cardiac surgery, assisted circulation in some circumstances. This will clarify the need for early communications with other medical staff, other services and other hospitals. However, the vast majority of patients require none of these and except under rare circumstances of patient needs and availability of special facilities, there is far more to be gained from good conservative management of the average shocked patient with acute cardiac infarction than through intervention including circulation assist, coronary arteriography and urgent aorto-coronary bypass surgery.

Oxygen

Most patients may benefit from oxygen administration and no important problems follow the use of high concentrations in patients with defective lung function as the arterial PO_2 rise is limited. Oxygen may be administered by mask, or spectacles in which case an inspired concentration of 40–50% may be reached (Collis, 1969). It should be noted that 'venturi' masks, delivering less than 30% O_2, although often better made, more comfortable and appealing to nurses, are often useless in raising arterial PO_2 in patients with cardiogenic shock. Endotracheal intubation with artificial ventilation is, of course, best soon after cardiac arrest and has additional advantage in the presence of acute pulmonary oedema, when a positive pressure cycle can often minimise oedema, clear the chest radiograph and aid arterial oxygenation. Where possible measurement of cardiac output should be used to exclude serious reduction in blood flow by pressure ventilation. Theoretical arguments as to the essential benefit or otherwise from oxygen therapy are legion. From a practical viewpoint arterial PO_2 of less than 100 mmHg should be regarded as in need of correction and higher levels as potentially beneficial by increasing diffusion gradients to poorly perfused tissues, especially ischaemic myocardium, and the brain. Hyperbaric O_2 may be considered when such specialist facilities are available (Cameron et al., 1966) although it remains to be determined whether any improvement in myocardial oxygenation occurs and, if so, whether it justifies the undoubted risk of oxygen toxicity.

Analgesics

Pain is often included in shock syndromes – more especially with trauma but also in certain forms of cardiogenic shock such as in acute myocardial infarction. Extreme pain contributes to vasoconstriction of the skin and may be associated with a 'visceral reaction' of nausea, vomiting, bradycardia and hypotension. Relief of pain can also rectify some of the adverse hypotensive mechanisms. On the other hand, most analgesics of sufficient power to alleviate this order of distress have important side effects. Morphine for instance leads to venous pooling and net vasodilation. Small doses, 3–5 mg slowly intravenously should be given at first if serious hypotension is to be avoided (Thomas et al., 1965). The consequence of idosyncrasy in terms of vomiting and hypotension can thereby be minimised.

Probably the best all round agent is heroin (diacetyl morphine) (McDonald et al., 1967), which seems to be less prone to cardiovascular depression. Again the initial dose should be small (e.g. 2 mg) and later doses incremental. Often pain may be sufficiently blunted for the patient to be able to put up with it at drug doses which are quite small. The principle of the smallest effective dose of drug carries many advantages; in particular allowing more latitude when other, potentially depressive drugs, such as antiarrhythmic agents, need to be given.

Analgesia may be needed together with light sleep or minimal anaesthesia for procedures such as DC shock treatment for arrhythmias, endotracheal intubation, preliminary care of external trauma etc. Here the services of a skilled anaesthetist are a priority – as again, the minimal drug impact, consistent with the effect desired, is the ideal.

Cardiac Arrhythmias

At the first opportunity in clinical evaluation the heart rhythm should be determined. Cardiac arrhythmias may easily be missed on clinical examination in very ill patients, especially in the presence in rapid heart rate – which, of course, may not seem out of place. Continuous ECG monitoring should be set up using an oscilloscope with wide screen and long traverse to enable the rhythm to be easily seen. In restless patients chest leads with wide stable electrode patches are recommended for ECG stability.

Cardiac arrhythmias are of paramount importance, as they provide one of the commonest causes of a shock state, especially in myocardial infarction; and unlike many causes, are subject to rapid safe reversal by the informed experienced therapist (Sandoe et al., 1970).

In cardiac infarction, arrhythmias occur in nearly all patients. They range in functional severity from occasional extrasystoles with transient fall in systemic blood flow to ventricular fibrillation with complete failure of the heart as a pump. Arrhythmias may be transient, requiring no treatment, or prolonged, when the possible risks of intervention need to be weighed against waiting for spontaneous reversion to sinus rhythm. All patients at risk should be regarded as most unpredictable and should be watched closely, both personally and with the aid of monitoring systems.

The most important arrhythmias are ventricular fibrillation, ventricular tachycardia, supraventricular tachycardia, atrial flutter and fibrillation, supraventricular bradycardia, nodal rhythm, ventricular bradycardia, heart block of various degrees and complete heart block. Since they are one of the most common practical therapeutic areas, a more extensive outline of individual problems and treatment is given.

Ventricular fibrillation (VF)

Following VF immediate mechanical failure of the heart leads to total loss of external work and systemic circulation. Arterial pressure falls to nearly zero in a few seconds and death rapidly supervenes. If VF is observed through ECG monitoring the first measure should be DC shock. Likely this will restore an effective beat: if not, general resuscitation measures, including artificial ventilation and external cardiac massage, and rapid intravenous administration of high concentration (e.g. 8.4%) of sodium bicarbonate should be initiated. Further DC shocks should then be given.

Ventricular tachycardia (VT)

VT often precedes the onset of ventricular fibrillation. Less serious than VF in haemodynamic terms, it may still result in a clinical 'collapse' indistinguishable from cardiac arrest when the heart rate is about 200/min. Less rapid rates are marginally less prone to VF but are still urgent problems. Two main haemodynamic factors are involved. The normal atrioventricular sequence of activation is destroyed by the ectopic pacemaker activity; atrial transport function is lost and the power of ventricular contraction diminishes. VT should be treated (Jewitt et al., 1968), first by intravenous injection of lidocaine 1–2 mg/kg over one minute, when sinus rhythm often returns. If ineffective, DC shock should be given. Procaine amide 250 mg i.v. may be given as an alternative to lidocaine but it is more likely to lead to hypotension. VT refractory to those two drugs and DC shock is a difficulty found especially in patients with seriously demaged myocardium. Other drugs such as diphenylhydantoin, quinidine, β-blocking agents, such as practolol, or ultimately tenormol can be effective but their use may result in general circulatory deterioration.

In all patients the presence of acute or chronic potassium depletion resulting from diuretic therapy should be borne in mind. Intravenous infusion of potassium may revert the arrhythmia 'per se' or may facilitate conversion by antiarrhythmic drug or DC shock. A useful sequence is to shock after any new pharmacological intervention, as soon as it is apparent that the drug by itself has not succeeded. When later choice drugs are used, heart block syndromes should be anticipated after DC shock and facilities for cardiac pacing put on stand-by.

Supraventricular arrhythmias

These are especially common. Most important are varieties of supraventricular tachycardia with different degrees of atrioventricular block and atrial fibrillation. Characteristically they are self-limiting but in chronically prone individuals may be very prolonged and lead to states of shock even in the presence of good ventricular function. Supraventricular tachycardia with one to one atrioventricular relation can be mild haemodynamically as atrial transport remains operative and overall heart function no worse than sinus tachycardia. Stroke volume may be reduced, but often only as an inverse result of tachycardia. When ventricular function is poor, however, stroke volume may fall further, especially in ischaemic heart disease. Atrial fibrillation also varies widely in the degree to which circulation deteriorates. Ventricular rates up to 150/minute may be tolerated well if ventricular function is good. Circulation is worse in the presence of high ventricular rate, and poor ventricular function.

Treatment of supraventricular tachycardia depends on the patients' tolerance of the arrhythmia. If deterioration requires action the rate of effect of treatment must be evaluated against the rate of deterioration of the patient. Tachycardia not caused by digitalis toxicity may be treated with ouabain i.v. (0.5 mg) followed by an oral regimen of digoxin 0.25 mg (new preparation) four hourly until heart rate is controlled. More rapid control can be achieved with a larger initial i.v. dose of ouabain (0.75–1.00 mg) but this may be followed by ventricular ectopic beats and is not without danger of some more serious rhythms.

DC shock should be used if reversion is thought to be necessary within the hour and of course if the patient is deteriorating rapidly. This is much safer than embarking on digitalis control and then being encouraged to DC shock by unanticipated rapid deterioration. DC shock in the presence of digitalis can be hazardous, but if unavoidable should be preceded with lidocaine i.v. 100 mg. Rare instances of resistant supraventricular tachycardias may require the empirical use of quinidine, verapamil or β-blocking agents (Sandoe et al., 1970; Lown et al., 1969).

Bradycardia

Slowing of the heart occurs in many rhythms but especially as supraventricular bradycardia. Very common in myocardial infarction on the back of the heart, it occurs also in relation to painful syndromes with other pathologies. Reduced cardiac output, low arterial pressure, pallor, sweating, nausea and vomiting often result. Loss of consciousness may follow and the general problem closely resembles an ordinary vasovagal faint. If haemodynamic effects are not severe, the arrhythmia can well be ignored, spontaneous acceleration of rate being the rule. The patient may feel better if the legs are raised somewhat and high elevation of the legs is a very useful acute measure if circulation fails rapidly. Acceleration of the heart with atropine i.v. 0.3–1 mg in increments of about 0.3 mg is a convenient maintenance policy (Thomas and Woodgate, 1966). Bradycardia associated with second degree heart block is often best treated by isoprenaline 0.05 mg slowly i.v.

Nodal rhythm

In nodal rhythm, atrial transport function is inoperative, making the effects of bradycardia more severe at any heart rate. The rhythm may be unstable and vary with atrio-ventricular dissociation. Treatment should be on the basis of the haemodynamic situation. Often no treatment is required, but where the rhythm gives way to idioventricular bradycardia, pacing facilities should be at hand.

Complete heart block

Complete heart block frequently leads to the clinical appearance of shock, through profound bradycardia (20–40/minute) or transient episodes of complete heart arrest. In some patients a higher rate (50/minute) with some stability may be tolerated well, when ventricular function is good and compensatory increase in stroke volume takes place. In myocardial infarction or chronic heart failure defective ventricular function may not allow increased stroke volume and when septal and anterior infarction leads to complete block the combined effects are devastating, often leading to arterial pressure around 50–60 mmHg, cardiac output around 1 litre/minute and loss of consciousness preceding death. Complete heart block is best treated by intracardiac pacing; but this categorical approach needs qualification. Temporary support of the circulation is often achieved by injection or infusion of isoprenaline (1 mg/l); overdose is dangerous, leading to ventricular arrhythmias and perhaps ventricular fibrillation. Close monitoring is mandatory and pacing should be instituted if control is not good. Transvenous pacing is now the routine technique. A bipolar catheter situated in the right ventricular outflow tract is preferred; pacing set to 'on demand' at an appropriate rate. Cut out when sinus rhythm returns is thus ensured because of the risk of a pacing shock in the vulnerable period, provoking ventricular fibrillation.

Pacing should not be regarded as an innocent procedure. Catheters are best placed in position by an experienced operator, especially in the presence of acute myocardial infarction, when other rhythms may be precipitated and a knowledgeable hand essential.

Cardiovascular Shock in Sinus Rhythm

When all first remedies are put in hand and their effects observed, patients will generally fall into two groups: those who have shown tangible signs of improvement and in whom time is mainly required to consolidate therapeutic gains, and those who remain seriously or desperately ill despite correction of safely reversible factors. These last patients, providing the 'hard core' of the shock problem, are then candidates for an escalation in therapeutic procedures. By their very selection their prognosis is bad and the return for an increasing commitment in time, skill, effort, personnel and finance becomes very much smaller.

When those conditions in which cardiac or major vessel surgery is the dominant consideration, as in leaking aortic aneurysm, dissecting aortic aneurysm, ruptured chorda papillae and ruptured intraventricular septum are segregated off, the majority of remaining patients have acute myocardial infarction as the primary lesion.

Cardiogenic shock, in sinus rhythm following acute myocardial infarction and persisting for several hours, is notoriously difficult to treat. Estimates of mortality range from 60–90% according to the precise terms of definition. There are no therapeutic regimens which are proven clearly superior in terms of overall patient survival. There are some which are reasonable and have physiological arguments in support. There are many which are interfering and dangerous.

One major issue is the maintenance of arterial blood pressure. For many years 'pressor' agents were routinely infused intravenously in patients when arterial pressure was below a certain value (often 90 mmHg systolic). Sometimes providing temporary benefit, doses were then increased, to be followed by rapid patient deterioration through further heart failure or cardiac arrhythmias. In using such agents it should again be appreciated that mean arterial pressure is merely the resultant of the interaction between flow (cardiac output) and resistance to flow (peripheral vascular resistance). While low arterial pressure commonly represents low cardiac output, it may also be the result of only moderate reduction in cardiac output and some reduction in peripheral vascular resistance. Similarly, reduced peripheral vascular resistance alone will lower arterial pressure markedly. The need for raising arterial pressure should not be judged by the level of pressure per se; rather the evidence for adequacy of regional perfusion should be assessed. Warm skin implies skin blood flow within acceptable range. Passing urine implies adequate renal blood flow. On the other hand, cold extremities, oliguria or anuria, cerebral confusion or stupor equate with inadequate regional perfusion generally, to the kidneys and the brain.

Drugs

Sympathomimetic and other 'pressor' agents. Each sympathomimetic 'pressor' agent has its own particular characteristics. Noradrenaline (Goldberg, 1960), is given by intravenous infusion 8–30 mg/l fluid. It is both an inotropic agent and a peripheral constrictor. Blood pressure rises comparatively easily. Vasoconstriction occurs dominantly in skin, splanchnic, muscle, renal arterial and venous circuits. Isoprenaline (Rosenblum et al., 1968), in contrast, is a powerful inotropic agent but reduces peripheral vascular resistance and has, therefore, some attraction in that increase in 'afterload' is less pronounced. This argument is taken further with dopamine (Goldberg et al., 1969) (3-OH tyramine), which has an inotropic effect, some vasoconstricting properties but an individual ability for renal vasodilation. Strong arguments have, therefore, been made for its wider use in shock states, where renal function may be one major factor limiting survival.

Other agents used with the object of increasing arterial pressure include substances acting through the endogenous catecholamines, such as metaraminol, and independently, such as glucagon. Glucagon can produce dramatic increase in cardiac output and was strongly favoured for a time. Experimental work suggests that the increased flow is largely splanchnic and therefore of little biological value (Katz and Mills, 1971).

Digitalis. There is an enormous literature on digitalis. Its actions in experimental circumstances, down to the level of cell wall ionic pump mechanisms have long been explored. Unfortunately the biological effects in various disease states have been less rigorously analysed notwithstanding the place of the drug in cardiac disease as a whole. In shock, digitalis has a variable effect. In patients more towards the range of congestive cardiac failure, stroke volume and cardiac output are often increased in line with evident clinical improvement. In those with more acute left heart failure the acute effects of digitalis may be limited to lowering the heart rate. In patients with an advanced shock syndrome due to acute myocardial infarction it is not common to see tangible improvement following digitalis except through an effect on cardiac arrhythmia. Studies with a catheter tip electromagnetic velocity meter in this group suggest in some patients an increase in the rate of cardiac work without improvement in mean blood flow.

Fluid loading and alpha-blockade. Inadequate distension of the muscle walls of the heart has been held to be a mechanism limiting heart work in cardiogenic shock (Nixon et al., 1966). Dependent on the assumption that the heart can continue to respond to a 'Starling-type' stimulus loading the patient with fluid is thought helpful in some circumstances. In practice fluid loading seems to offer more clinical profit in some patients after heart surgery than in those with acute myocardial infarction; although dramatic improvement in the latter condition has been shown in patients with bradycardia and posterior infarction, when accelerated heart rate following infusion alone leads to improved cardiac output (Nixon et al., 1966). Proof that fluid loading is beneficial in all patients with shock is not available, and detailed measurements of left atrial pressure show that left heart pressures are very delicately susceptible to small increases in fluid loading (Bradley et al., 1970). In such cases the improvement in cardiac output is not marked, but the beneficial effect of optimising left atrial pressure on pulmonary oedema may be great. Implicit in this is the potential danger of fluid loading in patients with selective left heart failure as in myocardial infarction. Central venous pressure is a poor guide to left atrial pressure (Forrester et al., 1971). It is easy to put fluid in; much less easy to get it out in the presence of poor renal function.

Linked with fluid loading, the use of alpha-adrenergic blockade (Bloch et al., 1965), has been portrayed as close to ideal therapy. Because of dilatation in capacity vessels, fluid can be more easily accommodated without precipitous rise of pressure in critical areas such as the left heart and pulmonary veins. Alpha-blockade can be difficult to stabilise in ill patients and drop in arterial pressure, incompletely supported by fluid infusion needs to be guarded against.

Mechanical Circulatory Assistance

With increasing recognition of the poor prospects of patients in extreme circulatory failure, various devices for relieving the heart of some of the mechanical work and also adding to the oxygenation of the blood have been devised and used. Their role is largely one of temporary life support pending definitive correction of the shock producing lesions. The problems of heart transplantation at present confine definitive action to more limited intervention such as excision of an inactive area of myocardium, emergency aorto-coronary bypass, valve replacement or ventricular septal defect repair.

Mechanical assist devices have often led to their own complications and so have not given safe support for an adequate length of time. Partial or complete heart bypass has been dogged by problems of blood damage. Less traumatic methods like synchronous body acceleration machines have not been haemodynamically successful. Two main advances have improved matters: membrane oxygenators (Carlson et al., 1972), and aortic balloon pulsation (Moulopoulos et al., 1962). Using membrane oxygenation, it is now possible to maintain an animal on partial bypass for several days without evident damage to its physiology. Under such circumstances sufficient time for spontaneous improvement of ventricular function following acute myocardial infarction is available and gives opportunity for less hurried appraisal of the more intricate cardiac faults, using cine angiography, coronary arteriography, etc. As a preliminary to surgery designed to improve myocardial blood supply aortic counterpulsation has been preferred by many. The principle of counterpulsation depends on the phasic inflation and collapse of a catheter mounted balloon in the aorta. Inflation is electrocardiographically triggered to coincide with ventricular diastole and collapse with systole. Thus ejection of blood by the heart is facilitated by a temporarily reduced aortic inflow impedance and increased mean diastolic aortic pressure has advantages in maintaining coronary perfusion. Various systems are available commercially and their use is probably more legitimate than any other assist device.

Committing a patient to mechanical assistance carries two main responsibilities: first, adding to the natural risk of the disease in some patients; second, the provision of high calibre cardiac surgical skill and facilities able to deal with the next stage of the problem. The whole matter is controversial since it is very difficult to predict precisely the clinical outlook in the shock syndrome in an individual patient. Various haemodynamic formulae have been proposed and they are certainly helpful. Even so, when approximately four out of five patients die small differences are very difficult to appreciate. A study of the results of aortic pulsation, coronary arteriography and bypass surgery at Massachusetts General Hospital (Dunkman et al., 1972), suggested some improvement over the natural history of the disease but certain of the patients committed had cardiac output values which suggested that they might have survived with conservative management. Thus it may be that almost as much is lost through the summated risks of mechanical assistance, arteriography and surgery in some patients as might be gained through determined therapy in others.

Metabolic and Mechanical Factors Influencing Myocardial Viability

Within the last few years the concept of 'idealising' the environment for ischaemic myocardium has been expanded. Largely originating from earlier work on 'stress' effects on vulnerable heart tissue (Raab, 1969), various proposals for metabolic care are on record. Infusions of potassium, insulin and glucose have been both used empirically and evaluated with some control (Sodi-Pallares et al., 1963). Unfortunately, although various striking experimental effects are known, there is no certainty that such remedies effect the clinical outcome of a patient with acute myocardial infarction (Medical Research Council, 1968); unless the major trouble be related to ventricular arrhythmias associated with chronic potassium deficiency.

Largely following on the demonstration by Raab et al. (1962) that sympathetic nerve stimulation increased ST segment elevation over ischaemic myocardium, the role of catecholamines, other inotropes and mechanical work load on ischaemic myocardium has been examined in the context of the patient with acute myocardial infarction. Essential to the approach is the concept of balancing oxygen demand with oxygen supply. When demand exceeds supply the tissue becomes ischaemic just as when supply falls below demand.

Metabolic work comprises external and internal work. External work is much more tangible than internal work and for inexact purposes may be equated with arterial pressure, neglecting kinetic and pulsatile considerations. Maintenance of high arterial pressure places needless demands on ischaemic myocardium, and while there is not yet a case to lower pressure in patients without serious haemodynamic failure after myocardial infarct, moderate reduction of pressure consequent on limited infarction should not be regarded as entirely bad in the short term. In hypertensive patients with acute myocardial infarction left ventricular failure can be offset by judicious control of arterial pressure and this may well carry secondary benefits for ischaemic myocardium. For seriously ill patients with cardiogenic shock, it could be that the lowest arterial pressure compatible with survival is the best. If a patient is passing sufficient urine to halt a rising blood urea, it may be wisest to avoid catecholamine support of the circulation whatever the arterial pressure, cerebral function allowing. Catecholamine infusion in such patients probably unnecessarily increases overall heart work both by direct effect on the heart and increase in external work through increased arterial pressure. Impending necrosis may be accelerated in critically perfused areas of myocardium. Since ultimate survival in cardiogenic shock following myocardial infarction is probably dominantly dependent on the net myocardial recovery, further necrosis induced by exogenous catecholamines may prevent recovery or reduce the available myocardial function in those who recover.

Beta-blocking agents lower ST segment elevation overlying acutely ischaemic heart tissue. The mechanism of this property is not entirely clear but a case has been presented for interpreting the ST segment reduction as indicating amelioration of ischaemia resultant on a fall in contractile work by the myocardium (Maroko et al., 1971). It is unlikely that increased blood flow provides any explanation (Becker et al., 1974), and beta-blockade does diminish myocardial work in normal myocardium. However, there are some difficulties in regarding this as the sole mechanism. From a practical viewpoint, lowering ST segment height by beta-blockade in patients without pulmonary oedema can be reasonably pursued in units with good monitoring facilities (Pelides et al., 1972), and this may also carry as yet unquantified benefit for ischaemic heart tissue. It should be strongly emphasised that beta-blockade has no place at all in patients with cardiogenic shock in sinus rhythm, since removal of adrenergic drive can rapidly lead to untreatable deterioration. For the future, the place of beta-blockade in association with mechanical support of the circulation in these patients will be an interesting prospect.

Acid base balance in seriously ill patients commands considerable respect. The most practical instance is following cardiac arrest, when consequent on complete loss of circulation, anaerobic mechanisms are activated, blood lactate rises and CO_2 accumulates in the presence of partially effective external cardiac massage and artificial ventilation. DC conversion of ventricular fibrillation may be difficult under such circumstances. In the presence of metabolic acidosis, treatment of ventricular arrhythmias in general can be adversely affected. Correction of pH can be temporarily achieved by rapid intravenous infusion of concentrated sodium bicarbonate solution (8.4%), when electrical conversion of arrhythmias is often facilitated. Likewise in the presence of extremely poor circulation, often associated with gross pulmonary oedema and the need for artificial ventilation, intravenous bicarbonate in sympathy with correct adjustment of ventilation rate, pressure and volume often aids in control of recurrent ventricular arrhythmias and is likely to be beneficial for ischaemic tissues generally. In such cases, the interest of an expert anaesthetist with regular measurement of blood gases, pH and base content should be encouraged (Robinson, 1969).

Special Care and Monitoring

Wherever local facilities and staff allow, nursing of patients with cardiogenic shock should be undertaken in a special care unit where continuous or intermittent personal observation can be given. At this stage in the development in 'special' or 'intensive' care, it is clear that a vast range of techniques is available and it is a matter for some judgement as to which are necessary, merely optional or where risk of intervention outweighs advantage. Given a general environment of continuing observation, simple measures carry most patient profit. Electrocardiogram monitoring, careful accurate fluid balance, close supervision during and after drug administration, particular attention to patient comfort and warmth alongside informed medical and surgical care are all basic.

Invasive methods, aligned particularly toward haemodynamic control start at central venous catheterisation for pressure monitoring and immediate access for drug administration. These catheters should ideally be radiopaque. Arterial catheterisation is helpful when sphygmomanometer readings are difficult, and advisable when agents such as isoprenaline and noradrenaline are infused in hypotensive patients if cuff pressure is uncertain. In patients with metabolic problems, especially involving respiratory dysfunction, multiple arterial blood samples are most conveniently taken from a small indwelling catheter. Arterial catheterisation always carries some risk of ultimate reduction or loss of arterial pulse and use of the radial artery is, therefore, to be preferred to the brachial. Short term (less than 12 hours) arterial catheterisation and intermittent flushing with heparinised saline can be a safe routine in experienced hands. 'Float' catheterisation of the pulmonary artery provides rather safe access for blood sampling, a means of measuring pulmonary artery pressure, and through the diastolic pressure, some representation of left atrial pressure. Pulmonary capillary 'wedge' pressure is also measurable using the Swan–Ganz catheter. Such pressure measurements are a most helpful guide if fluid infusion therapy is pursued. Cardiac output determination is facilitated by right side catheters either as a means of dye injection for arterial cuvette densitometry or for use in thermal dilution methods.

Left heart catheters, although giving direct values for left ventricular diastolic pressure, escalate the level of expertise and experience necessary for safe routine monitoring. Possible with miniature catheterisation techniques, they are best reserved for instances where it is thought mandatory to have certain knowledge of left heart values. When surgery is contemplated, for instance in acute pulmonary oedema associated with marked mitral incompetence, full assessment of myocardial failure and valve incompetence is better made in the catheter-angio laboratory as an elective procedure.

Body temperature is a useful adjunct to other monitoring information. Apart from the standard need for general temperature changes, skin temperatures can point out changes in skin blood flow in patients with varying degrees of peripheral constriction. Of course such data are only a general guide as many factors are involved; not least being environmental temperature and whether the patients limbs have been recently covered or uncovered. In the unconscious patient, core temperature from a rectal probe is more certain and convenient than most other methods of general temperature monitoring.

References

Becker, L., Ferreira, R. and Thomas, M. (1974): Effect of propranolol and isoprenaline on regional left ventricular blood flow in experimental myocardial ischaemia. *Cardiovasc. Res.*, (in press).

Bloch, J.H., Pierce, C.H., Manax, W.G. and Lillehei, R.C. (1965): Treatment of experimental cardiogenic shock. *Surgery, 58*, 197.

Bradley, R.D., Jenkins, B.S. and Branthwaite, M.A. (1970): The influence of atrial pressure on cardiac performance following myocardial infarction complicated by shock. *Circulation, XLII*, 827.

Cameron, A.J.V., Hutton, I., Kenmure, A.C.F. and Murdoch, W.R. (1966): Haemodynamic and metabolic effects of hyperbaric oxygen in myocardial infarction. *Lancet, 2*, 833.

Carlson, R.G., Lande, A.J., Ivey, L.W., Starek, P.J., Rees, J.R., Subramanian, V.A., Twichell, J.,

Baxter, J., Bloch, J.H. and Lillehei, C.W. (1972): Total cardiopulmonary support with disposable membrane oxygenator during aortocoronary artery-vein graft operations. *Dis. Chest, 62*, 424.
Collis, J.M. (1969): Respiratory therapy in physiological and practical aspects of shock. In: *International Anaesthesiology Clinics, Vol. 7, No. 4*, p. 799. Editor: J. Freeman.
Dunkman, W.B., Leinbach, R.C., Buckley, M.J., Mundth, E.D., Kantrovitz, A.R., Austen, A.G. and Sanders, C.A. (1972): Clinical and haemodynamic results of intra-aortic balloon pumping and surgery for cardiogenic shock. *Circulation, XLVI*, 465.
Forrester, J.S., Diamond, G., McHugh, T.J. and Swan, H.J.C. (1971): Filling pressures in the right and left sides of the heart in acute myocardial infarction. *New Engl. J. Med., 285*, 190.
Goldberg, L.I. (1960): The direct effects of norepinephrine, epinephrine and methoxamine on myocardial contractile force in man. *Circulation, 22*, 1125.
Goldberg, L.I., Talley, R.C. and McNay, J.L. (1969): The potential role of dopamine in the treatment of shock. *Progr. cardiovasc. Dis., 12*, 40.
Guyton, A.C. and Crowell, J.W. (1961): Dynamics of the heart in shock. *Fed. Proc., 20*, 59.
Ingvar, D.H. (1968): The pathophysiology of cerebral anoxia. Aspects of resuscitation. *Acta anaesth. scand., Suppl. XXIX*, 47.
James, T.N. (1961): Posterior myocardial infarction. *J. Mich. med. Soc., 60*, 1409.
Jewitt, D.E., Kishon, Y. and Thomas, M. (1968): Lignocaine in the management of arrhythmias after acute myocardial infarction. *Lancet, 1*, 266.
Jewitt, D.E., Mercer, C.J., Reid, D., Valori, C., Thomas, M. and Shillingford, J.P. (1969): Free noradrenaline and adrenaline excretion in relation to the development of cardiac arrhythmias and heart failure in patients with acute myocardial infarction. *Lancet, 1*, 635.
Katz, R.L. and Mills, C.J. (1971): Use of a catheter tip electromagnetic velocity meter to determine the cardiovascular effects of glucagon. *Cardiovasc. Res., V/1*, 62.
Lassen, N.A. (1959): Cerebral blood flow and oxygen consumption in man. *Physiol. Rev., 39*, 183.
Lown, B., Kosowsky, B.D. and Klein, M.D. (1969): Pathogenesis prevention and treatment of arrhythmias in myocardial infarction. *Research on Acute Myocardial Infarction.* Editor: S. Bondurant. American Heart Association Monograph No. 27.
MacKenzie, G.J., Taylor, S.H., Flenley, D.C., McDonald, A.H., Staunton, H.P. and Donald, K.W. (1964): Circulatory and respiratory studies in myocardial infarction and cardiogenic shock. *Lancet, 2*, 825.
McDonald, H.R., Rees, H.A., Muir, A.L., Lawrie, D.M., Burton, J.L. and Donald, K.W. (1967): Circulatory effects of heroin in patients with myocardial infarction. *Lancet, 1*, 1070.
Maroko, P.R., Kjekshus, J.D., Sobel, B.E., Watanabe, T., Covell, J.W., Ross, J. and Braunwald, E. (1971): Factors influencing infarct size following experimental coronary artery occlusion. *Circulation, 43*, 67.
Medical Research Council (1968): Potassium glucose and insulin treatment for acute myocardial infarction. Report of the Working Party on the Treatment of Myocardial Infarction. *Lancet, 2*, 1355.
Moulopoulos, S.D., Topaz, S. and Kolff, W.J. (1962): Diastolic balloon pumping (with carbon dioxide) in the aorta – a mechanical assistance to the failing circulation. *Amer. Heart J., 63*, 669.
Nixon, P.G.F., Ikram, H. and Morton, S. (1966): Infusion of dextrose solution in cardiogenic shock. *Lancet, 1*, 1077.
Pelides, L.J., Reid, D.S., Thomas, M. and Shillingford, J.P. (1972): Inhibition by beta-blockade of the S.T. segment elevation after acute myocardial infarction in man. *Cardiovasc. Res., 6*, 295.
Raab, W. (1969): Myocardial electrolyte derangement: crucial feature of pleuricausal, so-called coronary, heart disease. *Ann. N. Y. Acad. Sci., 147*, Art. 17, 627.
Raab, W., Van Lith, P., Lepeschkin, E. and Herrlish, H.C. (1962): Catecholamine induced myocardial hypoxia in the presence of impaired coronary dilatability independent of external cardiac work. *Amer. J. Cardiol., 9*, 455.

Ratshin, R.A., Rackley, C.E. and Russell, R.O. (1972): Haemodynamic evaluation of left ventricular function in shock complicating myocardial infarction. *Circulation, 45*, 127.

Robinson, J.S. (1969): Acidosis in low flow states in physiological and practical aspects of shock. In: *International Anaesthesiology Clinics, Vol. 7*, p. 895. Editor: J. Freeman.

Rosen, S.M. (1969): Renal failure during and after shock. Physiological and practical aspects of shock. In: *International Anaesthesiology Clinics, Vol. 7*, p. 861. Editor: J. Freeman.

Rosenblum, R., Berkowitz, W.D. and Lawson, D. (1968): Effect of acute intravenous administration of noradrenaline on cardiorenal haemodynamics in man. *Circulation, 38*, 158.

Sandoe, E., Flensted-Jensen, E. and Olesen, K.H. (Editors) (1970): *Symposium on Cardiac Arrhythmias*. A.B. Astra, Sodertalje, Sweden.

Sodi-Pallares, D., Bisteni, A., Medrano, G.A., Testelli, M.R. and De Micheli, A. (1963): Polarising treatment of acute myocardial infarction: possibility of its use in other cardiovascular conditions. *Dis. Chest, 43*, 424.

Thomas, M., Malmcrona, R., Fillmore, S.J. and Shillingford, J.P. (1965): Haemodynamic effects of morphine in patients with acute myocardial infarction. *Brit. Heart J., 27*, 863.

Thomas, M., Malmcrona, R. and Shillingford, J.P. (1966): Circulatory changes associated with systemic hypotension in patients with acute myocardial infarction. *Brit. Heart J., 28*, 108.

Thomas, M. and Woodgate, D. (1966): The effect of atropine on bradycardia and hypotension in acute myocardial infarction. *Brit. Heart J., 28*, 409.

Valentine, P.A., Fluck, D.C., Mounsey, J.P.D., Reid, D., Shillingford, J.P. and Steiner, R.E. (1966): Blood gas changes after acute myocardial infarction. *Lancet, 2*, 837.

Valori, C., Thomas, M. and Shillingford, J.P. (1967): Free noradrenaline and adrenaline excretion in relation to clinical syndromes following myocardial infarction. *Amer. J. Cardiol., 20*, 605.

Subject Index